Readers share the

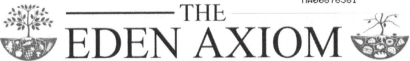

—— THE ——
EDEN AXIOM

MW00876381

"During our visit I appreciated your enthusiasm for healthy eating and Biblical stewardship of our bodies. Thanks for your book. With your motivation as well as other influences, I've been eating quite a bit more healthy as of late." – B.H., South Dakota

"My husband is having fun investigating new veggies, mostly raw. He introduced me to raw beets, and I'm surprised that I like them so much! Thanks, Kirk; I'm thrilled that my darling has made a 180 U-turn. He has been 'all in' on eating healthier, thanks to your book. Thank you!" – Jill Hook, Kentucky

"My wife used to argue with me, trying to persuade me to eat healthier. I would argue back that my diet was fine. Now, because of your book, the argument goes the other way. I'm eating better than she is and I tell her about why the things she is eating are bad for her!" – Michael Hook, Kentucky

"Uncle Kirk, because of you my dad has gone crazy!" – Selina Hook, Kentucky

"Thanks for sharing the 'Eden Axiom' book. We're about 1/3 into it. Looks good! We'll share the info with our Mexican coworkers. Thanks for your time and energies to help us all be better stewards of our bodies!" – R. & E. J., California

"Your research has inspired me enough to pursue these lifestyle changes. I'm glad that you took the time to write the book. It is a blessing!"
– Danielle Wells, West Virginia

"Really appreciate your fellowship and ministry to us concerning our diet. My wife found a sugarless tea that I can drink and last night instead of cookies I grazed on fruit. Little changes like this, but I think they will pay big dividends." Later… "I am making headway with my diet change. Still not quite where I want to be, but a 5 lb. loss sure looked good as I weighed in yesterday."
– Dave Lanham, Missouri

"The mcworst read ever. You deserve a break today, so get up and get away from this book!"
– Ronald McDonald, McDonaldland

"Absolutely finger lickin' devastat'n! So glad I sold the business when I did." – Col. Sanders, Kentucky

THE
EDEN AXIOM
A RADICAL LIFESTYLE OF BODY STEWARDSHIP

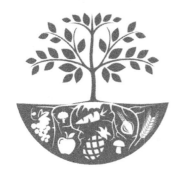
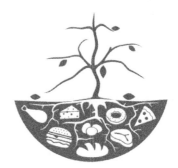

Version 6.7 – Print version 2 – April 2015

Copyright 2015 by Kirk Evan Rogers

TheEdenAxiom@faithwriters.net

Cover design and artwork by Colton Rogers

Available through Amazon and Kindle.

Dedication

This book is dedicated to my mom, Sharon Rose, who early on set me on a course toward choosing a healthy lifestyle.

Note to the reader: I have written this book primarily for Christians who know and love the Lord Jesus Christ, and who have an interest in living a healthy lifestyle pleasing to Him. If you are not a Christian, you will still find much of value here. But achieving good health and long life on this earth is of little value if the question of where you will spend eternity is not settled. So please consider seeking spiritual guidance through the study of the Bible, God's message to us, and by asking those around you who know God how you can know Him too.

Kirk Evan Rogers

Disclaimer: Please note that in this book the author shares information and gives suggestions in a sincere attempt to help people achieve better health. But keep in mind he is not a doctor or other medical professional. Please consult your own doctor or medical professional when addressing any medical issue you may have. Follow the advice in this book at your own risk. It will likely only be at the risk of achieving the optimal health you desire. The author believes the only risk of harm lies in ignoring the plain facts about how our lifestyle choices impact our health.

The statements in this book have not been evaluated by the FDA (aren't you glad?) and are not intended to diagnose, treat, or cure any disease.

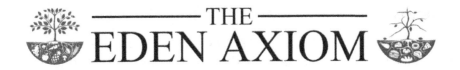

THE EDEN AXIOM

Foreword

I grew up eating lots of junk food, as well as regular meals high in fat and sugar. My parents' and extended family history is replete with heart disease, diabetes, and hypertension. I assumed it was genetic – and inevitable.

As I approached middle age, I felt a sense of dread that I would naturally inherit these chronic diseases my family suffered from. But I had an idea that eating healthier might improve somewhat my chances of avoiding them. So I would try to add some healthy foods to my plate. But I would still eat the junk food as well. I didn't really understand what a healthy diet was, and I had no idea of the powerful impact it could have.

Now I'm fighting back! Within 12 hours of beginning to read The Eden Axiom I committed **fully** to a whole food plant based diet. The facts gleaned from diverse authoritative sources, assembled in one place, and documented in Kirk's book supplied the motivation and the tools I needed to make a complete change.

Armed with these facts, I have no desire to eat the unhealthy foods I had been eating before. I only wish I had known these things years ago! I feel healthier and enjoy the delicious new food options recommended in the book. I'm glad to know I'm doing what I should to halt and reverse the onset of any of a host of preventable diseases, including the dreaded killers that have plagued my family for generations.

In addition, in this book several myths about certain supposedly "healthful" foods are shattered. I never realized what a powerful impact our food choices can have. Now I know how to choose the **best** foods for the optimal nutritional and health-preserving results.

Kirk's book helped me to see the big picture. The scriptural points he makes, along with the healthy lifestyle information, have provided me with a much clearer understanding of what it means to be a good steward of the life and health that God has given us.

Now I look forward to going to the grocery and exploring all kinds of healthful fruits, vegetables, nuts, whole grains, and beans that I previously ignored in favor of my pizza, ice cream and cookies! I praise the Lord for this book and trust you too will find it to be eye-opening and attitude-transforming.

Michael Hook

Missionary church planter

Louisville, Kentucky, January 2015

"MEN OCCASIONALLY STUMBLE OVER THE TRUTH, BUT MOST OF THEM PICK THEMSELVES UP AND HURRY OFF AS IF NOTHING EVER HAPPENED."
WINSTON CHURCHILL, BRITISH POLITICIAN (1874-1965)

"LET FOOD BE YOUR MEDICINE AND MEDICINE BE YOUR FOOD."
HIPPOCRATES, GREEK PHYSICIAN (460-377 BC)

"IT IS NO MEASURE OF HEALTH TO BE WELL ADJUSTED TO A PROFOUNDLY SICK SOCIETY."
JIDDU KRISHNAMURTI, INDIAN SPEAKER AND WRITER (1895-1986)

"THE GERM IS NOTHING. THE TERRAIN IS EVERYTHING."
LOUIS PASTEUR, FRENCH CHEMIST AND MICROBIOLOGIST (1822-1895)

"THE DOCTOR OF THE FUTURE WILL GIVE NO MEDICINE, BUT WILL INSTRUCT HIS PATIENT IN THE CARE OF THE HUMAN FRAME, IN DIET AND IN THE CAUSE AND PREVENTION OF DISEASE."
THOMAS EDISON, INVENTOR (1847-1931)

"LOOK! I HAVE GIVEN YOU EVERY SEED-BEARING PLANT THROUGHOUT THE EARTH AND ALL THE FRUIT TREES FOR YOUR FOOD."
GOD, CREATOR (∞B.C.- A.D.∞)

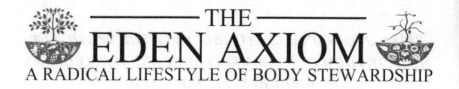

THE EDEN AXIOM
A RADICAL LIFESTYLE OF BODY STEWARDSHIP

Contents

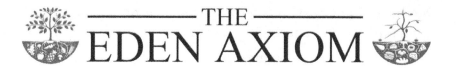

THE EDEN AXIOM

Introduction:

A Matter of Stewardship

A health crisis has snuck up on us. We who live in the United States and other Western countries have over the past few generations been increasingly plagued by an insidious and growing epidemic of chronic degenerative disease. It has happened gradually, so that most of us don't even know what is going on.

- We don't realize that our ancestors from previous generations **did not** suffer and die in large numbers from these diseases.

- We don't realize that in many societies contemporary to ours the people **do not** suffer and die in large numbers from these diseases.

- We don't realize that these diseases are largely **preventable**.

Many of us know this danger is a reality. We have seen our loved ones suffer and die of horrible chronic diseases, and many of us live in fear that we too could be stricken at any time. What most of us don't know is that we can make a few lifestyle choices which really will have a major impact on reducing the likelihood of chronic disease, and thus reduce the fear as well.

A surprising discovery

Chronic diseases are preventable? Absolutely. But only if we know and put into practice a few basic principles of good health. Some of these principles fly in the face of our prevailing cultural beliefs and practices. But they are founded on creation truths from the book of Genesis:

- how God created our bodies,
- the original environment which God made for humans to live in,
- the food which God made as the perfect fuel for humans to live on,
- the activities God originally commanded the first humans to engage in,
- and the relationships God created for human wholeness and fulfillment.

I see it as axiomatic that if we would seek to model our lifestyle after the pattern discernable in the early chapters of Genesis, rejecting as much as possible the aspects of modern life and culture which violate that pattern in ways that erode our physical wellbeing, we would experience much more abundant health and long life than we now do. This self-evident truth is what I call **The Eden Axiom**.

I didn't come to recognize this axiom on my own, simply by studying the Bible. I needed some help.

In the summer of 2013 I began making a serious study of what a healthy lifestyle actually entails, and whether it was possible to prevent and even cure certain chronic diseases without drugs or surgery. As I examined the data, I slowly came to a surprising realization. A pattern began to emerge.

Over and over the conclusions of the medical studies and the recommendations of doctors and researchers as to the lifestyle we should choose for optimal health settled on a common theme. And that theme was consistent with the Biblical pattern seen in Genesis 1-3.

At first I found this to be quite remarkable. But really, is it? It should be quite unsurprising, actually. God created things to be the way they were in the perfect-for-humankind original environment, and He prescribed the original lifestyle for humans to follow. Should we be surprised that science in our day has

Axiom (ăk'sē-əm) n. A self-evident or universally recognized truth

Ignaz Philipp Semmelweis was a Hungarian physician who practiced medicine in the mid 1800s. At that time the germ theory of disease was as yet unknown.

Giving birth to a baby in a hospital or maternity clinic in Europe in those days was very dangerous. From 10 to 30 percent of women contracted fatal puerperal fever. There were many theories as to the cause, but no one knew what it really was, or how to prevent it.

In the maternity clinic where Semmelweis worked, he noticed that the women who were examined by medical students who came directly from the dissecting room got the disease, but women cared for by midwives did not. He ordered the students to wash their hands in chlorinated lime solution before each examination. The rate of fatal puerperal fever immediately dropped from 18% to 1%.

Semmelweis attempted to promote his new technique among the medical community, but doctors refused to accept the possibility that hand washing could make any difference. He was denounced, persecuted and eventually died in an insane asylum.

Today it is a universally recognized truth, which we consider to be self-evident, that doctors must wash their hands between patients, that such practice saves lives. Perhaps one day it will also be widely considered axiomatic that in order for the human body to function properly we must seek to live the lifestyle prescribed by God for the first humans in Eden.

discovered that approximating that environment and that lifestyle, insofar as it is possible, would be the most healthy course to take?

This book is about the principles which arise out of the Eden Axiom, how the prevailing culture violates these principles with devastating results, and how we can turn the situation around and embrace a truly healthy lifestyle, the kind of lifestyle God originally intended for humans to follow.

What diseases?

So, what are the preventable yet debilitating and deadly chronic diseases I referred to above? Here are a few of the biggies:

- Heart disease, America's #1 killer
- Cancer
- Stroke
- Alzheimer's
- Diabetes
- Parkinson's
- Rheumatoid arthritis

And there are many more, as we shall see. These diseases cause untold suffering for literally billions of people, not to mention untold billions of dollars in health care costs. Who will be the next to be stricken down by one of these? You? Or someone you love?

I used to think these diseases could strike just about anyone, anytime – at least as they got older. But that's just not true. We really can dramatically reduce our chances of suffering from any of them with some very **doable** lifestyle changes.

A spiritual issue

I believe this is an issue which impacts more than just our life on this earth. It is also a spiritual issue. The Apostle Paul wrote,

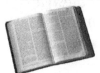

> Moreover, it is required of stewards that they be found trustworthy.   1 Corinthians 4:2 (ESV)

In the immediate context Paul is speaking of the stewardship of "the mysteries of God" with which he had been entrusted. But this important principle may be applied to the stewardship of our physical bodies as well.

Out of His love for us, and in accordance with His purposes, God specially created our bodies and entrusted them to us. We have been given a stewardship to care for them so that we might serve and worship Him to the fullest until He takes us home to Heaven.

So, in light of the fact that we can actually choose to reduce or even eliminate the threat that many chronic diseases will ever hinder our service and worship of our Creator while on this earth, the question must be asked: **Will He find us faithful and trustworthy stewards of our bodies?**

I pray you will read on and see how you have the power to improve your health and your prospects for living a long life, free of suffering from chronic disease. Do it for your sake, for the sake of your family, and as a faithful fulfilment of a stewardship from God.

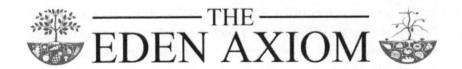
Part 1: The Problem

Chapter 1:

Journey Toward Understanding

When I was a child, my sister and I would go shopping with our mother. The best part was when mom would let us loose in the breakfast cereal aisle, where we could pick out whatever cereal we wanted. Froot Loops, Cap'n Crunch, Super Sugar Smacks, and Lucky Charms were some of our favorites. Nothing beats candy marshmallows for breakfast!

But then mom started reading about diet and health, and telling us that we needed to stop eating so much sugar. Gone were the joyous romps down the cereal aisle. Enter home made granola. Yuck. But we got used to it, and learned to like it.

With that background, as I grew up I was usually more health conscious than others around me. During my teen years I decided God must not exist, and as an atheist I believed I had only one shot at life. Since there is no afterlife, I reasoned, it seemed pretty important to try to make my time on earth last as long as possible. So it became my goal to stay healthy. And while I paid attention to my diet somewhat, my main way of pursuing the goal of living a long time was staying in good physical shape, primarily by running and participating in other sports.

But then at age 21 I became a Christian. As I studied the Bible and grew in my faith I began to understand the extent of God's claim on my life and my responsibility to obey Him and live for His purposes. I learned about the concept of stewardship, and considered how it relates to seeking to maintain good health. God gave me this body, and he wants me to use it for His glory. Now I had a new and better reason to aim for the same goal of good health. But still I had no understanding of the Biblical principles which provide clues to what a truly healthy lifestyle is.

Fuzzy understanding

The years rolled on. I married, began having kids, and started a career as a missionary church planter. All the while I considered myself to be health conscious, and to have a healthy diet. In fact, one of the major adjustments we had to make in our married life was the conflict between Yolanda's Cajun cuisine, loaded as it is with meat, oil, fried stuff, and sugar, and my desire to cut down on such fare.

But I never really looked into the issues of diet and health in depth, I never bothered to dig out the truth regarding what a truly healthy diet consists of, because I thought I already had a pretty good handle on it. I never consulted God's Word on this subject in a serious way. And I never knew about the reliable research which shows just how critical the role of a proper diet is

I didn't understand the extent of the damaging effects which sugar, refined flour, meat, oils and dairy actually have on the human body.

in achieving and maintaining good health. I never knew how easily the wrong diet can lead to the chronic degenerative diseases which kill most of us in the developed world.

I knew I shouldn't drink too much soda pop, that I should avoid fatty meats, that I shouldn't eat too much fried food, and that I should keep my ice cream portions small. But I just had fuzzy, nebulous ideas of why this was so. **I didn't understand the extent of the damaging effects which sugar, refined flour, meat, oils and dairy actually have on the human body**, and that a much more radical dietary approach was needed if I wanted to significantly increase my chances of avoiding major health problems in the future. I didn't realize I was being a poor steward of the body God had graciously provided for me.

Enter prostatitis

Then, at the age of 51 I was diagnosed with prostatitis. It appeared that this inflammation and enlargement of the prostate[1] was causing a cascade of problems including, among other things, urinary tract infections and damage to a kidney. Drugs and surgery were recommended. But I tend to be suspicious of drugs and surgical interventions. I know they are sometimes necessary and helpful, but I also know they often cause unhealthy side effects. So I wasn't comfortable with just accepting that course of treatment. I determined to find out if some alternative existed, a more natural way of restoring my health.

I started searching the Internet for information. I was amazed to discover that prostate problems, which men in Western cultures commonly suffer from, including benign enlargement (BPH) and cancer,[2] are rare in some cultures where the people eat radically different diets than we typically do.[3,4]

---

[1] The prostate is an organ only men possess. It sits below the urinary bladder, and surrounds the urethra, the tube which drains the bladder. When the prostate is enlarged, the space where the urethra passes through gets smaller (picture the hole in a fat doughnut), and thus the passage of urine out of the bladder is restricted. This can cause urinary retention (too much urine staying in the bladder all the time), and other problems.

[2] In the U.S. an estimated 50% of men in their 50s have BPH, 80% of men in their 80s. The American Cancer Society estimates that in 2014 there were 233,000 new cases of prostate cancer in the U.S., and 29,480 deaths from the disease.

[3] See the chart at this link for specific prostate cancer rates by world region: http://healthsciencedegree.info/prostate-cancer-statistics/

[4] Chinese-American men living in San Francisco, for example, are 19 times as likely to have prostate cancer as Chinese men living in China. Dr. Colin Campbell, Ph.D., The China Project (booklet, p25), Paracelsian, Inc., Ithica, NY

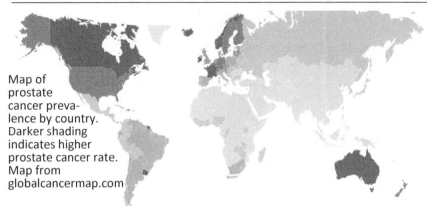

Map of prostate cancer prevalence by country. Darker shading indicates higher prostate cancer rate. Map from globalcancermap.com

In fact, the observed trend indicates that the more plants and less meat and dairy a man consumes, the less likely it is he will develop prostate problems. Not only that, but I learned that for those with prostate enlargement, a totally plant based diet has a good potential to correct the problem – at least as good as drugs and/or surgery, and without any harmful side effects.

Could this be the natural cure I was looking for? I had expected some exotic supplement to be the answer. Could it really be as simple as adjusting my diet? I had to give it a try. So I started avoiding all meat, eggs and dairy, eating only veggies, fruits, whole grains, beans, nuts and seeds.

A multiple benefit diet

As I learned about prostate health, I also came across information regarding heart disease, cancer, diabetes, and other chronic conditions. What soon became clear was that **the same diet therapy which is effective for BPH is also effective at preventing and sometimes even treating many of those other common and deadly chronic diseases which plague people in modern times** – with no negative side effects. This reinforced my determination to stick with the radical changes to my diet, not because I have these chronic diseases, but because I don't want to get them.

I also started to see the correlation between what I was discovering in the scientific literature, and the perfect plan for humankind's lifestyle hinted at in the Eden narrative of Genesis

1-3.

Earlier we briefly touched on what some of these preventable chronic diseases are. We'll look at a slightly expanded list in **Chapter 3**, and cover many of them in more detail later in the book.

The rest of the story

So how has my whole food plant based diet affected my prostate issue? Well, over the course of the next year or so, according to subsequent exams, **my prostate went from being enlarged, to just a little enlarged, to normal size.**[5] This is exactly what the research I had read said should happen.

So, have I seen any other health benefits personally? What about my weight? Well, I was already at an ideal weight while an omnivore. Since beginning eating only plant foods I have lost 5 pounds, so now I am at a slightly trimmer ideal weight. So nothing dramatic there. However, many who do need to lose weight find they realize dramatic benefits in this area when they limit their diet to whole plant foods. We'll discuss issues of weight loss later in the book.

This lifestyle did have a dramatic effect on my total blood cholesterol level, which we will also discuss later. But first, let's take a look at a few Biblical principles which speak to the issue of diet, health and the stewardship of our bodies which God expects of His children.

---

[5] However, I still needed surgery, because it turned out that a problem unrelated to my enlarged prostate, and unrelated to my diet, was the primary cause of my symptoms.

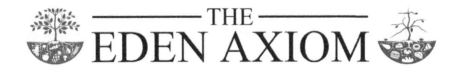

THE EDEN AXIOM

Chapter 2:

A Lifestyle Given By God

Questions of diet and other lifestyle factors impacting our health strike most of us as touching only on this world, and not being particularly relevant to our walk with God. But for the ancient Israelites under the law, diet was very important; dietary prohibitions and requirements were a key part of the law of Moses. These provisions were partially intended to help the Israelites stay healthy and prosper physically. Moses, speaking to the Israelites, summed up one of God's purposes in giving them the law:

> And the LORD our God commanded us to obey all these decrees and to fear him so he can continue to bless us and preserve our lives, as he has done to this day.   Deuteronomy 6:24

If Israel followed the law, including the dietary provisions, it would lead to them being **blessed** and their lives being **preserved**.

There were many provisions of the law which appear to be concerned, at least in part, with preserving the health of the Israelites. These included the regulations concerning hygiene, the quarantine laws for those with certain contagious diseases, and the dietary laws. It was a whole lifestyle.

Among the foods prohibited them were pork, birds of prey and scavenger birds, scavenger and bottom feeder fish, and shellfish. Consuming any of these has identifiable negative health implications, more so than consuming the permitted meats such as venison, beef and mutton.

21

As New Testament believers, we are no longer under the law as the Jews were. However, that doesn't mean God now doesn't care what His people eat, that it is just fine with Him if we eat loads of foods which cause disease, and engage in other unhealthy lifestyle habits.

We must be careful to not compartmentalize our lives, as if there is a spiritual realm which God cares about, and a physical realm which He is indifferent to. No. We are whole persons, body, soul and spirit. God cares about our complete, whole persons. He wants us to be healthy in all respects, at least insofar as it depends on us.[6]

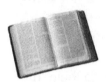 [16] Don't you realize that all of you together are the temple of God and that the Spirit of God lives in you? [17] God will destroy anyone who destroys this temple. For God's temple is holy, and you are that temple.

1 Corinthians 3:16-17

The church here is called "the temple of God." And the church is made up of saved people. They are spiritual people, having trusted the sacrificial work of Christ on the cross as payment for their sins, thus receiving forgiveness from God, and becoming His own dear children. But they are physical people as well, with physical bodies.

Intentional destruction of God's church, whether via the teaching of false doctrine, through division, or immoral conduct, or physical assault on its members, will, according to verse 17, be repaid in kind by God. It is a serious thing to cause injury to God's children.

Our bodies have great value, and how we conduct our lives has great importance:

---

[6] Of course, at times God does call on His children to expose themselves to danger. But always it is because there is a more important goal than good health in view. Running into a burning building to save someone, or living in a dangerous place for the purpose of doing missionary work, would be examples of this.

[19] Don't you realize that your body is the temple of the Holy Spirit, who lives in you and was given to you by God? You do not belong to yourself, [20] for God bought you with a high price. So you must honor God with your body.   1 Corinthians 6:19-20

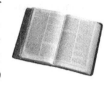

This indicates we should make lifestyle choices which are consistent with God's will, which bring honor to Him.

Please think carefully about this point. In discussions with believers about this topic, I find this is often the most difficult concept for them to come to terms with. They have been told their whole Christian lives that they need to focus on their spiritual walk, and that is true as far as it goes.

But the message often communicated by Bible teachers, by their words or their lifestyles or both (and by doughnuts, sweet rolls, and lattes between services each Sunday at church), is that God isn't much concerned with physical health. After all, "bodily exercise is only of little profit," and the "health and wealth gospel" has been thoroughly debunked, right?

"Whatever you do…"

It can be clearly demonstrated from the Scriptures that it is not necessarily God's will that we be healthy all of the time, and that sickness isn't necessarily a result of sin. But that doesn't mean that sickness is never a result of sin (see for example 1 Corinthians 11:27-30), or that we may make whatever lifestyle choices we please and God really doesn't care one way or the other.

So whether you eat or drink, or whatever you do, do it all for the glory of God.   1 Corinthians 10:31

Think about it: God clearly calls us Christians to honor Him with our bodies. And part of that is honoring God in how we eat and drink, as well as the other lifestyle choices we make.

The immediate context of this verse is avoiding giving offense to others by what we eat. But still, I believe there is a principle here which is directly applicable to our present discussion. Whatever we do should be for the purpose of honoring God, to whom all honor is due.

So we can ask, is it honoring to God when we feed our bodies substances which we know will erode our health? Is it honoring to God when we give priority in our food choices to that which is appealing to the physical appetites, regardless of the inevitable sickness which will eventually result? Do our choices to eat food which causes disease, and to engage in other unhealthy lifestyle practices, not impact our spiritual walk with God? Do they not grieve Him?

The seventh deadly sin

Wikipedia isn't generally to be relied upon as a source of spiritual truth, but whoever wrote the article on "the seven deadly sins" did a good job in the following snippet:

> …the sins are usually given as wrath, greed, sloth, pride, lust, envy, and gluttony. Each is a form of Idolatry-of-Self wherein the subjective reigns over the objective.[7]

Idolatry-of-self indeed. In gluttony the subjective "it-feels-good-so-I-do-it" attitude controls and enslaves. The objective, rational approach, which considers the facts about wise food choices, as well as other lifestyle factors, and acts accordingly, is disdained.

Since early times Christians have regarded these seven sins as particularly grievous, since they seem to be such common manifestations of the sin nature, so toxic to relationships with man and God, and so injurious to good health.

It seems to me that, though the modern church rightly condemns the first six, the seventh is all too commonly given a pass. We choose to not address it, really. In fact, I don't think I have ever heard a sermon on this subject. Whatever gluttony is, surely it isn't something *we* do!

This convenient overlooking of a certain sin which we are loathe to address because we can't fathom actually forsaking it reminds

---

[7] *Wikipedia,* Seven Deadly Sins,
https://en.wikipedia.org/wiki/Seven_deadly_sins

me of the religious leaders in the villages where we work in Africa. There are many "sins" which they denounce regularly to their congregations, such as drinking alcohol, or failing to fulfil their obligations to perform prayer rituals. Yet they let other sins pass by without comment, such as performing sacrifices to dead ancestors, and the corruption of village leaders. These are "taboo" subjects which not only the laypeople, but also the religious leaders are loathe to forsake.

Gluttony in the Bible

Sadly, our own Christian culture is little different. We, too, have our pet sins which it is relatively easy for us to avoid, and so we, and our religious leaders, happily denounce them. But what about the sin of gluttony? What about hedonism, a devotion to pleasure, including culinary pleasure, without regard for the consequences? Let's review a few Scriptures which deal with this subject.

Solomon warns his son:

> [20]Do not carouse with drunkards or feast with gluttons, [21]for they are on their way to poverty, and too much sleep clothes them in rags. Proverbs 23:20-21

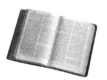

We usually think of a glutton as one who eats to excess. The Hebrew word has the general meaning of being "loose morally, worthless, or prodigal (recklessly wasteful)" (Strong's). So in this context the word glutton is appropriate.

We should note that the glutton's fundamental focus is not on eating a lot, but rather on physical pleasure. In seeking to satisfy that drive, he eats to excess.

But he also has a poor standard for discerning what he should eat. His paradigm is pleasure, not nutrition and wise body stewardship. He doesn't know or doesn't care what health-damaging effects his food choices might have, nor what God might have to say about taking care of his health.

God had strong words of rebuke for Eli and his sons who had become fat thanks to their eating of excessive amounts of meat

(1 Samuel 2:29). They valued their "fleshly pleasures" more than honoring God. Eli's obesity contributed to his death (1 Samuel 4:18).

Paul advised the Roman believers:

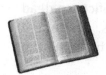

> Instead, clothe yourself with the presence of the Lord Jesus Christ. And don't let yourself think about ways to indulge your evil desires.   Romans 13:14

The word "evil" translates the Greek word meaning "flesh, physical body; human nature." Thus this verse speaks of the natural desires which we have as human beings, but which we seek to fulfil in selfish, sinful ways. Gluttony is one manifestation of this.

Paul said this about the enemies of the cross of Christ, those who opposed the church and the preaching of the Gospel:

> They are headed for destruction. Their god is their appetite, they brag about shameful things, and they think only about this life here on earth.   Philippians 3:19

"Their god is their appetite" is explained by commentators in these terms:

- It is as though they worship their stomachs.
- They obey their stomachs as they would obey God.
- Their stomach is their highest concern.

Again, a focus on the pleasure of eating. Here it is characterized as idolatry, indicating that their drive to satisfy a sensual desire for culinary pleasure fills their hearts to the point that it has displaced God and His will as the main priority.

Paul warns the Galatians about the consequences of living for sensual pleasures:

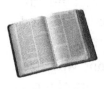

> [7] Don't be misled—you cannot mock the justice of God. You will always harvest what you plant. [8] Those who live only to satisfy their own sinful nature will harvest decay and death from that sinful nature. But those who live to please the Spirit will harvest everlasting life from the Spirit.   Galatians 6:7-8

The phrase "decay and death" translates one Greek word, which also may be translated "corruption" or "ruin." The Translator's Handbook, an exegetical resource I use in my work, has this comment:

> (S)ome take (the word) to refer primarily to moral and spiritual decay. It is likely, however, that it also refers to physical decay and therefore should be understood as a term for death in a general sense.[8]

The moral and spiritual decay, which has been actively at work since the fall of mankind, typically leads to self-destructive behavior, resulting in physical decay and death.

So I believe this verse is a good description of what happens to a person physically as a result of living a life bent on satisfying the sinful nature. Whether the drive to satisfy the lust of the flesh goes in the direction of drugs, alcohol, licentious behavior, indulgence in the "rich" yet health-damaging diet of excess meat, dairy, sugar, oil and other processed foods, or whatever, the result is decay and death.

This is simply cause and effect. Sowing and reaping, planting and harvesting. It is God's natural laws working as He designed them to.

God tells us that we will reap what we sow. So why do we think we can sow an unhealthy lifestyle and yet reap good health? And then when the unhealthy lifestyle results in sickness we pray that God would heal the sick. But He already told us we would reap what we sow. We haven't obeyed this precept of His Word, heeding His warning, so why should He answer our prayer when we start reaping?

Our churches keep long prayer lists of the sick. And well they should. We should pray for the sick. But if we have the means to do something about the problem, don't we believe God would have us to pursue that as well, in addition to praying? Prayer alone is not causing the lists to get shorter.

---

[8] Daniel C. Arichea, Jr., Eugene A. Nida, A Translator's Handbook on Paul's Letter to the Galatians, United Bible Societies, New York

Some may conclude that our continuously long prayer lists indicate it is God's will for all those people to be sick. That's possible. But it's also possible He has given us the means to shorten the lists, yet we refuse to take the necessary measures. I prefer to blame a disobedient church rather than God.

We who are God's children, of all people, should know better than to fall into the gluttony trap. So how very tragic that we indulge in culinary hedonism and thus suffer from the resulting decay and death as much as the world does.

To be sure, most believers aren't consciously aware of the clear connection that exists between what they eat and the chronic diseases which will likely strike them as a result. I pray this book will be a wake-up call to many.

Created with a specific fuel in mind

Right at the beginning God gave us a pretty obvious hint as to the type of fuel mankind was created to run on:

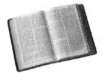

> Then God said, "Look! I have given you every seed-bearing plant throughout the earth and all the fruit trees for your food."   Genesis 1:29

In the original creation the eating of whole plant food was God's perfect prescribed method of providing all of the nutrients needed by the human body. This is the heart of **The Eden Axiom.**

Think of that for a moment! The perfect diet God provided for man in His original perfect creation consisted only of whole plant foods. No milk, no meat, no added sugar, no added oils, no white flour, no artificial ingredients.

But the Eden Axiom isn't just about food. Other aspects of a healthy lifestyle can be seen in the early chapters of Genesis as well.

Created for physical activity

God didn't just create Adam and Eve and then tell them to

lounge around watching TV, playing video games, surfing the Net, reading magazines or playing bingo. He gave them a purpose and physical work to do:

> ^{1:28}Then God blessed them and said, "Be fruitful and multiply. Fill the earth and govern it. Reign over the fish in the sea, the birds in the sky, and all the animals that scurry along the ground."
>
> ^{2:8}Then the LORD God planted a garden in Eden in the east, and there he placed the man he had made.
>
> ¹⁵The LORD God placed the man in the Garden of Eden to tend and watch over it.   Genesis 1:28, 2:8,15

God told Adam and Eve the activities they were to engage in. They were to "be fruitful," "govern" earth and all its inhabitants, and "tend" the Garden. They were to be active and busy! They had purpose.

The word rendered "tend" means "to be in charge of and responsible for." In the garden context in means "to cultivate, to garden." Adam and Eve were to be gardeners, or farmers.

So God prescribed specific physical activities for the first humans, activities which promote good health. It is well known that gardening is an excellent form of exercise.

Later, in Genesis 3, we read of the Lord God paying Adam and Eve a visit, "walking in the garden." Commentators have speculated that before Adam and Eve sinned it may have been God's custom to visit them like this regularly. Perhaps they even took strolls together through the Garden, as they interacted and got to know God better. So here we have another very healthy physical activity they likely engaged in: regular walking.

This reminds us of Jesus' example as He went about His ministry and taught His disciples. He was what theologians call a "peripatetic teacher," derived from the Greek adjective meaning "walking about." He was itinerate, almost constantly on the move, walking about with his disciples in tow, teaching them as they actively moved through life together. A very healthy modus operandi indeed, both from a physical and a spiritual point of view.

It is clear that God didn't create us to sit around most of the day. This principle of moderate physical activity is another important aspect of The Eden Axiom.

Created for relationships

God created humans for a purpose: that He might have a relationship with them, that they might know, love and honor Him. The whole Bible is full of stories of God relating to people, and of people relating to each other and to God.

We find much instruction in this regard. The ten commandments is an example of this. Each one supports maintaining good relationships with God and with others. Good health depends largely on these good relationships.

We see this in Eden. God created people, He spoke with them, and they spoke with Him. They spent time together. He created marriage, the human relationship most foundational in society. As long as God and Adam and Eve were rightly related to each other, all was well. Rupture of relationship resulted in the disaster of disease and death.

In the last section we saw that God gave mankind purpose in a physical sense, work to accomplish. We see here that God also gave mankind purpose in that we are to pursue good relationships with God and others. We have something important to work toward, a purpose to look forward to pursuing each day.

When your relationships are right, your health and longevity is enhanced. Harmonious relationships are another important principle of The Eden Axiom.

A low-stress environment

I suspect that life in the Garden of Eden before the fall was fairly stress free. Adam and Eve had all their needs met, no dangers to be concerned about, no fears, no disease, close fellowship with each other and with God.

Perhaps the most stress they felt was when they had a little difficulty communicating as husband and wife! Or perhaps there was a bit of stress when they walked past a certain tree with fruit which was beautiful and looked delicious, but which they weren't allowed to eat. Otherwise there were likely very few things to ruffle their peaceful existence.

But all that changed when they sinned. As mentioned above, that fateful day, as sin entered the human race, their relationships with each other and with God were severely damaged. The result was intense stress. This stress of knowing they had disobeyed God, blaming others for their sin, the fear and shame they felt, must have been a crushing agony. Especially since previously they had known only peace and joy. That stress could only be relieved by a way of salvation provided by God, by faith and repentance, and by a realization of His forgiveness and a restored relationship.

As we look to God's Word to determine what a healthy lifestyle for us should be today, the issue of stress is an important consideration, a significant aspect of the Eden Axiom.

Simplicity

Adam and Eve's lives were relatively simple. I'm sure they never gave maintaining good health a second thought. They didn't need to learn how to combine foods or count calories, or a lot of facts about physiology and nutrition, what each vitamin does in the body, or what supplements they should take, how much, and when. They didn't have to try to remember long lists of foods to avoid in order to stay healthy. (There was such a list, but it contained only one item!) Neither did they need to try to carve out time in their day for a workout. They simply ate the foods God had provided, engaged in the activities God had prescribed, and related to each other and to God harmoniously.

It wasn't till they stepped outside of this lifestyle, eating food God had not given them, and in fact had forbidden, that they got into trouble (Genesis 3). That's when life started getting complicated!

Is it possible?

So we have seen that God gave Adam and Eve a perfect, nourishing and health-giving diet of whole plant foods. Adam lived for 930 years on that diet. And we also know that the other pre-flood humans lived long and apparently healthy lives on that same diet.

In light of these facts, it seems prudent to consider carefully whether the foods we are feeding ourselves, which are by-and-large so markedly different from the foods we were created to eat, might be at least part of the reason so many in Western countries are sickened and have their lives cut short by chronic disease. Likewise regarding the other healthy lifestyle factors which God established for humans in the beginning. We have forsaken all of them to one degree or another.

As you will see in these pages, **virtually all features of a diet and lifestyle which depart from the principles we can glean from the early chapters of Genesis have indeed been proven to contribute to the most common deadly chronic diseases**. And the further the departure, the more the disease.

Is it possible that the same God who created a specific diet for the first humans, and later prescribed a specific diet for His people, the Israelites, might also have a preference as to the dietary choices His people make today? After all, He loves His children. Would we not expect that He should want us to make lifestyle choices which would minimize painful and deadly disease? Wouldn't that be what you would want for *your* children?

God hasn't given the church specific commands regarding specific foods we should or should not eat. But if He wants us to glorify Him with our lives, which are lived in physical bodies, I think we can agree that He would have us make lifestyle choices which promote rather than degrade good health. It is evident that God is pleased with such choices, as they are in accord with the wise body stewardship He expects of His children whom He loves.

Trusting God for good health

Of course, I am not suggesting that every case of sickness or death is a result of poor lifestyle choices. God may allow or even cause sickness for any number of reasons. Whatever it is that brings about suffering in our lives, good will come out of the experience which far surpasses whatever discomfort and

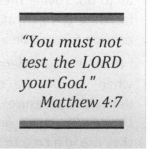

"You must not test the LORD your God."
Matthew 4:7

sorrow we have endured. He will teach us important lessons which we may never have learned otherwise, or bless us in some other way.

This book is based on the premise that certain lifestyle choices can make a dramatic difference in improving our health and the stewardship of our bodies. But with that emphasis I do not intend to minimize the importance of prayer, and trusting in God's sovereign working in our lives. No matter what lifestyle measures we adopt to achieve good health, we must always be trusting God, that He will work through our efforts, or even outside our efforts, to give us the measure of health He desires.

What we must beware of, however, is putting the Lord to the test by knowingly living in a way which will tend to bring on disease, all the while praying to God to protect us from our unhealthy, hedonistic choices. God will not bless such an attitude.

I do not contend that a certain lifestyle will guarantee a certain result. I seek rather to urge believers to be good stewards of their bodies, living in accordance with what the Biblical pattern, as well as the scientific evidence, indicates is most healthful, all the while trusting God to work to bring healing and physical well-being.

Loving others

I close this chapter with one more thought which is very important to me. It has to do with the matter of loving our spouses, children, and others around us, as Scripture commands us to do. Loving them includes making choices which will likely facilitate us being alive and able bodied enough to take care of, provide for, and be a blessing to them.

I think this consideration really shines a light on our selfishness when we declare our freedom and intention to indulge in unhealthy pleasures. Based on the dietary and other lifestyle choices Christians make every day, one might wonder whether they are in a race to be the first into the nursing home, the mind clouded by Alzheimer's, or the first to be chained to a dialysis machine, or the first to suffer the pains of chemo and radiation treatments, or the first to the morgue.

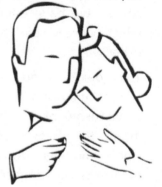

For me, the goal of being alive, healthy and able-bodied so that I can take care of my wife for her whole life, the goal to outlive her, motivates me to maintain a healthy lifestyle. That is one way I obey God's command to love her.

Ephesians 5: Husbands, love your wives

[25]For **husbands,** this means **love your wives,** just as Christ loved the church. **He gave up his life for her**… [28]In the same way, **husbands ought to love their wives as they love their own bodies.** For a man who loves his wife actually shows love for himself. [29]**No one hates his own body but feeds and cares for it,** just as Christ cares for the church.

Notice that Ephesians 5 says that God "feeds and cares for" his body, the church. We would do well to meditate on this Scripture as we ask God to lead us into the proper feeding and caring for our own physical bodies.

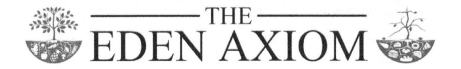

THE EDEN AXIOM

Chapter 3:

Diet-Induced Chronic Disease

Now let's get into a little more detail about just what diseases are caused by an unhealthy diet.

In 2012 Dr. Michael Greger, M.D. gave a very entertaining and informative lecture explaining the latest scientific evidence which proves that almost all of the leading causes of death in the U.S. can be prevented and even cured by plant based nutrition. At that time, the top 15 killers, in order, included 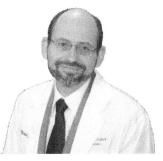 heart disease, cancer, healthcare, emphysema (COPD), stroke, accidents, Alzheimer's, diabetes, kidney failure, flu and pneumonia, suicide, blood infection, liver disease, high blood pressure, and Parkinson's. See the **Appendix** for the link to this talk, as well as links to other talks, by Dr. Greger.

The category "healthcare" in the list above may surprise you. This includes death due to adverse drug reactions, medical mistakes, and hospital acquired infections. In other words, **requiring medical care can be dangerous, as it puts one at risk of dying from a cause wholly unrelated to the original problem.**

Though we who live in the developed world have every reason to be thankful for the high level of medical care available to us, and for the caring doctors who sincerely seek to address our health needs effectively, **the obvious conclusion from the data at hand is that to stay alive it is important to stay out of the**

medical system as much as possible.

As Dr. Greger demonstrates, well-documented scientific studies show that a properly balanced plant based diet can prevent at least 14 of these 15 top killers, and can arrest the progress of and even reverse several of them as well. "Accidents" would be the only one apparently lacking solid evidence for this connection. (Though of course, someone on a plant based diet won't be making any midnight ice cream runs to the market, thus reducing their chances of having accidents.)

To Dr. Greger's list could be added a host of other diseases which have been linked to the consumption of animal fat and protein, though not all of them are necessarily deadly. These include obesity, gallstones, kidney stones, osteoporosis and cataracts, as well as many others, some of which are listed in **Chapter 6: Red meat**.

Cleaning up the wreckage

*I graduated from medical school back in the early 70s, and I thought I was going to be seeing six cases of leprosy every week, and four cases of typhoid fever... And in 40 years of medicine I have never seen a case of leprosy, I've never seen typhoid, thank God. **And what I have spent 40 years doing is cleaning up the wreckage of the North American 20th century diet.***   — *Dr. Michael Klaper*

Deadly cultural beliefs and practices

A diet which eliminates meat, dairy, added sugar, fat and oil, and refined flour, and replaces these things with whole plant foods including veggies, fruits, whole grains, beans, nuts, and seeds, is quite different from what most people in our westernized, advanced countries practice. To adopt such a diet goes against the grain of our culture, but it is consistent with the Eden Axiom.

So will we follow the principles of good health we find in God's Word and which are confirmed by medical science, or will we follow our dangerous cultural practices, because "we've always done it that way," or "I must have the foods I have always eaten"? Do we fear missing out on some pleasure or violating cultural norms (Romans 12:1-2), or are we more concerned with stewardship?

As missionaries in Guinea, West Africa, we have seen many deadly aspects of the culture of the people with whom we work. For example, when we first began living in the village in 1992, we saw that when a baby was born, the umbilical cord was cut with a knife or razor blade which had not been sterilized. As a result of this, all too often the baby would get tetanus, and die a painful death at about a week old.

Through education and government vaccination programs, this area of the culture has changed, and now infant tetanus deaths are quite rare. The people became convinced that what they were doing was not healthy for the baby, and many of them changed their practice.

The current (at this writing) Ebola epidemic is another example. The culture of the Africans resists the germ theory of disease. Health measures which would quickly stop the progress of the disease should they be believed and practiced are discounted. Many of the people believe instead that sorcery is the cause, and/or that the health workers who seek to visit their villages are trying to spread the disease. These are deadly beliefs, resulting in untold suffering and thousands of otherwise preventable deaths.

It is tempting to look down on such cultural beliefs and pity the poor, ignorant people who are in such a hopeless situation. **But are we any better?** In our own culture we have deadly beliefs and practices as well, and just as with the Africans, we are unaware of it. My goal is to increase your understanding of these issues so that positive change can happen for you, your family, and for others you love.

In the U.S. millions suffer from the painful and debilitating effects of heart disease, and hundreds of billions of dollars are spent each year to treat patients.[9] It is our #1 killer, accounting for one in every four deaths. **That's 600,000 deaths each year. Yet the whole food plant based diet supported by scientific and clinical research, promoted by many doctors, and recommended in this book, could prevent the large majority of those deaths.**

This diet also prevents prostate enlargement and prostate cancer. Likewise, as indicated earlier, suffering and death from diabetes, many cancers, stroke, obesity, Alzheimer's and many other diseases, would be largely prevented if we would adopt this diet.

Of course other positive, healthy lifestyle changes such as exercise and lowering stress are helpful as well. But it is clear that diet is the most important factor in avoiding chronic disease and maintaining good health.

We must realize that the Standard American Diet (SAD) is a cultural practice. It is not something that is universal, or that can't change. We *can* change our health damaging eating habits. If we do, we will have no reason to fear an otherwise likely future of pain and suffering.

And if you are already in the middle of that future, a change of lifestyle, especially focused on a change in your diet, can help you put it largely behind you, since it can actually stop the progression of, and even reverse, many chronic diseases.

A SAD way of life

Just what is this Standard American Diet that is so deadly? Do *you* eat this diet? This pie chart summarizes the four main types

---

[9] In 2010 the cost of treating heart disease patients was about $444 billion. R. Morgan Griffin, *WebMD*, Heart Disease: What Are the Medical Costs? http://www.webmd.com/healthy-aging/features/heart-disease-medical-costs

of foods of the SAD, showing the proportion of each which the average American eats:

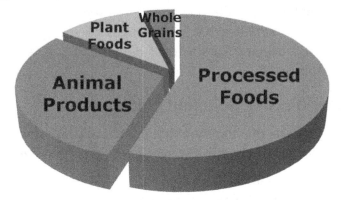

In the SAD, Whole Grains make up about 4% of the diet; unprocessed Plant Foods, 11%; Animal Products (meat, eggs, dairy), 30%; and Processed Foods[10], 55%.

The two small wedges at the top, which total only 15% of the SAD, represent what we call **whole plant foods**. As you read on you will see how it is that these are the foods which promote good health. The two large pieces of the SAD pie represent the unhealthy foods which promote deadly and debilitating chronic diseases.

What does your own personal dietary pie chart look like? What about the dietary pie chart of your children, and others you love? Are they similar to the SAD pie above?

You hold in your hands the information which will help you reshape your dietary pie chart in a way which could protect you from chronic disease and prolong your life.

Do you want good health? Do you want to avoid chronic disease? Do you want to be a good steward of the body which

---

[10] Processed foods include foods which typically come in a package with an ingredients label, and don't contain only whole foods. E.g., canned soup, crackers, granola bars, candy and breakfast cereals. Rolled oats and 100% whole wheat flour, though they have been minimally processed by "rolling" or milling, and may come in a package with a label, are considered by most to be whole foods.

God created especially for you? Do you want to help those you love to be healthy and live long lives of worship and service to God as well? If so, as you read on you will see the importance of expanding the **whole plant food** wedges of your pie until the animal and processed food wedges diminish in size, and maybe even disappear.

Chronic disease deficient cultures

In many cultures our common modern chronic diseases are rare or unknown. Why? **It's not a genetic issue. It's their diet.**

Dr. John McDougall, M.D., has been researching the connection between diet and disease for nearly 40 years, and has used his

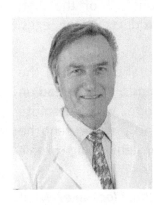

findings to successfully treat thousands of diseased patients, getting them off their medications and enabling them to lose literally tons of weight. The core of his dietary philosophy is that humans are by nature starch eaters. That is, for proper nutrition and good health we require a diet consisting largely of high-carbohydrate vegetables in their whole food form. He points out that

> All large populations of trim, healthy people, throughout verifiable human history, have obtained the bulk of their calories from starch (i.e. corn, rice, potatoes, sweet potatoes, manioc, etc.).[11]

For example, Dr. Denis Burkitt, M.D., served as a missionary surgeon in Africa for 20 years. In his entire time there, treating thousands of patients, he only knew of one case of cardiovascular disease, and that in a judge who had been educated in the West and was eating a diet similar to the SAD. Dr. Burkitt said,

> "In Africa, treating people who live largely off the land on vegetables they grow, I hardly ever saw cases of many of the most

---

[11] Dr. John McDougall, M.D., <u>The Starch Solution</u>
https://www.drmcdougall.com/misc/2009nl/feb/starch.htm

common diseases in the United States and England, including coronary heart disease, adult-onset [type 2] diabetes, varicose veins, obesity, diverticulitis, appendicitis, gallstones, dental cavities, hemorrhoids, hiatus hernias, and constipation. In 20 years of surgery in Africa, I had to remove exactly one gallstone."

Dr. McDougall added that

While serving as head of the governmental health services of Uganda, (Dr. Burkitt) witnessed more than 10 million people flourish on grains and tubers, eating almost no meats, dairy products, or processed foods.[12]

Yet Dr. Burkitt noted that, tragically, when people from such cultures move to the west and adopt our lifestyle, they get our chronic illnesses at similar rates.

The Blue Zones

The "Blue Zones" are a fascinating study. American explorer, educator and author Dan Buettner, together with National Geographic, identified five communities around the world where the citizens tend to live the longest. These people live in Ikaria, Greece; Sardinia, Italy; Okinawa, Japan; Nicoya, Costa Rica; and Loma Linda, California (Seventh Day Adventists).[13,14]

In these Blue Zones, people typically reach 100 years of age at rates 10 times greater than the U.S. average. Teams of scientists visited each of the Blue Zones with the goal identifying "lifestyle characteristics that might explain longevity." They found common factors which characterized the residents of each locale. I will summarize some of them here:

- Their daily routines keep them **physically active** throughout the day, but they don't do exercise "work outs."

---

[12] McDougall, Denis Burkitt, MD Opened McDougall's Eyes to Diet and Disease https://www.drmcdougall.com/misc/2013nl/jan/burkitt.htm

[13] Blue Zones, Explorations http://www.bluezones.com/about-blue-zones/explorations/

[14] Dan Buettner, How to live to be 100+ https://www.youtube.com/watch?v=ff40YiMmVkU

- They have a **purpose** for living, specific tasks to do and goals to achieve each day, including into old age; they don't "retire."

- Their lifestyles naturally and effectively manage **stress**.

- Their diet centers on **plant foods**; meat is typically eaten only five times per month.

- They are **religious**, attending faith-based services four times per month (found to add up to 14 years of life expectancy).

- The have strong family **relationships**, they are committed to their spouses, they invest in their children, and they care for their old folks; often three or more generations live under one roof. Healthy relationships and support outside the family are fostered in social circles which they choose or are born into, and which last for their entire lives.

Did you notice something unexpectedly missing from the above list? If you were to ask a typical westerner what factors are important for longevity, don't you think they would include near the top of the list a good healthcare plan, ready access to state-of-the-art medical care and drugs, and regular medical checkups? Yet the Blue Zones project appears to have found such things irrelevant.

Imagine that. Doctors, nurses, hospitals, and drug and insurance companies seem to be relatively unimportant to the longest lived people. Of course Blue Zone citizens do avail themselves of healthcare services, whether Western-based or "folk remedies." But it is interesting that these things did not stand out to the researchers as particularly significant factors in enabling them to live so long.

It is very significant that typically the older Blue Zone citizens live into their 90s and beyond in fairly good health, often working at their profession, or actively assisting in the home (such as caring for great-great-great grandchildren!) till the day they die of old age. And quite often they die suddenly and peacefully in their sleep.

Consider the above listed Blue Zone factors in light of our Western culture. It is easy to see why, in spite of the most advanced medical system in the world, we are sorely lacking in truly good health. Our system continues to increase our average life spans, but at the same time it increases the number of years spent decrepit, disabled, and dysfunctional.

And as you can see, the Blue Zone factors parallel to a large extent what we have already discussed in the previous chapter regarding the Biblical principles of the Eden Axiom.

A deadly export

The SAD is spreading across the globe at a rapid rate. McDonald's, KFC, Coca Cola, processed meats, sugar-added foods, unnatural vegetable oils, refined grains, etc., are rapidly moving in and spreading their gospel of dietary hedonism.

Dr. Daphne Miller, M.D., in her lecture The Wisdom and Science of Traditional Diets[15], tells of a summer she spent lecturing medical students on the subject of nutrition at Chubu University in Okinawa, Japan. She found the dieticians at the hospital giving healthy eating advice to patients such as "eat low sodium Spam." The message of American corporate food giants was getting across loud and clear, while the amazing testimony of the longest living population in the world, living just a few miles away on the same island, was ignored.

Many years ago I took a bus ride from the Casa Blanca, Morocco, airport to a hotel. I was shocked to see several McDonalds restaurants along the way.

More recently, an older first generation Chinese immigrant woman told me that in the old days in China chronic diseases were rare, but now they are increasing rapidly. She told how when she was young they used to walk to the market twice a day to buy produce, and they ate very little meat – they couldn't afford it. But now, when she returns for a visit her young

---

[15] Dr. Daphne Miller, M.D., The Wisdom and Science of Traditional Diets (minute 57:45) https://www.youtube.com/watch?v=Z_VC4Ya6iII

relatives are always whining about how they want to go to McDonalds. She fears for their future.

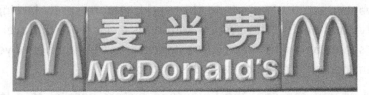

Sadly, tragically, the medical and mortality history in many countries is beginning to mimic our own, with alarming rises in chronic disease over the past few decades.

This proves it's not genetic. Our culture's propensity toward a sugar sweetened, fat laden, animal product heavy diet has been killing us for years, and now it is killing untold millions more around the globe. Yes indeed, cultural beliefs and practices can be deadly!

So what are we going to do? Are we going to go on living the way we have, eating what we have "always" eaten, not getting the exercise we should get, living with chronic stress and sleep debt because that is our culture? Are we going to do this in spite of the known dangers of this lifestyle?

If so, what makes us any different from an African who refuses to buy into the truth that it's a germ, not sorcery that causes Ebola or tetanus? Both we and the African have true and verifiable information which if believed and put into practice would save countless lives. But both typically refuse to believe and act, and immense suffering results.

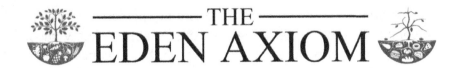

Chapter 4:

Background

So far I have made a lot of undocumented assertions regarding the power of diet to either promote or destroy health. **Chapters 5 thru 8** contain a more detailed discussion about specific foods and partial foods, and the effect they have on the body, whether for good or ill. I have included there extensive documentation to show these aren't my original, unsubstantiated notions, nor are they fanciful theories promoted by a few wing nuts hawking diet books. While there are many experts in the fields of medicine, diet and health who disagree with the conclusions I have come to, those who support my position are numerous and authoritative, and their views are founded on substantial scientifically verifiable evidence.

But before getting into those specifics, we will discuss the genesis of and rationale for this book, we will look a little more in detail at the basic guiding principles upon which my study of these issues is based, we will discuss some terminology used, and perhaps delve into a few other mundane topics.

Why this book?

Why would I think anyone would want to read this? Ever since my wife and I started making serious diet changes toward whole food plant based we have had many conversations with friends and family, explaining what we have learned and why we live the way we do. Some asked me to write down the findings of my research for them. In answer to that request I started doing that, and the work grew and grew till it turned into this book.

The amount of research I did to satisfy my personal desire for understanding of these things is considerable. I know most people will never make such an effort, and thus may never learn the valuable information which has changed my thinking and improved my life. For this reason I felt it would be worthwhile to distill what I have learned into one document, making the information accessible, and useful, to more people.

There are many books on diet and health, even many with similar emphases and conclusions to this present work. This book is unique in at least three primary ways.

First, it marshals a significant amount of reliable scientific evidence which I find most interesting and compelling, and so I think will similarly interest others and compel them to respond as I have.

Second, I combine the presentation of that evidence with a briefly developed Biblical theology of the importance of a healthy lifestyle and wise body stewardship. I explain the Scriptural rationale for why it matters that we who believe in Jesus pay careful attention to the science of diet and chronic disease, as well as other topics related to health. And why we should not only pay attention, but actually live our lives accordingly. This theological content is primarily in **Chapters 2** and **13**.

The **third** way in which this book is unique is really why writing it was important to me. I have a strong desire to share this life-changing, even life-saving information with those I know and love. I share personally with any who are interested in the subject. But there is so much more to say than can be shared in a normal conversation.

I could give people a list of good books on the subject, or website articles and videos they should take in. But I know of none which cover both the spiritual and scientific aspects of the subject as I would wish. And I fear that few would go to the trouble of following through and actually reading the materials I recommend.

However, if I could hand them a book that I myself wrote, I think most would be interested enough to actually read it, even if just because someone they know was the author. Thus the opportunity to publish this book gives me great satisfaction.

But at this point you are probably still skeptical, unconvinced that it is necessary to make such a radical change in your lifestyle. You may be thinking, "I love meat, milk, ice cream, fried foods, etc. I could never change my diet that radically."

Fine. I hear you. But whatever you currently believe about these things, whatever your response is so far, please keep reading, and see if your understanding of this important subject doesn't grow in significant, life-changing ways.

I know I won't convince everyone on every point. All I ask is that you read with an open mind, and make wise choices based on the light you have. And if you doubt the truth of what I have shared, please check out the links for more information, and do further research of your own as needed. If you can come up with refutations of what I have written in these pages, please let me know so I can get back to my hamburgers and cheesecake!

But seriously, I hope and pray that you will join me in rebelling against the dangerous lifestyle aspects of our culture, in considering the principles of the Eden Axiom, and adopting at least some of these lifestyle perspectives and habits. **It's a matter of stewardship. It's a matter of life and death.**

Some basic guiding principles

Much of what I discuss in this book is controversial. Beyond a few basic universally recognized facts, there is consensus on few things in the area of nutrition. I have listened to all sides I am aware of on each point, and made my best judgment call based on what seems to accord most consistently with the facts as I

The human body was designed to derive 100% of its sustenance from plants.

understand them.

Usually my conclusion on an issue is heavily influenced by some basic guiding principles which arise out of the Eden Axiom. I consider these principles to be self-evident, especially if one believes the Bible, and understands some basics of human physiology. These guiding principles are:

- **The human body was designed to derive 100% of its sustenance from plants** (Genesis 1:29), and thus animal products, should not normally be necessary in order to maintain good health.

  o This principle does not necessarily mean that non-plant foods should never be consumed, but it suggests that we should be suspicious of non-plant foods, that consuming them, at least in excess, may be unhealthy.

  o A lot of time has passed since that perfect environment existed on earth. Plants and their nutritive properties have changed much over the millennia. The ravaging effects of sin have affected all organisms. Modern crops are often grown in nutrient depleted soils, such that the produce no longer provides the life-sustaining nutrition it once did. Thus it may be that deviating from the dietary pattern of Eden is warranted in some way, or under certain circumstances. Scientific research will tell us if and when this is the case.

- The original diet humans were created to consume consisted of *whole* plant foods, and thus that is the healthiest form in which they should be eaten.

  o This principle is confirmed by multiple scientific studies indicating that non-whole foods, i.e. processed foods, have a negative impact on health.

  o This principle does not necessarily mean that extracts or supplements or even synthetic drugs should never be consumed. Specific health conditions may warrant their use if a whole food solution is not available.

- Nutrients which are in their natural context, in plants, should be preferred for nourishment and therapy over extracts or synthetic chemical drugs, vitamins, minerals, etc.

  o God created our bodies to function as they normally function. They are complex and intricate, both in make-up and in function, far beyond our understanding. Drugs are often used to alter a natural process in the body in order to relieve a symptom (e.g. pain relievers) or achieve a desired lab result (e.g. statin drugs).

  But this tinkering with the normal chemical processes of the body is based on only a very imperfect understanding of how these processes work. It is impossible to predict the full effects of a drug, and research studies, while helpful, have limited ability to do this. As Dr. Klaper says regarding this, "You can't do just one thing." A drug intended to correct one problem in one area of the body will actually set off a whole cascade of unintended side effects. So it is counterintuitive that using a drug to mess with God's design regarding how the body should function would normally be a good thing to do.

  When experiencing pain or some other sign of disease, the body is giving a signal that something is wrong. It could be that there is nothing wrong at all that should be corrected by a drug, and taking the drug will just be unnecessary and dangerous tinkering. The root cause of the pain or other symptom should be identified and treated, rather than masking the symptom. Often the source of the problem is a toxic diet, stress, and/or other lifestyle factors.

  o Again, this is a guiding principle; specific health conditions may warrant the use of certain specific nutrients or synthetic drugs when a natural dietary alternative is not available. This of course was not an issue in Eden, before the effects of the fall had taken hold.

- There were no toxic substances in Eden, where humans were created to exist. Thus if we are to attempt to live healthy lives, we should make a reasonable effort to avoid toxins.

   o Of course avoiding all toxins is impossible. But we can avoid many by choosing to reject animal products, which provide most of our toxin exposure, and choose instead whole plant foods, which are relatively free of toxins, and in fact protect us from toxins.[16]

- Being physically active with work and other activities, getting a moderate amount of exercise throughout the day, is ideal for good health.

   o This is exemplified by the lifestyle God intended for the first humans. Thus I tend to believe scientific study findings which corroborate this principle.

- Simplicity.

   o This principle is basic to the Eden Axiom. Simply stated, life in Eden was simple. And, especially when it comes to staying healthy, I prefer simple, straightforward solutions, whenever possible, over complex, confusing ones.

   If simplicity is so important, why is such a long book needed, with so much complicated information? Because there is so much confusion out there regarding the subject of health. We need to be convinced of the importance of making changes, re-educated in order to know which of the gazillion messages we receive are true, which are false, which are just complicating and confusing the issue.[17] Then we can reject the false and focus on the few simple truths we need in order to live the best, most healthful, and most God-honoring

---

[16] Dr. Michael Greger, M.D., <u>What to Eat to Reduce Our Toxic Exposure</u>
http://nutritionfacts.org/2014/10/09/what-to-eat-to-reduce-our-toxic-exposure/
[17] Of course, this book is just my attempt to sort these things out and present them clearly. Many other opinions exist, and I encourage the reader to do further study and decide for him or herself where the truth truly lies.

lifestyle.

Evaluating evidence

Not everything I believe about human health has been confirmed by randomized double blind placebo controlled crossover studies. In many cases this sort of scientific rigor is not possible, or such studies may never be performed due to their high cost and the fact that those who have the means to allocate the needed funding, such as drug companies or the government, lack motivation to pursue such lines of investigation. **There is no money to be made, and much to be lost, when study results prove certain drugs are more harmful than helpful, or that eating healthy food is the most effective measure one can take to prevent disease.**

Additionally, in many cases it is either unethical or impractical to do a rigorous case controlled study. After all, it's rather difficult to feed one group of study subjects kale and sweet potatoes, another group steak and eggs, and a third group a placebo, such that none of the groups nor the researchers know who is eating what.

No randomized double blind placebo controlled crossover studies have been done to prove the health-damaging effects of tobacco use, yet other available evidence is so clear on this topic that no one doubts what the results would be were it possible to do such a study. Similarly, no rigorous studies have been done to test the hypothesis that drinking a lot of water can prevent dehydration.

The same is true regarding much of the truth we can know about lifestyle factors such as diet and exercise. Though rigorous studies are sometimes lacking, adequate data is in, and the results are plain for any objective person to see and accept.[18]

Doctors regularly prescribe smoking cessation and increased fluid intake for their patients. If they were to be consistent, and

---

[18] Greger, Preventing Alzheimer's Disease with Plants
http://nutritionfacts.org/video/preventing-alzheimers-disease-with-plants/

ethical, they would also prescribe diet and other lifestyle changes – not just suggest them, but educate their patients and strongly impress on them the importance of following this advice lest they suffer serious debilitating and painful consequences. And the doctors need to follow the same advice themselves, modeling the road to healing for their patients! More on that in **Chapter 15: Doctors' motives for prescribing drugs instead of diet**.

So my approach is that if scientifically rigorous studies are not available regarding a certain issue, I am generally satisfied when it is clear to me that **the preponderance of the evidence** points in a given direction, especially if the conclusion is consistent with my guiding principles. And especially if the alternative therapy is a synthetic, side effect laden drug.

For example, if it is true that most or all cardiovascular disease patients so far that have adopted a certain diet have experienced an improvement in their health, and none suffer any ill effects, rigorous scientific studies are not needed for me to be convinced that the diet is effective, even if the sample size is only a few dozen individuals. The control group, heart patients eating the SAD, taking drugs, and submitting to invasive surgical procedures, is exceedingly large, and contains no individuals in the process of getting well. And I am not concerned that we tease out just how effective the diet is, whether 90% or 99% or 99.7% or whatever. No drug or surgical therapy comes close, so the best course of treatment is obvious.[19] More on how this "heart attack proof diet" works later.

In evaluating evidence I also try to evaluate the potential biases of those who promote it, recognizing that everyone has some bias, that no one is completely objective (including me). I tend to be skeptical of studies funded by drug companies, for example; they will almost always spin the results in their (financial) favor. Even the FDA and other federal agencies have this tendency,

---

[19] Greger, <u>Evidence Based Medicine or Evidence Biased?</u>
http://nutritionfacts.org/video/evidence-based-medicine-or-evidence-biased/

since often they are funded by the industry they are supposed to be overseeing, and typically led by former Big Pharma and Big Food CEOs and other industry officials. More on this in **Chapter 15: Misleading authorities and "experts."**

I am also skeptical of websites which tout the benefits of some therapy, but also sell that therapy. What they say may in fact be true, but I look for more objective sources to verify their claims.

In my studies on this subject and in making conclusions I have tried to be as objective as I can, to be influenced neither by our prevailing cultural dietary norms, nor by what my personal lifestyle has been, nor by what I like to do or the foods I like to eat. I enjoy the taste of yummy junk foods with lots of fat and sugar. But I don't want to let those pleasure-focused food preferences influence my conclusions on what is healthy and what I should eat.

> *I don't want to let pleasure-focused food preferences influence my conclusions on what is healthy and what I should eat.*

My views are evolving, and always will on some finer points, no doubt, as I continue to learn more. I will try to note the more important areas where experts disagree with my conclusions. And I would appreciate anyone reading this book letting me know of any errors they detect, or of anything I should add.

I have cited many references, but have not taken the trouble to do so for every significant assertion I make in these pages. You can easily find out more information about specific issues by searching the web. In fact, you would do well to use this book as a springboard for your own investigation, and check out anything stated herein of which you are not firmly convinced.

Terminology

A few notes about terminology. I often use the term "**whole food plant based diet.**" This is the most common designation I have seen in the literature for the diet my research has determined is the most healthful.

Note that "plant based" does *not* mean that plants are merely central, and from there one may branch out into non-plant foods and still expect a healthy result. Because of this possible confusion I prefer the term "whole plant food diet." However, I will defer to the preponderance of the usage by the experts, and usually I will use "whole food plant based."

> Junk food vegans tend to suffer from the same chronic diseases as the SAD population.

This is a diet with no animal products, that is no meat (beef, pork, fowl, fish, shellfish, insects, etc.), eggs, or dairy products (milk, cheese, yogurt, etc.), **and as few partial foods or food extracts as possible** (sugar, oil, refined flour, chemicals, etc.).

This diet is similar to many **vegan** diets. But I am not primarily motivated out of concern for animal rights, as vegans often are. Some extreme vegans will not use leather, down, wool, or any other products in which animals or animal products were used. I definitely don't agree with this position. Though I am grieved by the excessive animal suffering that goes on in factory farms and through the utilization of cruel slaughtering methods, that is not my focus.

Vegan diets are often focused on what is most healthy for animals. Thus they may include much oil including in fried foods, white bread, and a lot of added sugar. As a result many vegans, while theoretically helping some animals, are definitely not helping themselves; junk food vegans tend to suffer from the same diseases as the SAD population, so I am not interested in that diet.

The diet I recommend is based solely on what is most healthy for humans. So it excludes unhealthful plant-derived products.

For these reasons I don't describe myself as a vegan, nor my diet as a vegan diet, even though many who call themselves vegans may have a diet very similar to mine.

Another term, **strict vegetarian**, can be useful, as it connotes a plant-only diet, but without some of the baggage the term vegan often carries. However, it doesn't necessarily indicate whole food only. Thus "whole food plant based" is more descriptively accurate, as well as being the term most commonly used.

Here are a few more terms and definitions which you may find interesting:

Vegetarian or **lacto-ovo vegetarian** – Those who eat no meat, but do eat eggs and dairy.

Semi-vegetarian or flexitarian – A vegetarian who occasionally consumes meat.

Pollotarian or **pollo-vegetarian** – Someone who eats chicken and other poultry, and dairy, but not other meats.

Pescatarian or **pesco-vegetarian** – Someone who eats fish and other seafood, and dairy, but not other meats.

Pollo-pescatarian – I bet you can figure that one out yourself!

Fruititarian – Someone on a plant based diet who eats primarily fruit, and lesser quantities of vegetables, nuts, and seeds.

Raw foodist – Someone who eats any of a variety of diets of foods which are not heated to over 120 degrees F. Some varieties of raw foodism are plant based, others may include dairy products and certain meats. Usually processed foods are not included in raw food diets.

How radical?

Though many would consider my diet radical, technically speaking what I follow in practice isn't always a 100% strict whole plant diet. In reading this book, some may get the impression that avoiding all the unhealthy types of foods identified in this book every day for the rest of your life is essential if you are to avoid the health problems associated with heavy use of these foods, or obtain the best health this diet can make possible. This is not my position. Occasional consumption of "off the menu" items is not a problem for healthy people.

For example, recently someone took me to a Chinese buffet restaurant. The only food available there which was truly whole food plant based was fresh orange slices. There were lots of veggies, but they were all bathed in tons of peanut or other cooking oil. I filled my plate with these veggies, some white rice, and the fruit, and enjoyed my meal. I knew that if I ate that way frequently, it would pose a health problem. But doing so semi-occasionally is no big deal.

However, for some, especially heart disease patients and those with other chronic diseases such as arthritis, eating this way even occasionally can be a problem; they need to be especially careful not to stray from whole food plant based.

See the section **Baby steps** in **Chapter 10** for more on this subject. Also see my rant near the beginning of **Chapter 14** for some perspective on the application of the term "radical."

The fine print

In this book I have tried to include information which I have found to be significant in helping me understand the most important aspects of this subject. You may notice some redundancy, similar statements made in different contexts. I have not attempted to remove all of this redundancy because some readers may jump around rather than reading the points sequentially. But I have tried to not be too wordy; I apologize for whatever extent I have failed to do this.

This book focuses on achieving and maintaining good health by consuming the right kinds of food and drink, and avoiding the wrong ones. This is because what you eat impacts your health more than anything else.

But, as indicated earlier, the principles of the Eden Axiom are broader than just diet. A very few other important topics relating to good health are covered briefly, including exercise, sleep, and healthcare.

You may find that you understand the material best if you read from the beginning to the end. But it can also be used as a reference book to provide quick info on whatever topics are covered. The detailed Table of Contents should be a help in this.

This book includes references to many web site addresses. Sometimes web pages change, so please let me know if a link no longer works so I can update future editions of the book to reflect that.

I quote from and cite extensively certain doctors and researchers. The first footnote citation of their works will include their whole name and title, while subsequent citations will only have their last name.

Now, on to the "meat" of the book. We'll start by discussing the benefits of whole plant foods, and then move on to the problems associated with animal products and partial, processed foods. Each of the following points is important. I believe the more each one impacts your health choices, the healthier you will be, especially over the long term.

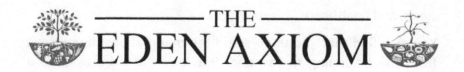

THE EDEN AXIOM

Part 2: The Data

Chapter 5:

Foods Which Promote Health:

Plants

It is good to consider that in our society, where the SAD is so unhealthy, good health is achieved both by eliminating certain things from your diet as well as by adding others. For example, it will help to add more vegetables to your diet, but it will help much more if you both add them and also cut down on or eliminate animals products and added sugar and oils.

In this chapter we will take a look at the foods which make up the healthy diet for humans, and learn some of the solid evidence which supports their inclusion. Then in **Chapters 6** and **7** we will learn about the foods which should not be eaten, and just how these foods cause disease.

Whole foods vs. processed foods

➢ **Importance of whole foods:** Plant foods have innumerable compounds which our bodies benefit from. Nutritional science only knows of a few of these (vitamins, antioxidants, protein, sterols, flavonoids, etc.). But there are many others that have not been identified, or it is unknown what they do for us.

What is clear is that when we rely on supposedly "nutrient enriched" processed foods and supplements to get the

nutrients we need, we will always miss many vital nutrients, and the ones the product is "enriched" with will be of inferior quality and efficacy. Even if some good nutrients are present, innumerable others will be missing.

Furthermore, the ones present may not be in the right form or ratios to be of benefit to the human body.[20] I believe this is one of the causes of the rise of chronic diseases in the past few generations, as we have gotten away from eating whole foods and moved toward more refined, packaged, processed foods, which are so often stripped of much of their goodness long before they get to our table.

Other essential nutrients are fiber, oils, and carbohydrates, including sugars. These also are present in whole plant foods in the right proportion so that when eaten together they may be properly assimilated and used by the body, promoting health rather than doing harm.

But sugars, oils, and/or fiber which are added to foods are processed substances, wrenched from their original whole food context[21] and altered from their original form. The quantities added to foods are relatively excessive. When we eat those foods, the unnatural nature and quantity of these substances does not nourish, but rather stresses our bodies, and when this diet is sustained over a long period, chronic diseases such as heart disease, diabetes, and cancer are often the result.

Another very important thing we must understand is that packaged foods are produced to make a profit. It doesn't matter what the label or ad says about how healthy the product is. **The manufacturer is not interested in your health**, at least not primarily. They want your money.

---

[20] For example, take a flake of your favorite iron-fortified breakfast cereal and crush it to a fine powder. Now take a strong magnet and pass it through the powder. You will probably find that some of the powder sticks to the magnet. This is because iron filings have been added to the cereal. This is not the form of iron which your body wants for optimum health! Your body needs the form of iron which naturally occurs in plant foods.

[21] Or non-food context, as in the case of wood pulp.

Whole foods do not make gobs of money for any big companies. Packaged, processed foods do, especially when their labels proclaim "Low Fat!," "High Fiber!," "Vitamin Fortified!," "Heart Healthy!" Artificial, often petroleum-derived vitamins may be added to them to get you to buy, but these are not what our bodies were designed to live on.

Vitamin and mineral supplements (pills, powders, etc.) are also often of questionable origin and efficacy. But this is not food, it is not nutrition. That's why it is so important to eat a variety of vegetables, fruits, grains, nuts, seeds, and beans. **So remember this rule of thumb: Eat whole plant foods; the fresher the better.**

➢ **Antioxidants:** This is a complicated subject, and I myself don't understand it well. But thankfully a basic understanding of a few simple concepts is all that is needed to know how to make healthy food choices in this regard. I will give a very brief summary in plain English.

As a normal part of cellular function some substances called free radicals are produced. They also invade the body from the environment, such as when we breathe any kind of smoke or other air pollution, or ingest toxins such as mercury, PCBs and dioxin.[22] These free radicals damage healthy cells. This damage can result in the cells becoming cancerous, multiplying out of control and becoming tumors. They can also lead to heart disease, Alzheimer's, Parkinson's, and other diseases.

Antioxidants are substances produced in your body which snuff out the free radicals' power to do damage. But your body can't produce enough antioxidants to deal with all the free radicals, so you need to get a lot of them from the food you eat.

Vitamins C, E, and beta carotene are antioxidants. Thus many health experts advise taking a lot of those vitamins. But this is a naïve approach. It's like saying since G and B flat are nice notes,

---

[22] Rachel Dickens, R.D., *The Conscious Dietician,* The Antioxidant Army – Understanding How We Can Fight Off Free Radicals and Oxidative Stress http://www.theconsciousdietitian.com/general-nutrition/antioxidants/

we should always listen to music with a lot of Gs and B flats. No, we need to recognize the importance of the other notes if we want to make beautiful music.

PCB concentrations in various foods

PCBs (polychlorinated biphenyl) are toxic chemicals which were used for many years by certain industries in manufacturing. They are a type of chemical known as "persistent organic pollutants" because they do not naturally break down in the environment. When ingested, PCBs are not easily eliminated from the body, and can cause many health problems. No level is considered safe.

Though production and use of PCBs is now pro-hibited in most countries, they are still being re-leased into the environment from old paint, wiring and other products, and industrial waste dumps.

PCBs tend to concentrate in animal flesh. The European Food Safety Authority tested over 11,200 food samples from 18 countries for PCB levels. Here are the results, in micrograms/kg:

Fish oil:	*117*	*Beef:*	*5*
Fish meat:	*35*	*Pork:*	*4*
Chicken eggs:	*17*	*Honey:*	*4*
Dairy:	*9*	*Vegetable oils:*	*3*
Wild meat:	*8*	*Chicken meat:*	*3*
Infant/baby food:	*6*	*Plant foods:*	*.08*

– EFSA Journal 2010, Results of the monitoring of non dioxin-like PCBs in food and feed

Our bodies, also, know that loading up on vitamin pills is not pleasant. They demand a much greater variety of antioxidants, each contributing their goodness in just the right way, a full symphony orchestra with thousands notes played in harmony, as found in whole plant foods. No supplements could ever come close to this.

The fact is that there are thousands of different antioxidants, and they deal with free radicals in a variety of ways. Jeffrey Blumberg, Ph.D., Professor of nutrition at Tufts University in Boston, said,

> We can't rely on a few blockbuster foods to do the job. You can't eat nine servings of broccoli a day and expect it to do it all. We need to eat many different foods. Each type works in different tissues of the body, in different parts of cells. Some are good at quenching some free radicals, some are better at quenching others. When you have appropriate amounts of different antioxidants, you're doing what you can to protect yourself.
>
> Fruits, vegetables, whole grains, legumes, and nuts contain complex mixes of antioxidants, and therein lies the benefit of eating a variety of healthy foods.[23]

Notice that Blumberg didn't mention meat, dairy, or eggs. Why not? Because though some animal products do have a few antioxidants, they pale in comparison to those found in plants. One study of nearly 2000 plant foods and a little over 200 animal products found that the plants had on average over 1000 units of antioxidant power, 64 times the animal product average of 18. The animal "food" with the highest value was ox liver, which scored a whopping 71. Even plain old iceberg lettuce, with a measly score of 17, beat out fish, chicken, eggs and yogurt.[24]

But not only do animal products contribute very little by way of antioxidants, consuming them often means getting an extra

---

[23] Jeanie Lerche Davis, *WebMD*, How Antioxidants Work
http://www.webmd.com/food-recipes/features/how-antioxidants-work1?page=3
[24] Greger, Antioxidant Power of Plant Foods Versus Animal Foods
http://nutritionfacts.org/video/antioxidant-power-of-plant-foods-versus-animal-foods/

dose of free radicals, in addition to those naturally produced in your body. When animal products are grilled, char broiled, fried, or otherwise cooked at high temperatures, free radicals are produced. And of course animal products contain many free radical toxins as well, regardless of how they are cooked.

Sadly, the SAD, with its paucity of whole plant foods, provides less than half the daily needs of antioxidants, and at the same time increases the need for more. Thus it is no wonder antioxidant-deficiency diseases are so common.[25]

So, what plant foods should you eat to ensure you are getting enough antioxidants? Frankly, if you are eating a whole food plant based diet, antioxidants are in the same category as fat, protein, calories, fiber, vitamins, minerals and all the other nutrients that SAD people have to stay awake nights wondering about. Whole plant food eaters don't have to worry about it. Just eat a good variety of yummy plant food and you will get all you need.

If you still want more details, here's a list of some of the foods with the highest antioxidant content:

- herbs and spices such as oregano, cloves, cinnamon, ginger and turmeric,
- beans and other legumes,
- fruits such as berries, prunes and plums, red apples, pecans, cherries,
- veggies such as artichokes, broccoli, kale, spinach, and potatoes.
- and tea, especially green tea and hibiscus tea.

➢ **Fiber:** Whole plant foods are naturally rich in fiber, and of a kind which is crucial to good health. Yet there is no fiber in meat or dairy products. Additionally, processed foods, such as breads,

---

[25] Greger, <u>Minimum "Recommended Daily Allowance" of Antioxidants</u>
<u>http://nutritionfacts.org/video/minimum-recommended-daily-allowance-of-antioxidants/</u>

cakes and crackers made with white flour, are usually low in fiber. If they are high in fiber, it may only be because cellulose, sourced from wood pulp, has been added to the food after the natural fiber has been taken out. And the more of these fiber-free and fiber-poor foods you eat, the less fiber-rich whole foods you will eat.

A diet rich in whole foods with their naturally occurring fiber is critical for bowel health. **And your bowel health affects the rest of your health as well, including your immune system,[26] and the proper absorption of nutrients and elimination of toxins and other wastes.[27]**

One sign of poor bowel health due to low fiber intake is constipation. Some doctors will advise their patients that it is okay if they have less than one bowel movement per day, that such a condition is not a risk factor. In fact, numerous articles on the Internet repeat the mantra that it is normal to have anywhere from three BMs per day to three *per week*.

But keeping the material from stagnating, keeping it moving along through the intestines at a good clip, is critical to maintaining a healthy bowel, and by extension a healthy body.[28] Some doctors now recognize that two to three bowel movements per day is much more healthy and should be considered normal.[29]

But how will you achieve that? By popping an extra prune or two

---

[26] Marge Dwyer, *Harvard School of Public Health News,* Bacterial metabolites regulate immune system function in the colon and may help reduce inflammatory bowel disease http://www.hsph.harvard.edu/news/features/bacterial-metabolites-regulate-immune-system-function-in-the-colon-and-may-help-reduce-inflammatory-bowel-disease/

[27] R. Morgan Griffin, *WebMD,* The Benefits of Fiber: For Your Heart, Weight, and Energy http://www.webmd.com/diet/fiber-health-benefits-11/fiber-digestion

[28] Greger, Stool size matters http://nutritionfacts.org/video/stool-size-matters/

[29] McDougall, Constipation, Hemorrhoids, Varicose Veins https://www.drmcdougall.com/health/education/health-science/common-health-problems/constipation-hemorrhoids-varicose-veins/

each day? By gulping down some Metamucil (along with its food coloring, artificial flavor, and sugar)? **No, but by replacing all that fiber-free meat and dairy in your diet, and all those fiber poor processed foods as well, with fiber rich fruits, vegetables, whole grains, beans, nuts, and seeds.**

So just how does BM frequency affect health? One way is through toxins. When fecal matter moves too slowly through the colon, some toxins which were sent there to be disposed of are reabsorbed into the body, where they may promote cancer and other diseases. Also, fiber in the colon can absorb some toxins such as heavy metals (e.g. lead, mercury) and bile acids, and convey them out of the body.[30]

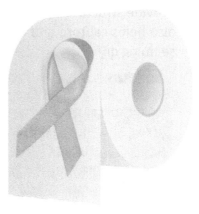

A study published on the National Institute of Health website found that **women who had on average three or more bowel movements per day were 46% less likely to get breast cancer** than women who had only one per day.[31] And you aren't going to get that kind of regularity eating animal products. Perhaps pink ribbons should be emblazoned on toilet paper packages rather than on fast food chicken buckets!

And as documented in these pages, a high fiber whole food plant based diet, with its associated larger stool mass and increased frequency of BMs, is protective from colon cancer,[32] type 2 diabetes, heart disease, diverticulosis, digestive disorders, and other ailments.

Having to use the restroom more often may not seem appealing.

[30] Greger, From Table to Able: Combating Disabling Diseases with Food http://nutritionfacts.org/video/from-table-to-able/
[31] Sonia S. Maruti, et al, A Prospective Study of Bowel Motility and Related Factors on Breast Cancer Risk http://www.ncbi.nlm.nih.gov/pmc/articles/PMC2848455/
[32] Greger, Stool size matters http://nutritionfacts.org/video/stool-size-matters/

But it is a good sign that you are on the path toward better health!

➢ **Sawdust in our food:** Sawdust is essentially fiber. Would you eat sawdust straight, or mix some into your coffee and drink it? No. But cellulose sourced from wood pulp,[33] which is essentially sawdust, is added to many foods from breakfast cereals to pancake mixes to chicken nuggets to ice cream sandwiches.[34] This enables the manufacturer to reduce the fat in the food without compromising taste or texture too much. It also serves as a "filler," adding bulk and reducing the cost of manufacture.

Small cellulose particles impart a smooth consistency, "mouthfeel" and stickiness to products such as salad dressings, barbecue sauces and, yes, ice cream. Longer fiber lengths provide structure and a firmer texture to baked goods. Cellulose also helps capture and retain moisture and keeps products from seeming dry.[35]

INGREDIENTS: SKIM MILK, WAFER (BLEACHED WHEAT FLOUR, ISOMALT*, MALTITOL*, CARAMEL COLOR, SORBITOL*, PALM OIL, COCOA, CORN FLOUR, MODIFIED CORN STARCH, SALT, BAKING SODA, NATURAL FLAVOR, SOY LECITHIN), MALTODEXTRIN, POLYDEXTROSE, SORBITOL*, CREAM, STABILIZER (MONO AND DIGLYCERIDES, CELLULOSE GEL, CELLULOSE GUM, CARRAGEENAN), SUCRALOSE (SPLENDA® BRAND), VITAMIN A PALMITATE, ACESULFAME POTASSIUM, NATURAL FLAVOR, ARTIFICIAL FLAVOR.

Treasure hunt: Can you find the sawdust in this ingredients list from an ice cream sand-wich?

McDonalds adds wood pulp to their fish filet, strawberry

---

[33] Note that strictly speaking the term cellulose refers to the substance which makes up plant cell walls, including the cells which make up the wood of trees. Essentially it is the same as fiber, however cellulose from wood has none of the phytonutrients of edible plant cellulose. In this section the term refers specifically to cellulose from wood pulp.

[34] Miriam Reimer, 15 Food Companies That Serve You 'Wood' http://www.thestreet.com/story/11012915/1/cellulose-wood-pulp-never-tasted-so-good.html?cm_ven=outbrain&psv=tscserps&obref=obnetwork

[35] Jennifer K. Nelson, R.D., L.D. and Katherine Zeratsky, R.D., L.D., Is cellulose the latest food additive? http://www.mayoclinic.org/healthy-living/nutrition-and-healthy-eating/expert-blog/cellulose/bgp-20056281

sundaes, and Caesar salad dressing. Additionally, some food manufacturers add wood pulp to cereals, cake mixes, and many other products. Look for "cellulose" on the label.

I know of no data which shows that eating this artificially-added wood pulp poses a health risk. But foods with this additive are unhealthy by definition, because they are highly processed, containing only partial foods, not whole foods, in addition to the fact that they contain non-food, i.e. wood pulp. Many of the other ingredients, such as sugar, oil, white flour, and chemicals are doubtless more unhealthy than the wood pulp itself.

Also, wood fiber is not a healthy substitute for fiber found naturally in food, because much of the benefit of fiber is not from the bare cellulose, but from the polyphenol nutrients bound to the fiber, which have many health promoting effects.[36] Wood pulp doesn't have these. The ingredients in a processed food may have their natural, healthy fiber removed, and then non-nutritious wood pulp is added back in. Thus it is accurate to say that foods with added cellulose, just like foods with added vitamins, minerals, sugars, and oils, are unhealthy.

➢ **Non-whole foods to avoid:** Eating only whole plant foods implies the following would be off the menu:

- ✓ oils and fats, including cooking oil, olive oil, margarine;
- ✓ fried foods such as snack chips, tater tots, French fries;
- ✓ sugar and other sweeteners;
- ✓ fruit and vegetable juices (see later discussions of juicing for possible exceptions);
- ✓ protein powders, whey protein, etc.;
- ✓ fake meats and cheeses such as chicken made from soy protein;
- ✓ white flour, including white bread, French bread, noodles

---

[36] Greger, Juicing Removes More Than Just Fiber
www.nutritionfacts.org/video/juicing-removes-more-than-just-fiber/

not made from 100% whole grain wheat flour,[37] etc.;

✓ added chemicals, including colors, flavors, vitamins, minerals, and preservatives.

"Hey, not so fast! That includes a lot of foods I eat every meal, foods I love! How could I ever stop eating all those things?!"

My answer to this objection is three-fold:

First of all, recognize that there is a lot more data for you to consider before deciding how you should respond. The information you will read in the rest of the book, considered objectively, may make the above suggestions sound pretty reasonable, even desirable. So be forewarned. You may want to play it safe and put this book down now!

Second, please understand that many in our modern society today actually are on diets which avoid these substances, at least to a substantial degree. I am among them. And we enjoy our food as well as better health. **It is possible!**

And **third**, you don't have to make a complete change all at once. As these new truths about healthy eating become more and more a part of your thinking, you will start to pay more attention to the unhealthy things you used to eat and drink without a second thought. And you will gradually start to eliminate the health eroding items from your shopping list, from your diet, from your home, and from your life.

And no one will force you to make this change. You will want to do it because you have come to know and believe the truth, that each of these partial foods has negative effects on your health – but only if you eat them!

➢ **"Enriched" and "fortified" foods:** Don't be fooled by these labels. The manufacturer has removed important nutrients in the processing of the food, making it practically non-food. Then

---

[37] Many find they also realize a health benefit by reducing or eliminating all wheat, and/or all flours, from their diet.

an attempt is made to add back in nutrients which will supposedly make the product food again, and which it is thought will encourage people to buy it. But this is dishonest, as these "nutrients" are often synthetic petroleum-derived versions of their natural counterparts, the nutritional value of which has not been proven (and in some cases has actually been disproven), and they may be harmful rather than healthful.

Furthermore, vitamins in their natural context of unprocessed food have been shown to be much more healthful than isolated, especially synthetic, nutrients. So try to avoid any packaged food which has "enriched" or "fortified" on the label. Such food is "fortified"

> *Avoid any packaged food which has "enriched" or "fortified" on the label.*

not to make you healthy, but to get you to buy it. Whole plant foods, on the other hand, are the ones which are truly enriched and fortified by God with just the right mix and amounts of the nutrients your body needs for optimal health.

➢ **Fresh, frozen, or canned:** Canned fruits and vegetables are generally not nearly as nutritious as fresh or frozen, so it is best to avoid them. Pumpkin, tomatoes, and beans (kidney, pinto, black, etc.) are said to be exceptions to this. Just be sure to check the label and reject if you see added preservatives or other chemicals, or a lot of salt. Aside from little nutritive value, canned fruits usually contain large amounts of sugar, so it is best to stay away from them. If you get used to eating only fresh fruits, canned fruits will lose their appeal anyway.

Fresh local produce when in season is usually best, full of more living nutrition than that which has been processed by freezing or canning. However, produce destined for the produce aisle is usually picked before it is ripe, and it may be several days before it reaches the store. During that time it can lose some of its nutritive value. That which is to be frozen, on the other hand, is more likely to be picked at its peak of ripeness, and frozen soon afterward; thus it may contain more nutrients. So sometimes frozen is better.

However, one study found no nutrient difference between fresh and frozen berries. The important thing is to eat lots of fruits and veggies, whether you purchase them frozen or fresh. And whatever you can grow yourself, or obtain from local growers, will be the very best.

Veggies

> **Dark green leafys: Some of the most nutritious foods are cruciferous and green leafy vegetables.**[38] A few of the most common are Swiss chard, spinach, dark green lettuce, kale, broccoli, cauliflower, cabbage, Brussels sprouts, and the like.[39] Numerous studies prove that these veggies promote good health and protect from cancer, heart disease, stroke, diabetes, etc.

Dark green leafy veggies are especially good at keeping the lining of your arteries healthy, preventing any artery-clogging plaque from developing, and ensuring that any plaque that is there doesn't come loose, causing a clogged artery and a heart attack or stroke. Of course the ability of such veggies to do this will be hindered by high meat, sugar, and oil consumption, which actively causes damage to your blood vessels.

Regular cabbage is very nutritious, but purple cabbage is even better. (Generally, the more color in a plant food, the better.) I try to make a point of eating some broccoli, spinach, purple cabbage and kale every day, as well as some of the others veggies listed above when possible.

Head lettuce is not bad for you, but it contains little by way of nutrition aside from water and fiber. If you want the maximum

---

[38] Winston Craig, MPH, Ph.D., RD., Health Benefits of Green Leafy Vegetables http://www.vegetarian-nutrition.info/updates/benefits-of-green-leafy-vegetables.php
[39] Cari Nierenberg, *WebMD,* Leafy Greens -- Ranked and Rated http://www.webmd.com/diet/healthy-kitchen-11/leafy-greens-rated

nutrition bang for your buck, your precious food money is more wisely spent on darker green and other colored veggies.

➢ **Sweet potatoes:** Many have called sweet potatoes a superfood because there are so many healthy benefits associated with their consumption. They are packed with vitamins and minerals.

The traditional diet of the people of Okinawa was primarily sweet potatoes, and they have the reputation of being the population with the longest living people of anywhere on earth.

A study was done comparing the nutritional value of many foods with their price per pound. Sweet potatoes came out the clear winner, providing the most nutrition bang for your buck.

Be sure and eat sweet potatoes without adding sugar, marshmallows, etc.! They are already sweet. (If you are used to eating them with loads of sugar and marshmallows added, they won't taste sweet. But give it time. As your taste buds adjust to your new diet you will find they are quite tasty.)

➢ **Starch: Throughout the ages starchy foods have been the cornerstone of the diets of all great civilizations.** Don't be afraid of eating lots of whole grains, potatoes, etc. See info from Dr. McDougall referenced at the end of this book.

This goes against what is becoming the conventional wisdom that carbohydrates are bad for you, or should only be consumed sparingly. This "wisdom" is not based on the best science. Carbohydrates from sugar and refined flour are indeed bad for your health. But when they come from whole plant foods, they are very good, and can be a staple in a healthy diet, as they have been for billions around the world since the beginning.

➢ **High carb/low carb and glycemic index:** This emphasis on plant foods and starch may raise the eyebrows of those who believe a low carb or paleo diet is the best path to good health. One reason has to do with what is believed by many to be the dangers of eating high glycemic index foods.

Starch-based diets in history

The most important evidence supporting my claim that the natural human diet is based on starches is a simple observation that you can easily validate for yourself: All large populations of trim, healthy people, throughout verifiable human history, have obtained the bulk of their calories from starch. Examples of once thriving people include Japanese, Chinese, and other Asians eating sweet potatoes, buckwheat, and/or rice, Incas in South America eating potatoes, Mayans and Aztecs in Central America eating corn, and Egyptians in the Middle East eating wheat. There have been only a few small isolated populations of primitive people, such as the Arctic Eskimos, living at the extremes of the environment, who have eaten otherwise. Therefore, scientific documentation of what people have eaten over the past thirteen thousand years convincingly supports my claim.

Men and women following diets based on grains, vegetables, and fruits have accomplished all of the great feats in history. The ancient conquerors of Europe and Asia, including the armies of Alexander the Great (356 – 323 BC) and Genghis Khan (1162 – 1227 AD) consumed starch-based diets. Caesar's legions complained when they had too much meat in their diet and preferred to do their fighting on grains. Primarily six foods: barley, maize (corn), millet, potatoes, rice, and wheat have fueled the caloric engines of human civilization.

– Dr. John McDougall, M.D.

The glycemic index (GI) is a measure of a food's effect on blood sugar. The higher the GI, the faster that food raises blood sugar. So some advise people with certain diseases such as diabetes to go on a low glycemic diet, choosing foods with low GIs. After all, having consistently high blood sugar causes and exacerbates diabetes, right?

It sounds logical. But there are many more factors which must be considered. First of all, it is true that high GI foods which contain refined sugar, flour and other non-whole plant foods should of course be avoided. However, some of the highest GI scores are assigned to certain whole plant foods, such as potatoes and watermelon. To my knowledge there is no real evidence that eating these foods is problematic. It really is hard to find something truly unhealthy about any whole plant food!

There are other things one should know about the GI picture:

- Fiber tends to lower the GI of foods, since the fiber slows the rate at which the sugars are released into the blood. Thus many plant foods with a lot of carbs (starch) will not spike the blood sugar much, since they also have a lot of fiber.

- Processed foods, on the other hand, have high GIs, since fiber is typically removed (not to mention sugar added) in processing. White rice, for example, has a GI of 89, brown rice, 50.

- Cooking and especially overcooking tends to raise the GI of foods. For this reason, generally raw or lightly cooked foods are better from a GI standpoint.

- Adding oil to a high GI food will tend to lower the GI, because the oil slows the absorption of the sugars.

This last fact leads some to recommend eating a baked potato with lots of butter, or dipping bread in olive oil. But this reflects a simplistic understanding of the true picture.

A baked potato has a GI of 111, while French fries score only 60. If all you know is that you should eat foods with lower GIs, you would conclude that French fries are better for you than a baked potato.

So is this addition of oil and fat really making the food more healthy overall? No. Oils and fats tend to cause obesity, raise inflammation, impair and harm the vascular system, cause and exacerbate diabetes, etc. This is covered in more detail in later chapters.

- Foods which do not contain carbs, or few carbs, will tend to have low GIs, even if they are very unhealthy.

For example, pizza may have a GI of 36. Peanut MMs score 33, ice cream 38, and most meat products have a GI of zero. So if a person has been told to limit high GI foods, they may have a hard time making healthy choices.

The whole plant food principle reminds us that whenever such a food is vilified, accused of being unhealthy, contributing to disease, we should be suspicious and dig deeper and find out what the truth really is. One question which comes to mind is, if all high GI foods are really so unhealthy, how can it be that large, healthy civilizations have thrived on foods like potatoes or rice, without epidemics of chronic disease?

Actually, high GI whole plant foods (starches) tend to satisfy hunger better than low GI foods, and thus they don't promote as much weight gain. And they contain the vast array of nutrients we were created to live on. The insulin response to them, even if they have a high GI, is normal and healthy. And in fact high carb consumption and low fat consumption are the factors which have been shown to prevent diabetes, not shunning high GI whole plant foods in favor of animal products and oils.[40]

It is clear that "eat whole plant foods" is a much more reliable guide to eating healthy than "eat low glycemic index foods."

It is true that some low carb diets may be superior to the SAD, particularly if they eliminate unhealthy things like sugar, oils and processed foods. But they are vastly inferior to a well

---

[40] McDougall, Glycemic Index – Not Ready for Prime Time
https://www.drmcdougall.com/misc/2006nl/july/glycemic.htm

balanced whole food plant based diet. See **Chapter 11: Diets to avoid** for more discussion of this subject.

➤ **Sea vegetables:** Sea vegetables such as nori, wakame, and kelp, contain many valuable nutrients such as protein, iodine, iron, vitamin A, niacin, folic acid, and antioxidants. There is evidence that long-term consumption of sea vegetables confers protection against estrogen-related cancers, such as breast cancer.[41]

I have found the best prices on large nori sheets on eBay. Nori can be eaten straight as a snack, used to make sushi, or torn or cut into small pieces and added to soups, stews and many other dishes.

Fruit

➤ **Whole fruits are great food:** Whole fruits are packed with good nutrients, and it is good to eat a lot of them. Moreover, eating fruit is the good way to satisfy your desire for sweets.

Because of the high sugar content of fruit, some health authorities say it is a best to limit fruit consumption somewhat. This would especially be true for those trying to lose weight, those with cancer, and diabetics. But for most of us I believe it is safe and beneficial to eat a lot of fruit, as long as it is the whole fruit (less any inedible skin, seeds, etc., of course).

Be sure to eat the skin of the fruit whenever possible (apples, grapes, etc.), because usually the skin has most of the nutrients. There is little nutrition in a skinned apple, for example, but much in a whole red apple (yes, red is more nutritious than green or yellow).

➤ **Avoid fruit juice:** Fruit juice is mostly water and sugar. Drinking fruit juice causes blood sugar to rise. For some types of juice the rise may not be as sharp as drinking sugar water or

---

[41] Greger, Which Seaweed to Help Prevent Breast Cancer? http://nutritionfacts.org/2014/05/15/which-seaweed-to-help-prevent-breast-cancer/

soda, thanks to the phytonutrients in the juice.[42] But it is still significant, and this is inflammatory and unhealthy if a lot of juice is drunk, especially if it is filtered. This is not surprising, since fruit juice is not a whole food.

The sugar in whole fruit does not cause blood sugar levels to rise sharply, however. The fruit sugar is released more slowly into the blood thanks to the fiber of the fruit and other factors.

➢ **Fruit and fructose:** Fruit contains fructose. When fructose is added to foods and eaten, it is damaging to the body.[43] But when fruit is eaten the body is able to handle the fructose just fine. This makes sense, since it is in the context of a whole food.

Table sugar (sucrose) contains 50% fructose, and high fructose corn syrup contains 55% fructose. The fructose in these substances is one of the main reasons they are bad for your health. Apple juice, however, contains about 66% fructose, so it puts that much more strain on the body as it struggles to metabolize it. In some respects, apple juice can be more unhealthy to drink than sugar water.[44]

➢ **Berries:** Berries get special mention among fruits. Research studies continue to find health benefits of eating berries: strawberries, blueberries, blackberries, raspberries, cranberries, etc. **The phytonutrients which give berries their dark blue and bright red colors are very beneficial to health.** (This is true of plant foods across the board – the more colorful they are the more of certain very healthy phytonutrients they contain.)

Berries are expensive, but consider the money an investment in your healthy future. After all, cancer is expensive, too! Studies have found that strawberries can combat esophageal cancer, for

---

[42] Greger, If Fructose is Bad, What About Fruit?
http://nutritionfacts.org/video/if-fructose-is-bad-what-about-fruit/
[43] Robert H. Lustig, M.D., *Advances in Nutrition*, Fructose: It's "Alcohol Without the Buzz" http://advances.nutrition.org/content/4/2/226.long
[44] Greger, Apple Juice May Be Worse Than Table Sugar
http://nutritionfacts.org/video/apple-juice-may-be-worse-than-sugar-water/

example.[45,46] Money spent on berries should count toward your health insurance deductible!

> **Dried and cooked fruit:** Fresh fruit is most healthful, but dried and cooked fruit is pretty good, too. But don't eat it if it has added sugar, as dried papaya, pineapple, banana chips, cranberries and other fruits often do.

We purchased a used food dehydrator at a second hand store, and have used it nearly every day since. It is great to have plenty of dried banana chips, pineapple, strawberry, apple, peach and orange slices, and other fruit, always on hand for snacking.

Dried bell peppers are good, too. After making thin slices, we mix them with seasoning, and then put them in the dehydrator.

Perhaps the yummiest food dehydrator item is "fruit roll." That was one of my favorite lunchbox items when I was a school kid. Just toss some fruit in a blender and make a little fruit smoothie. Smear a very light coating of coconut oil on a piece of baking parchment paper, place it on the dehydrator tray, and pour the blended fruit onto the paper. In 12-24 hours you have your fruit roll. Berries probably make the tastiest fruit rolls, but try it with various mixes of whatever fruits you have on hand to find your favorite combination.

Grains

As mentioned earlier, grains have formed the nutritional foundation of many great civilizations throughout history. Including a variety of whole grains in your diet is a great idea.

> **Whole grains:** Always insist on whole grains. There really is a significant nutritional difference between whole and refined grains. Refined grains such as white flour not only don't provide nearly the nutrition as whole grains, but are known to cause

---

[45] Kathleen Doheny, *WebMD Health News,* Strawberries May Help Prevent Esophageal Cancer Small Study Shows http://www.webmd.com/cancer/news/20110406/strawberries-may-help-prevent-esophageal-cancer
[46] Greger, Strawberries Versus Esophageal Cancer http://nutritionfacts.org/video/strawberries-versus-esophageal-cancer/

disease.

➢ **Whole grains and blood pressure:** In one study the consumption of whole grains was found to lower blood pressure and researchers concluded this effect could decrease the likelihood of coronary artery disease and stroke by 15% and 25%, respectively. This is the same result expected from drug therapy, but of course without any negative side effects.[47]

> *Consumption of whole grains cuts the risk of cancer; refined grains increase the risk.*

➢ **Whole grains and mouth cancer:** A study found that consumption of whole grains cut the risk of mouth cancer in half, while the consumption of refined grains (white bread, bagels, etc.) increased the risk by six times.[48]

➢ **How to get whole grains into your diet:** Whole wheat flour is the most common way whole grains are eaten in the U.S. But it is much better to get as much of your whole grains as possible in a less processed form. You can prepare a variety of whole grains the way you prepare rice. Then serve them with beans, lentils, or some sauce over them. You can also put them in soups and stews. And of course oatmeal is great for breakfast – or anytime, for that matter. More on oats later.

➢ **White flour: It is best to try to avoid foods with white flour in them.** This includes most commercially sold breads, rolls, bagels, biscuits, muffins, doughnuts, etc.

For those who are accustomed to baking their own bread, it is often difficult to get used to baking without white flour. But it is possible. The results might not be as light and airy as what you are used to, but before long you will be used to the new, more

---

[47] Greger, <u>Whole Grains May Work As Well As Drugs</u>
http://nutritionfacts.org/video/whole-grains-may-work-as-well-as-drugs/
[48] Greger, <u>Stop Cancer Before It Starts</u> (minute 26:00)
https://www.youtube.com/watch?v=dYxpgwFip2M

wholesome taste and texture. There are many good whole grain bread recipes available online.

White flour has had the most nutritious parts of the grain removed in order to "improve" color and texture, and to lengthen shelf life. **Eating white flour, like eating meat, oil and sugar, is damaging to the endothelium of your veins and arteries, and thus promotes heart disease as well as other vascular diseases.**[49] It also harms your health in other ways, like unnecessarily raising your blood glucose levels and promoting type 2 diabetes, and causing inflammation.

Read labels carefully. "Wheat flour" doesn't necessarily mean it doesn't contain white flour. After all, white flour is, technically, wheat flour. Look for "100% whole wheat flour," and then verify that "wheat flour" or "white flour" doesn't appear later on the label.

➢ **Problems with eating whole grain flour:** Believe it or not, consumption of 100% whole wheat flour has health drawbacks as well. It is certainly much better than white flour and other partial foods, and much better than animal products. Dr. McDougall describes the result of the grain milling process:

> The intact cell wall of the kernel has been destroyed and now the digestive enzymes (amylase) easily digest the inner nutrients. In addition, the flour has a much larger surface area to volume ratio than did the whole grain, making digestion and absorption much more rapid. For you this physical change may translate into easier weight gain, and higher blood levels of glucose, triglycerides, and cholesterol. The amount of insulin released by the pancreas into the blood is also increased as grains are processed from whole grains to cracked grains to coarse flour to fine flour. More insulin can mean more weight gain, and maybe, more risk of diabetes and heart disease. However, compared to animal-foods, free-oils, and plant-parts processed beyond recognition, whole wheat bread is definitely health food.[50]

---

[49] Dr. Caldwell B. Esselstyn, Jr., M.D., Is the Present Therapy for Coronary Artery Disease the Radical Mastectomy of the Twenty-First Century? http://www.dresselstyn.com/Esselstyn_Caldwell_Article.pdf
[50] McDougall, Grains
https://www.drmcdougall.com/misc/2008nl/jan/grains.htm

➤ **White rice/brown rice:** Some say white rice is just as healthy or healthier than brown. Many health authorities disagree, including Dr. McDougall:

> Milling whole-grain, natural rice to remove its outer coating does not make it a more nutritious food. Processing removes 50% of the dietary fiber, 84% of the magnesium, 74% of the manganese, 80% of the thiamin, 85% of the vitamin B-6, and 69% of the total essential fats. These factors are known to be important for health, including improving bowel function, and blood sugar and cholesterol levels.[51]

Researchers found that regular consumption of white rice was associated with a higher risk of type 2 diabetes. Brown rice intake, on the other hand, lowered the risk. Other whole grains, such as barley and oats, were found to be even better than brown rice in this regard.[52]

So brown rice is better, and to me tastes much better, with a much better texture, than white rice.

Even so, Dr. McDougall says that, while brown rice is better for your health, studies indicate that choosing white over brown will have minimal impact on your health compared to issues like consuming meat and dairy. In other words, your chances of having problems with chronic diseases such as diabetes and heart disease decrease so significantly by being off meat and dairy, the difference between brown rice and white becomes not nearly as important.

The point is that one shouldn't make the color of one's rice be a deal breaker when it comes to the big picture of dietary choices. If sticking with white rice will help you stick to a meat-free diet, go for it. But make an effort to sneak more and more brown rice into your diet!

➤ **Oats:** Oats have some special properties which make them

---

[51] McDougall, <u>White Rice Works for Most People</u>
https://www.drmcdougall.com/misc/2012nl/jan/fav5.htm
[52] Greger, <u>Whole Grains May Work As Well As Drugs</u>
http://nutritionfacts.org/video/whole-grains-may-work-as-well-as-drugs/

extra nutritious. The high quality fiber in oats is very healthy for your gut, and can prevent colon cancer. Eating a bowl of oatmeal every day confers significant protection against cancer, in fact.

Eating oats regularly also lowers triglycerides, cholesterol, and blood sugar.[53]

As mentioned earlier, eating whole oats, including rolled oats and steel cut oats, will dramatically lower your chance of getting type 2 diabetes. Many other health benefits are rolled up in oat consumption as well.

Cooked or raw, oatmeal is great with some berries or bananas on top, along with some non-dairy "motherless" (and sugar free) milk, such as almond or soy. You would do well to make it a daily breakfast habit.

➢ **Bread:** Bread is a real weak spot for many trying to eat healthier. Many forms, such as muffins, cake, and doughnuts, are especially bad for the body, as they contain a lot of oil and sugar, as well as white flour.

Finding truly healthy whole wheat bread for sale can be very difficult. Read labels and look for a brand which doesn't have sugar, artificial colors, preservatives, and other chemicals. And as mentioned earlier, be sure the ingredients label only has "100% whole wheat flour," not "white flour," "enriched flour," "bleached flour," or "wheat flour." Baking your own bread is of course best, as then you have total control over what you are eating.

Beans

➢ **Beans/legumes: All legumes** (soybeans, lentils, chick peas, mung beans, kidney beans, black beans, split peas, etc.) **are part of a healthy diet, and strongly linked to reduction in chronic illness and increased longevity.** One study done in several

---

[53] Greger, Stop Cancer Before It Starts (minute 26:40)
https://www.youtube.com/watch?v=dYxpgwFip2M

countries found an 8% reduction in risk of death for every 20 gram (2 tbsp.) increase in daily bean consumption.[54]

Dried and canned beans are both good, but choose canned beans with no added sugar (dextrose, etc.), no chemical additives, and very little or no salt. All beans are good, but lentils, mung beans, and soybeans are especially nutritious.

➢ **Soybeans: Consumption of soybeans is associated with decreased breast cancer.**[55] This may partially explain why while on a traditional Japanese diet, which includes tofu and other soy, Japanese women have very low rates of breast cancer. But when they move to the U.S. and start eating what we typically eat, their breast cancer rates shoot up to nearly match the U.S. average. (There are many other possible reasons, such as decreased consumption of sea vegetables (seaweed), and certainly an increase in meat consumption plays an important role.)

Some authorities believe soybeans are not healthy. They cite the presence of plant estrogens in soybeans, and estrogen is implicated in breast cancer. However, if this were truly a danger, one wouldn't expect to find low rates of breast cancer among populations which consume a lot of soy. And I believe the research that shows soy's benefits to health most compelling.[56]

Of course the more "whole food" and least processed your soy foods are, the better. Tofu is processed a little, but is still a healthy food in moderation. But there is evidence that products made from isolated soy protein, such as fake "vegan" chicken and cheese, promote cancer and should be avoided.[57]

➢ **Dried beans:** Dried beans are less convenient than canned,

---

[54] Greger, Eat Beans to Live Longer http://nutritionfacts.org/2014/09/16/eat-beans-to-live-longer/

[55] Greger, Can Eating Soy Prevent Breast Cancer? http://nutritionfacts.org/2014/09/18/can-eating-soy-prevent-breast-cancer/

[56] Breastcancer.org, Soy http://www.breastcancer.org/tips/nutrition/reduce_risk/foods/soy

[57] McDougall, Soy – Food, Wonder Drug, or Poison? https://www.drmcdougall.com/misc/2005nl/april/050400pusoy.htm

but are a good choice since they don't have ingredients added which you don't want to be eating. You have to think ahead, as the larger varieties such as kidney and pinto take a long time to soak and cook. However, lentils, mung beans, field peas and split peas don't take long to cook. In fact, you can cook lentils together with brown rice and they will be done at the same time. **There is some evidence that small beans like lentils and mung beans are easier to digest and more nutritious than large beans.**

The larger bean varieties should be soaked overnight. Then be sure to pour off the water and rinse the beans before adding water for cooking.

➢ **Beans and protein:** Beans have a lot of protein. Thus many people think that if you don't eat meat you must eat a lot of beans. That is not true. All veggies have protein, as do grains, nuts, seeds, and to a lesser extent fruits. A whole plant food diet free of beans can easily provide you with adequate protein. However, beans have lots of great fiber and other valuable nutrients, and many authorities recommend eating them several times a week. See more on protein in the **Nutrients and supplements** section in **Chapter 15**.

➢ **Beans, fiber, and gas:** Many fear that increasing their fiber intake, especially beans, will result in them suffering from more intestinal gas. (Perhaps they are more concerned that those in close proximity to them will suffer.) While it is true that many notice this problem when first increasing their intake of beans, once the population of gut bacteria adjust to the new diet, the amount of gas should subside. Don't let this fear prevent you from upping your bean intake! But if you are especially concerned about this issue, just increase your bean intake gradually.

Spices

➢ **Packed with nutrients:** Most spices are packed with health-promoting compounds. **Pound for pound some spices have the**

most antioxidants of any food.[58] Some have a powerful anti-inflammatory effect in the body. Oregano, black pepper[59], cloves, ginger, cumin, cayenne, rosemary, etc. all add a great nutritional kick to any dish, and can really spice up your bean, vegetable soup, and spaghetti sauce recipes. And try to add cinnamon to any food where it is appropriate, such as your morning oatmeal.

➢ **Turmeric:** This spice deserves special mention. Turmeric is one of the spices found in curry. **It contains curcumin, which has strong anti-inflammatory effects in the body.**[60] It has been shown to suppress cancer, causing cancer cells to self-destruct.[61]

Note this interesting correlation: India, where turmeric is consumed much more heavily than in the U.S., has far less cancer (1/23rd as much prostate cancer, for example). This is no doubt due to partially to other lifestyle factors as well, such as higher intake of plants and lower intake of meat, but the likelihood that turmeric and other spices play a prominent role in the statistic is consistent with the known science.

Turmeric is also effective at combatting osteoarthritis[62], rheumatoid arthritis[63], Alzheimer's[64], ulcers, and a host of other ailments.[65] Add some turmeric to your food as often as possible,

---

[58] Greger, Antioxidants in a Pinch http://nutritionfacts.org/video/antioxidants-in-a-pinch/

[59] Some claim black pepper is unhealthy. In fact this is not true, except for those who should be on a low-oxalate diet (oxalates tend to encourage kidney stone formation in some people).

[60] Greger, Which Spice Fights Inflammation? http://nutritionfacts.org/video/which-spices-fight-inflammation/

[61] Greger, Turmeric Curcumin Reprogramming Cancer Cell Death http://nutritionfacts.org/video/turmeric-curcumin-reprogramming-cancer-cell-death/

[62] Greger, Turmeric Curcumin and Osteoarthritis http://nutritionfacts.org/video/turmeric-curcumin-and-osteoarthritis/

[63] Greger, Turmeric Curcumin and Rheumatoid Arthritis http://nutritionfacts.org/video/turmeric-curcumin-and-rheumatoid-arthritis/

[64] Greger, Treating Alzheimer's with Turmeric http://nutritionfacts.org/video/treating-alzheimers-with-turmeric/

[65] Go to www.nutritionfacts.org and search for Turmeric for a list of other videos and articles on this amazing spice.

sprinkled on salads or added to soups or other dishes. It can be expensive in the tiny containers sold in grocery stores, but you can get it relatively cheaply online if you buy it in 16 or 18 oz. containers. Some local stores may sell it in bulk as well.

Seeds

➢ **Seeds and nutrition:** Seeds are very nutritious. Raw is best, and un-shelled when possible. (Obviously for some, like sunflower and coconut, they need to be shelled.)

Many studies indicate the health benefits of seeds. One of the main benefits comes from many seeds' high content of α-linolenic acid (ALA). ALA is the only essential omega-3 oil, the only one your body needs to obtain from dietary sources. See below under **Oils and fats** for more on this subject.

Good food seeds include flax, sesame, chia, hemp, sunflower, pumpkin/squash, coconut and poppy. When you eat a fruit, such as an orange, apple or watermelon, try to eat the seeds. Chew them up good! Once you get used to it, it becomes second nature.

➢ **Flax, hemp, chia and sesame seeds:** These seeds especially are natural multivitamins + multi-minerals + fiber + protein + healthy fats. But they are whole food, and so contain a much better balance of nutrients, and many more much higher quality nutrients, than a multivitamin multi-mineral pill.

It is best to grind a small amount at a time (up to a few cups) in a coffee grinder, and store in the fridge or freezer. If you eat them whole, many seeds will pass through you whole, and it will be a waste of money (possible exception: apparently you don't need to grind up chia seeds in order to get the full benefit).

Sprinkle the ground seed meal over salads, stir into soups, use as thickening agent in sauces, add to chunky smoothies. Some nutrition authorities recommend getting 1 to 4 tbsp./day of any or all of these.

If you don't like these seeds, or have a hard time obtaining them, don't let that worry you; you can still do well on a whole food plant based diet without them.

➢ **Flax seeds:** These deserve special mention, as they are especially important to good health. They support a healthy urinary tract, and one study found flax seed consumption to be as effective as the drug Flomax in helping men with urinary retention, but of course without the drug side effects.

Studies have shown that daily flax seed meal can also prevent and slow progression of breast and prostate cancers, improve blood sugar levels and thus possibly prevent type 2 diabetes, improve cholesterol levels, blood pressure, and hot flashes, and lessen joint pain. And flax is a good source of boron, which is an important mineral for bone health. It also has heart healthy precursors to omega-3 fatty acids, thus giving you the expected benefits of omega-3s without the downsides of eating fish, with all its fat, toxins, etc.[66]

> *Daily flax seed meal can prevent and slow progression of breast and prostate cancers.*

Some experts recommended consuming at least 2 tbsp. of ground flax seeds per day to get the maximum advantage of this little health powerhouse. When purchased in bulk flax seeds are very inexpensive – a couple dollars worth could last you a month or two. Not a bad buy considering all the expensive and painful health problems it is able to help prevent.

➢ **Cocoa:** There are many health benefits to consuming cocoa. It contains polyphenolic flavonoids, and there is evidence that these antioxidants reduce blood pressure, increase blood vessel health, and are heart healthy. Consumption of cocoa is associated with reduction in the risk of diabetes.[67]

---

[66] Greger, Just the Flax, Ma'am http://nutritionfacts.org/video/just-the-flax-maam/

[67] Bill Hendrick, *WebMD Health News,* Cocoa Consumption May Decrease Blood Pressure, Improve Cholesterol, Researchers Say http://www.webmd.com/diabetes/news/20110323/cocoa-rich-in-health-benefits

But note that we're talking about plain, unadulterated cocoa here, not sugary chocolate! Consuming sugar is dangerous, so be careful how you get your cocoa. Powdered baking cocoa, such as Hershey's, is probably the most available, inexpensive, and convenient form. But it is bitter, so getting it down without consuming a lot of milk and sugar can be a challenge. You can put some in a blender with some almonds, dates and cold water to make a chocolate smoothie (bananas, vanilla and coconut are yummy optional additions to this recipe).

➢ **Sprouts and microgreens:** We have seen that seeds are very nutritious. And we have seen that leafy veggies are very nutritious also. But sprouted seeds and "microgreens" (sprouts which are allowed to grow several inches tall) are even more nutritious than either, at least in some respects.

When seeds are sprouted the antioxidant level increases dramatically, from doubling to up to 20 times what the seed contained.[68] Dr. Greger also notes that, even though red (or purple) cabbage is extremely healthful,

> red cabbage microgreens have a 6-fold higher vitamin C concentration than mature red cabbage and 69 times the vitamin K.

And the cost of microgreens? Dr. Greger continues:

> Homemade sprouts are probably the most nutrition-per-unit-cost we can get for our money.[69]

He recommends broccoli and lentil sprouts most highly, and warns against alfalfa sprouts, as salmonella infection has been connected to them (though known cases number only in the hundreds, not the hundreds of thousands attributed to contaminated chicken).

Nuts

➢ **Nuts:** Nuts are of course a type of seed, and like other seeds they are good sources of healthy fats, protein, vitamins, minerals

---

[68] Greger, Antioxidants Sprouting Up
http://nutritionfacts.org/video/antioxidants-sprouting-up/
[69] Greger, Are Microgreens Healthier? http://nutritionfacts.org/2013/05/02/are-microgreens-healthier/

and fiber. Cashews, almonds, walnuts, pecans, brazil nuts, etc. are all good food for most people.

A very large study showed that daily nut consumption results in fewer cancer deaths, fewer heart disease deaths, fewer respiratory disease deaths, and lengthens lifespan.[70] At least one study determined that eating a handful of nuts every day is as effective at preventing heart disease as 60 minutes of daily moderate exercise. (Don't do one or the other, do both!)[71]

On the other hand, Dr. Caldwell Esselstyn of the Cleveland Clinic, who has successfully helped many patients stop and reverse their heart disease by adopting a whole food plant based diet, has a different view. He says nuts are not healthy for heart disease patients, and others should only eat limited quantities, due to the high fat content. He sees evidence that this fat, even though it is in a whole plant food, contributes to heart disease because it damages the cells lining the blood vessels. As indicated earlier, other evidence supports the notion that nut consumption is heart-healthy.

Another thing to consider is that if you are overweight and want to try a whole food plant based diet to improve your health and lose weight, it is probably best to avoid nuts (and avocados as well), at least until you reach your healthy weight goal. While some research seems to suggest that nuts have a negligible effect on weight gain,[72] others dispute these conclusions.[73]

While nuts are a yummy source of essential nutrients, it is important to understand that you can get all the nutrition you need from other whole plant food sources. So if you have heart

---

[70] Greger, Nuts May Help Prevent Death http://nutritionfacts.org/video/nuts-may-help-prevent-death/
[71] Greger, Halving Heart Attack Risk http://nutritionfacts.org/video/halving-heart-attack-risk/
[72] Greger, Nuts and Obesity: The Weight of Evidence http://nutritionfacts.org/video/nuts-and-obesity-the-weight-of-evidence/
[73] Jeff Nelson, Nuts & Weight Gain: It's Worse Than We Thought http://www.vegsource.com/news/2012/08/nuts-weight-gain-its-worse-than-we-thought.html

disease or need to lose weight, and are concerned about eating nuts, be assured that you can get along fine without them.

➤ **Peanuts:** Peanuts are actually in the bean family, but their nutritional profile is closer to that of nuts, so they can properly be referred to as nuts. Peanuts (and peanut butter) are a good source of protein and other nutrients.

Some claim that toxins from mold which sometimes grows on peanuts are dangerous, and can lead to cancer. This risk seems to be very small, however, especially when eaten in the context of a whole food plant based diet, which, it appears, confers protection from such toxins.[74]

➤ **Coconut:** Coconut is a very healthy food. Fresh is best, but not so convenient if you aren't skilled at getting the meat out. Pre-shredded dried coconut is most convenient, but you should not eat sweetened coconut, as the sugar content is high. It is very hard to find unsweetened dried coconut in stores, so the best sources of coconut flakes and chips are online. The best, most nutritious and most delicious dried coconut is that which is dried at the lowest temperature.[75]

Whole plant foods: No downside!

I hope it is clear by now that consuming whole plant foods promises only benefits to the body; there is no downside as far as good health goes. As we shall see, the alternatives, processed foods, partial foods, and animal products, while often providing some nutrition, carry a great amount of baggage, dangerous substances which work to erode health.

---

[74] Greger, Eating Greens to Prevent Cancer
http://nutritionfacts.org/video/eating-green-to-prevent-cancer/
[75] www.wildernessfamilynaturals.com has the best quality I have found, though it is expensive. www.nuts.com is also a good source, though theirs is dried at a much higher temp. www.amazon.com currently sells a 10 kilo sack of organic coconut flakes at a good price, but this is also apparently dried at a high temp, as the flavor is much less strong than the good stuff from Wilderness Family Naturals.

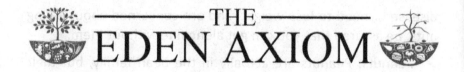

THE EDEN AXIOM

Chapter 6:

Foods Which Promote Disease:

Animal Products

In the last chapter we saw some of the wonderful ways plant foods promote good health and long life. In this chapter we will look at animal products and see some of the reasons their consumption promotes chronic disease, thus rendering them poor dietary choices.

Dairy

➢ **Dairy propaganda:** Dairy products have always played a large role in most Western diets. For most of us it is almost axiomatic that consuming dairy is an important part of staying healthy. And the dairy industry has promoted this idea through slick advertising, which is often misleading.

For example, the slogan I grew up with: "Every body needs milk." Really? I guess so, if you mean human breast milk and if we're talking infants. Otherwise, not so much. Not at all, really. The American Dairy Council got into legal trouble for that slogan, since it was a lie, so they came up with a new one: "Milk has something for every body." Right. For some bodies it has acne, digestive trouble, cancer, heart disease. "Milk does a body good." Really? That's not what the science says. "Got milk?" Well, I guess one good way to avoid telling a lie is to just ask a question. Please don't be fooled by slick advertising. Make dietary choices based on the true facts about nutrition.

The dairy industry plays up the supposed positive nutritional value of their products. According to them we need dairy in order to get enough calcium. The protein content of dairy products may also be promoted as beneficial. However, one has to ask, **where do adult cows get calcium and protein from?** From plants. Doesn't it make sense that we also could get these nutrients from plants? Indeed it does, and indeed we can. See **Chapter 15: Nutrients and supplements** for more on the subject of calcium and protein.

God designed the mother's milk of each species to be the perfect food, with the perfect unique combination of nutrients, for the young of that species. In nature no baby animal in the world, much less an adult animal, drinks the milk of another species. But we humans have manufactured a pretend "need" for the milk of cows. The USDA choosemyplate.gov website says

> How much food from the Dairy Group is **needed** daily? The amount of food from the Dairy Group you **need** to eat depends on age. Recommended daily amounts are shown in the chart below. [Emphasis added.]

The chart goes on to indicate that everyone nine and older needs three cups of milk a day. They don't explain why humans need milk from an animal (milk which has a balance of nutrients appropriate for calves, but not at all for humans of any age), while no adult animals have such a need. And of course they can provide no sound scientific evidence that this need exists. It only exists to keep the money flowing into the Big Dairy coffers, and subsequently on to the USDA and the politicians which support and are responsible for this insanity.[76]

➤ **Dairy and protein:** One cup of milk provides 8 grams of protein, which is 16% of the amount we supposedly need each day. However, this is mostly the animal protein called casein. And various studies indicate that casein in high levels can cause cancer in rats. Such studies cannot be duplicated in humans, of course, but human population studies suggest strongly this link

---

[76] Of course it comes back to us, the voters; we have the leaders we choose.

is a concern, as research by Dr. Colin Campbell, author of *The China Study*, shows.[77]

This is further supported by data from Japan. Between about 1950 and 1995 their consumption of dairy, meat, and eggs increased 20-, 10-, and 7-fold respectively (the rest of their diet not changing much at all), while their prostate cancer rate increased 25-fold over the same period.[78]

The conclusions suggested by these correlations have been confirmed by several high quality case-control[79] and cohort[80] studies. Such studies are so conclusive that Dr. Campbell calls milk protein a significant carcinogen (cancer-causing substance). Of course, there are many who would dispute that this is a valid characterization.

The consumption of animal protein, including milk protein, has been shown to damage the endothelium, or inner lining, of blood vessels. See the discussion of this under the topic **Red meat** later in this chapter.

➢ **Dairy and constipation:** Even a little bit of dairy can cause problems. Dr. McDougall noted,

Avoiding proteins from milk and milk products is very important. I

---

[77] Dr. Colin Campbell, Ph.D., The Remarkable Health Benefits of Nutrition https://www.youtube.com/watch?v=XEuRMm-a6mo. For more interesting information about casein and its potential function as a mild narcotic, see Dr. Neal Barnard, M.D.'s lecture Chocolate, Cheese, Meat, and Sugar – Physically Addictive (minute 10:20) https://www.youtube.com/watch?v=5VWi6dXCT7I

[78] Greger, Prostate Cancer and Organic Milk vs. Almond Milk http://nutritionfacts.org/video/prostate-cancer-and-organic-milk-vs-almond-milk/

[79] In case-control studies researchers look "back" at the diets of patients with cancer and compare those diets to the diets of controls, that is people without cancer.

[80] In cohort studies researchers work with preselected groups, or cohorts, of study subjects going forward. For example, one cohort may be individuals who consume a lot of dairy, while the control cohort would be those who consume no dairy. Researchers would then be interested in comparing the health outcomes of the two groups over time. Such studies may take many years to complete.

have seen some people who have made nearly a complete change to a health supporting diet. But they couldn't give up the little bit of skimmed milk in the morning on their dry cereal–and their bowels didn't work very well. A little dairy protein can literally jam up the works for most people who are sensitive to it.[81]

Of course this won't be the experience of everyone, since many can tolerate dairy fairly well without immediately noticeable effects. However, many have problems with constipation, and for some even a small amount of dairy intake could be the reason. Of course, a low fiber diet, one with too much meat and not enough whole plant foods, will always contribute to this unhealthy condition as well.

➢ **Low fat and nonfat dairy:** For many years the fat in dairy was considered to be the thing to avoid. So it was widely promoted that consuming dairy is good, but you should make the "healthy choice" for the low fat or nonfat products.

However, the scientific literature seems to show increasingly that the protein in dairy is actually more dangerous than the fat. And whole milk is 21% protein, while skim milk is 41% protein. For this reason, skim milk may in fact be more dangerous to your health than whole or low fat milk. This conclusion is supported by studies which have found that men who drink skim milk are more likely to get prostate cancer than men who drink whole milk – or no milk at all.[82,83]

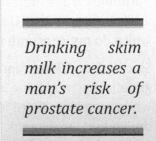

Drinking skim milk increases a man's risk of prostate cancer.

➢ **Dairy and industrial waste:** Analysis of toxins in milk found

[81] McDougall, Constipation, Hemorrhoids, Varicose Veins
https://www.drmcdougall.com/health/education/health-science/common-health-problems/constipation-hemorrhoids-varicose-veins/
[82] Ryan Devon, Does Skim Milk Cause Prostate Cancer?
http://www.livestrong.com/article/524487-does-skim-milk-cause-prostate-cancer/
[83] Barnard, Chocolate, Cheese, Meat, and Sugar – Physically Addictive (minute 15:20) https://www.youtube.com/watch?v=5VWi6dXCT7I

PCBs and many other contaminants – over 100 times as much PCB chemicals as that present in plant foods! The FDA estimated that 30% of adults' daily intake of toxic dioxins is from dairy. For children it is 50%.[84] Want to cut your children's dioxin intake in half? Well, there's an easy way to do that.

➢ **Dairy and hormones:** Milk and other dairy sold in the U.S. usually have added hormones. One is rBGH – bovine growth hormone, given to cows to boost milk production. It has the effect of increasing the amount of pus, antibiotic residues, and the cancer-accelerating growth hormone IGF-1 in the milk. Yuck.

But even if hormones aren't given to the cows, the milk can have hormones in it, because most milk on the market comes from pregnant cows. The pregnant cows have a lot of hormones running through their bodies, and many of these get into their milk. **It is not normal or natural for calves to drink such hormone-laden milk, much less for people to do so.**

When people drink this hormone-laden milk, the hormones can cause problems in the drinker's body. Studies show that milk hormones are responsible for acne, a condition suffered by most adolescents in the U.S., but almost unknown in populations which do not consume milk.[85]

Since the 1960s and 70s, when milk producers started genetically modifying cows to enable them to produce milk while pregnant, there has been a dramatic increase in estrogen-dependent malignant diseases – ovarian, prostate, uterine, breast, and testicular cancers. This is not a rigorous proof. It is a correlation, but it is very likely there is a connection.

Also, consuming dairy from hormone-laden pregnant cows is implicated in the tendency toward early sexual maturation. Early sexual maturation is associated with increased likelihood of breast cancer and shorter lifespan. **Note that skim milk contains**

---

[84] Greger, Dairy, Estrogen and Male Fertility
http://nutritionfacts.org/video/dairy-estrogen-and-male-fertility/
[85] Greger, National Dairy Council on Acne and Milk
http://nutritionfacts.org/video/national-dairy-council-on-acne-and-milk/

more hormones than fat milk.[86] For an excellent video lecture on the dangers of milk consumption, see the link on this topic in the **Appendix** under Dr. McDougall.

➤ **Milk and SIDS:** A breastfeeding mother who drinks cows milk can pass certain compounds from the milk on to her child, which can cause infant apnea and SIDS.[87]

➤ **Milk and twins:** Milk drinking women bear 5 times the rate of twins as those on a plant food only diet.[88] This is probably related to the hormone content of the milk. What other funny stuff are those hormones perpetrating in our bodies?

➤ **Milk and pus:** I mentioned above pus in milk. Yes, all milk has pus in it. Bovine growth hormone only increases the amount. The maximum level allowed is 750,000 pus cells per milliliter.[89] Yes, per milliliter. And there are 237 milliliters in every cup. Yuck.

➤ **Cheese and saturated fat:** Americans' cheese consumption continues to rise, till now we eat an average of 30 lbs. of cheese per year. This is considered to be a serious public health issue. Cheddar cheese is 74% fat. Cutting down on cheese consumption, preferably to zero, can have a significant positive impact on your health.[90]

> *Cheese is probably the most fattening food that people include in their diets.*
> *— Dr. Neal Barnard*

---

[86] Greger, Hormones in Skim vs. Whole Milk
http://nutritionfacts.org/video/hormones-in-skim-vs-whole-milk/
[87] Greger, Cow's Milk-Induced Infant Apnea
http://nutritionfacts.org/video/cows-milk-induced-infant-apnea/
[88] Greger, Dairy & Sexual Precocity http://nutritionfacts.org/video/dairy-sexual-precocity/
[89] McDougall, Dairy Products - 10 False Promises
https://www.drmcdougall.com/misc/2003nl/apr/PDF030400NL.pdf
[90] *Center for Science in the Public Interest,* Don't Say Cheese
http://www.cspinet.org/new/cheese.html

➢ **Cheese and aluminum:** Aluminum is added to processed cheese to improve its texture. (That is, "processed American cheese," or "cheese food" products.) But aluminum is highly toxic to the human body, thought to cause Alzheimer's,[91] for example. One source claimed that 45 grams of processed "American cheese food," the amount in a cheese sandwich, contains 428% of the FDA's provisional tolerable daily intake of aluminum, meaning it contains 4 times as much aluminum as one can safely consume in a day. Apparently other cheeses don't have aluminum.

➢ **Dairy and sugar:** Dairy naturally contains a sugar called lactose. Whole milk is 30% lactose, while skim milk is 57% lactose.

Of concern here is that 75% of African Americans, over 80% of Asians, 51% of Hispanics, and 21% of North American whites are lactose intolerant.[92] For these people, quite possibly including you, the digestive system is not able to properly digest lactose. That is because the bodies of lactose intolerant people does not produce *lactase*, the enzyme critical for lactose digestion.

It is important that humans be capable of digesting lactose as infants, since it is the sugar in mother's milk as well. So why do most people become lactose intolerant later in life? Genetic evidence indicates that normally a human's genes should switch off the production of lactase after weaning. After all, it should normally no longer be needed then. A mutation is responsible for leaving the lactase-producing gene switched on, and thus some of us are capable of digesting lactose into adulthood.

Given that 75% of African Americans are lactose intolerant, it is quite ironic – and tragic – that milk ads feature black athletes and other celebrities with their white milk mustaches, ads at

---

[91] McDougall, <u>Alzheimer's Disease</u>
<u>https://www.drmcdougall.com/health/education/health-science/common-health-problems/alzheimers-disease/</u>
[92] Itan Yuval, Ph.D., <u>Lactose Intolerance by Ethnicity and Region</u>
<u>http://milk.procon.org/view.resource.php?resourceID=000661</u>

least partially aimed at encouraging milk consumption among blacks.

Lactose intolerance by ethnicity:

Asian	80-100%
Native American	80-100%
African American	75%
African	70-90%
Indian	30-70%
French	17-65%
Jewish North American	60-80%
Hispanic	51%
Anglo North American	21%
Italian	20-70%
German	15%
British	5-15%
World average	**65%**

Dairy contains a lot of sugar at the outset, but then sugar is added to many dairy products, such as yogurt, ice cream, and chocolate milk. Even plain milk raises your blood glucose level, but adding more sugar makes it even more dangerous. It is best to not consume these products. Nutritionally they are not needed by the body.

➢ **Raw grass fed dairy:** If in spite of the above info you still want to consume dairy, you would do well to insist on raw grass fed.

Raw dairy is usually hard to obtain. The FDA regulates it heavily, ostensibly to protect consumers from disease-causing products. But in reality it is apparent that their main goal is to protect Big

Dairy interests.[93] The FDA has even gone so far as to have some farmers arrested for selling raw milk.

While it is true that raw dairy may have more potential to contain disease-causing bacteria than pasteurized products, the pasteurization process destroys or diminishes the vitamin content of milk and destroys good bacteria. Some say it actually promotes harmful pathogens, and that more than raw milk it is associated with increased tooth decay, colic in infants, osteoporosis, heart disease, and cancer.

Pasteurization also destroys enzymes which naturally occur in milk, including the enzyme lactase. Lactose intolerant individuals no longer produce lactase in their bodies, but lactase is available in raw milk, and thus it is claimed that many who cannot tolerate pasteurized dairy are able to consume raw dairy without a problem. Some studies, however, suggest there is no difference, that symptoms of lactose intolerance persist even when raw dairy is consumed.

Homogenization is done to prevent the cream from separating from the rest of the milk. Some claim this is problematic, because this process reduces the size of the fat globules in the milk, and as a result when it is consumed the fat is more readily assimilated into the body. Thus it is claimed that weight gain is promoted by the consumption of homogenized milk more than it is by the consumption of raw, non-homogenized milk.

In any event, the best science clearly shows that it is ill advised to consume dairy in any form. Even raw, grass fed, non-homogenized dairy contains animal protein (casein), cholesterol, cow hormones, lactose, saturated fat, pus, and sometimes, dangerous bacteria. It still promotes inflammation and disease. To be sure, it is the perfect food for taking a healthy calf from 60 lbs. to 600 lbs. in eight months, but not so good for human consumption. Certainly it has no essential nutrients not available

---

[93] If the FDA operated consistently in light of the available science, to fulfil their mandate to protect consumers they would have to warn against all dairy consumption.

in plant sources, which have no associated health hazards.

➢ **Dairy and rotting teeth:** Everyone knows we need dairy for strong, healthy teeth, right? Well... One day in Guinea, West Africa, my wife and I happened to be visiting a mission hospital while they were conducting a special dental clinic to provide cheap or free dental care for several different ethnic groups from the area. We volunteered to help out for a few hours.

We mentioned to the Guinean dentist how appalled we were at the number of teeth many of the Africans had to have extracted, some in the double digits, due to cavities and unhealthy gums. The dentist told us that during his career he had noticed a strong correlation between the ethnic group and the degree of dental decay. The Fulanis were the group with the most dental problems, he said.

It wasn't till recently that we were considering this, and realized that this correlated with their culture. Raising cattle and consuming dairy are central to the Fulani culture. And note that the dairy which apparently produces gum and dental disease is raw, grass-fed, and non-homogenized. Interesting that **the people group drinking the most milk have the worst teeth.**

Eggs

My opinion of the advisability from a health standpoint of eating eggs has shifted back and forth quite a bit over the years. In my youth I ate eggs freely. Then when I was found to have high cholesterol, my doctor told me to avoid high cholesterol foods, including eggs. So I did. But then a few years later I did some looking around on the Internet and found a bunch of articles citing studies which supposedly showed egg consumption had no link to heart disease, and so was safe. I immediately began eating 10-14 eggs per week. Yum. However, in my latest research, I have discovered that what I had read was egg industry propaganda. Eggs are in fact not a part of a healthy diet.

➢ **Egg studies:** Many scientific studies have shown that animal sourced dietary saturated fat, cholesterol, and protein promote heart disease and other chronic health problems, and this has been shown repeatedly to be true for eggs specifically.[94]

A study found a link between egg consumption and prostate cancer progression.[95]

Another study found a significantly increased risk of cardiovascular disease, type 2 diabetes, and heart disease in people who ate only four eggs per week, compared with those who didn't eat eggs.[96]

Egg consumption is associated with increased chance of developing type 2 diabetes and of a person with diabetes dying. Women who eat eggs and get pregnant are twice as likely as those who abstain to contract gestational diabetes.[97]

The 20 year long Harvard Physician's Health Study looked at the effect of egg consumption on 20,000 physicians. The finding was that those who consumed an average of 7 eggs or more per week were significantly more likely to have a shorter life than those who consumed no eggs.[98,99]

➢ **Eggs and health claims:** The American Egg Board is appointed by the U.S. government to promote the consumption of eggs as a help to the egg industry. They dole out $10 million per year to egg producers to be spent on advertising. (Wow. Ya think some lobbyists were involved in getting that one started? What business is it of the Feds to have any such involvement? Using my tax money to promote a health eroding product. But don't get me started.)

The Egg Board and those who utilize their advertising dollars try

---

[94] Greger, How the Egg Board Designs Misleading Studies
http://nutritionfacts.org/video/how-the-egg-board-designs-misleading-studies/
[95] Greger, Why the Egg-Cancer Link? http://nutritionfacts.org/2014/08/21/why-the-egg-cancer-link/
[96] Greger, Debunking Egg Industry Myths
http://nutritionfacts.org/video/debunking-egg-industry-myths/
[97] Greger, Bad Egg http://nutritionfacts.org/2011/08/31/bad-egg/
[98] Ibid.
[99] Greger, Whose Health is Unaffected by Eggs?
http://nutritionfacts.org/video/whose-health-unaffected-by-eggs/

to paint quite a rosy picture about the health benefits of egg consumption. But by law the use of the advertising subsidy has an inconvenient string attached: subsidized ads must not contain lies. They must make only truthful claims about eggs. (Ads which don't receive federal funding can legally be full of lies, of course.)

Since these subsidized ads must be truthful, and the science is so clear about the dangers of eating eggs, they cannot claim eggs are "nutritious," "healthy," or "good for you." Instead they have to use terms such as "fresh," "nutrient-dense" and "can reduce hunger."[100] Imagine that. You eat food, and it reduces your hunger. One could similarly label candy bars, Fruit Loops, chips, doughnuts and French fries.

Similarly, because eggs contain so much fat and cholesterol, the United States Department of Agriculture (USDA) does not allow egg sellers to put "Eggs are an important part of a well-balanced, healthy diet" on an egg carton.

Egg industry spokespersons insist that one shouldn't tell people they shouldn't eat eggs just because they contain so much saturated fat and cholesterol. After all, they contend, if people are frightened into not eating eggs they won't get the benefit of many important nutrients found in them, such as choline, and the carotenoids lutein and zeaxanthin.

Actually, a study on choline from eggs indicated that it may increase the risk of stroke, heart attack and death. And the carotenoids, important for eye health among other things, are only present in eggs in very small quantities. **In fact, you would have to eat nine eggs to get the quantity of these carotenoids**

> *You would have to eat nine eggs to get the quantity of eye-healthy carotenoids found in one spoonful of spinach.*

---

[100] Greger, Who Says Eggs Aren't Healthy or Safe? http://nutritionfacts.org/video/who-says-eggs-arent-healthy-or-safe/

found in one spoonful of spinach.[101]

The egg industry has attempted to snooker the public with their false and misleading advertising much the same as the tobacco industry.[102]

➢ **Eggs and salmonella:** Not only may eggs not be billed as "healthful," but they can't even be touted as "safe" by the egg industry because, according to the USDA, over 100,000 Americans are infected with egg-born salmonella each year. In fact, the Egg Board's own research results said that **"The sunny-side up method (of cooking) should be considered unsafe"** when they found salmonella bacteria surviving on such cooked eggs. Other studies indicate none of the normal methods of cooking eggs will be certain to kill all the salmonella.[103]

Interestingly, when there were 100 cases of salmonella poisoning from alfalfa sprouts reported, there was quite a stir, and the FDA warned the public against eating sprouts. But 100,000 cases from eggs get no press. The egg lobby has a lot more influence than the sprout lobby, apparently.

➢ **"Free range" and "pastured" chickens and eggs:** This section is for those who, in spite of the above information, absolutely refuse to give up eggs.

When we think of "free range" chickens we probably get a picture in our minds of a flock of chickens scratching around in a farmyard all day. But in reality this is often not the case. **That "free range" labeled chicken may have spent most of his life cooped up in cramped quarters, much like factory farm chickens.** But in order to earn the "free range" label, the chicken had the option of going out and stretching it's legs in what may have been a small patch of grass, dirt or gravel.

---

[101] Greger, Does Cholesterol Size Matter? http://nutritionfacts.org/video/does-cholesterol-size-matter/

[102] Greger, Eggs and Cholesterol: Patently False and Misleading Claims http://nutritionfacts.org/video/eggs-and-cholesterol-patently-false-and-misleading-claims/

[103] Greger, Total Recall http://nutritionfacts.org/video/total-recall/

Additionally, the access to outside may be at the end of a huge building housing thousands of birds. Some of them may never even know that going outside to get some "free range" is an option. So it seems you really can't depend on the "free range" label to indicate chickens or eggs significantly more healthful than factory farm products.

"Pastured" eggs are from hens who really do live outside every day of their adult lives, and they have an opportunity to scratch and eat their natural diet, supplemented with commercial chicken feed. Eggs and meat from these chickens would definitely be less damaging to health than those from factory farms. So if you feel you must eat eggs, look for ones with the "pastured" label.

The best thing to do is to seek out local farmers and get to know them so you can verify personally their livestock raising practices. And remember, the chickens should have a diet which includes grass and other plants, insects, etc., with grain being only supplemental. They also should be raised free from hormones, arsenic and other chemicals.

Fish and shellfish

➤ **Fish and health:** For most of my life I believed that fish was the healthiest meat one could eat. However, many of the unhealthy aspects of other meats are the same in fish. **Fish contain a lot of fat, animal protein, cholesterol and toxins.**

➤ **Fish and omega-3s:** This topic is covered in **Chapter 7** in more depth, so I will be brief here. The much celebrated healthy omega-3 oils in many fish have been shown to not actually be needed for arterial health. One of the main reasons given for consuming more omega-3 oils is to offset the dietary omega-6 oils so prevalent in the SAD, and thus improve the ratio from the typical unhealthy 16/1 to be closer to the target of 4/1. But if one simply reduces the intake of omega-6 oils by avoiding added oils (cooking oil, fried foods, oily salad dressings, etc.) and omega-6 laden grain fed meat altogether, and eats only healthful whole plant foods, one can get all the omega-3s one needs without having to deal with the problematic issues of consuming fish.

I wonder if those who promote the eating of fish in order to improve heart health ever stop to think how ridiculous their view really is. Sure, the fish contains omega-3 oils, and there is some evidence that these oils may promote heart health in that they counteract some of the toxic effects of the high omega-6 intake of people on the SAD. However, fish contains a lot of fat, including saturated animal fat, which has been proven repeatedly to be detrimental to heart health, as well as promoting a host of other chronic diseases such as diabetes. Fish also has a lot of unhealthy animal protein and dietary cholesterol. The Physicians Committee for Responsible Medicine stated,

> While fish are frequently referenced as good sources of essential fatty acids, the high amounts of other fats and cholesterol and the lack of fiber make fish poor dietary choices. Fish are also often high in mercury and other environmental toxins that pose dangers to the consumer.[104]

It is quite evident that boosting omega-3 intake in the context of eating a meat-rich diet is useless, as so many people who do so still die of heart disease. On the other hand heart disease patients who ignore omega-3 recommendations but switch to a whole food plant based diet see remission and in some cases reversal of their disease, and experience no more symptoms.[105]

➤ **Fish and toxins:** An article in the Journal of Pediatrics asserted that "Almost all fish contain some mercury."[106] Some are concerned about the possible harmful effects of mercury in vaccines, and rightly so. However, a half can of tuna has as much

---

[104] *Physicians Committee for Responsible Medicine,* Essential Fatty Acids
http://www.pcrm.org/health/health-topics/essential-fatty-acids
[105] Esselstyn, et al, A Strategy to Arrest and Reverse Coronary Artery Disease: A 5-Year Longitudinal Study of a Single Physician's Practice
http://www.dresselstyn.com/site/study01/
[106] *My Wellness Warriors,* Current Research: 'More Specifics About Fish'
http://www.mywellnesswarriors.com/food-nutrition/caution-foods/current-research-more-specifics-about-fish/

mercury as 100 thimerosal-preserved vaccines.[107,108] Fish and shellfish may contain other heavy metals as well, such as cadmium, arsenic and lead.

> *While fish are frequently referenced as good sources of essential fatty acids, the high amounts of other fats and cholesterol and the lack of fiber make fish poor dietary choices.*
> — *Physicians Committee for Responsible Medicine*

Fish and shellfish flesh also contains PCBs, the highest level of any food; over 1400 times as much as plant foods! Other chemicals such as flame retardants are also present.

Industrial pollutants eventually make their way into the oceans where fish consume them and concentrate them in their bodies. **It is estimated that over 90% of persistent organic pollutants consumed by humans, which includes many toxic chemicals, come from animal products**, of which fish is a significant contributor – along, of course, with beef, chicken, pork, processed meats, etc.[109]

Mercury in fish is of special concern to pregnant women or women who may become pregnant, because if the mother's body is contaminated with high levels of mercury, it increases the risk of abnormal brain development in the baby. And it can

---

[107] Greger, Mercury in Vaccinations vs. Tuna
http://nutritionfacts.org/video/mercury-in-vaccinations-vs-tuna-2/
[108] Note that injecting mercury into a vein is probably more dangerous than eating mercury – but not ingesting it at all is better! Also, the specific form of mercury is different (ethylmercury in thimerosal vs. methylmercury in fish). Both forms are known to be powerful toxins, but they may not produce the same toxic effects. Greger, Mercury in Vaccinations vs. Tuna
http://nutritionfacts.org/video/mercury-in-vaccinations-vs-tuna-2/
[109] Greger, How Long to Detox from Fish Before Pregnancy
http://nutritionfacts.org/video/how-long-to-detox-from-fish-before-pregnancy/

take over a year of no mercury intake from fish or other sources for the body to adequately detox itself.[110]

So if you are a woman who eats two or more servings of fish per week, you would do well to have your level of mercury tested, and abstain from fish, shellfish, and any other possible mercury contaminated food for a year before considering getting pregnant. And of course it will be necessary to keep up the habit at least till you stop bearing children (and your last one is weaned).

➢ **Farm-raised fish:** Wild fish consumption is dangerous enough, but the consumption of farm-raised fish is even worse. **Toxins are present in higher concentrations in farm fish environments than in oceans, rivers and lakes.** The fish ingest these toxins and they are concentrated in their flesh. For example, in one survey 95% of farm raised catfish sold in the U.S. were found to contain dioxins.[111]

What are dioxins? Dioxin is

> a highly toxic compound produced as a byproduct in some manufacturing processes, notably herbicide production and paper bleaching. It is a serious and persistent environmental pollutant.[112]

What do ingested dioxins do to humans?

> Dioxins are highly toxic and can cause reproductive and developmental problems, damage the immune system, interfere with hormones and also cause cancer.[113]

In addition to the problems posed by toxins, farm fish are not fed a natural diet. Commercial farm fish feed is usually composed of wheat, corn, soy and other ingredients that fish

---

[110] Greger, Hair Testing for Mercury Before Considering Pregnancy
http://nutritionfacts.org/video/hair-testing-for-mercury-before-considering-pregnancy/
[111] Greger, Dioxins in U.S. Farm Raised Catfish
http://nutritionfacts.org/video/dioxins-in-u-s-farm-raised-catfish/
[112] *Oxford Dictionaries,* Dioxin
http://www.oxforddictionaries.com/us/definition/american_english/dioxin
[113] World Health Organization, Dioxins and their effects on human health
http://www.who.int/mediacentre/factsheets/fs225/en/

were never created to eat. This has a negative effect on their nutrition profile. Since they are eating omega-6 rich grain instead of their naturally omega-3 rich aquatic diet, their flesh has the opposite balance of these oils than what you want. So people trying to follow dietary recommendations of their doctors by eating "oily fish" which supposedly have lots of omega-3s may be wasting their money, not to mention contributing to their own chronic diseases.

You think grain-based fish food is bad? Prepare to be grossed out. **A common ingredient in fish feed is chicken feces.**[114] In fact, some fish farms deliver the feces to the fish directly, utilizing "poultry-over-fish farming," which consists of chicken cages suspended over fish tanks! Combining factory farming of poultry with factory farming of fish – what a wonderful idea.

Farmed salmon may be fed unnatural pigments to ensure their flesh is salmon pink, rather than the dull gray it would otherwise be due to their unnatural diet. And pesticides may be added to the fish pens to reduce algae growth.[115]

Just as with factory farm chickens, farm fish are raised in crowded conditions, and thus diseases spread through the populations quickly. So, just as with poultry, cattle, and other livestock, antibiotics are fed to the fish to control disease, including sea lice, and these antibiotics of course end up in your body if you eat the fish.

As the populations of wild fish continue to decline, and the fish farming industry continues to grow, farm-raised fish are becoming more and more common in supermarkets and are often served at restaurants. **Do you know where that yummy fishy you are eating came from?** You can be sure it wasn't from

---

[114] Michael Snyder, There Is A Staggering Amount Of Feces In Our Food
http://www.infowars.com/there-is-a-staggering-amount-of-feces-in-our-food/
[115] Dr. Joseph Mercola, M.D., Farmed Fish Production Overtakes Beef
http://articles.mercola.com/sites/articles/archive/2013/07/24/farmed-fish-production.aspx

a pristine, toxin free environment.

➤ **Big fish:** Remember that 30 lb. salmon you caught during your Alaskan vacation last year? Best to take a quick pic and then toss it back. The larger the fish, the more toxins they contain, since they have had longer to consume and concentrate them in their flesh.

Also, many commonly consumed fish such as salmon, snapper, and tuna are predatory, dining primarily on other non-plant sea life. Why is this significant? They are higher in the food chain than smaller fish which eat algae and other plants. For this reason they tend to concentrate more toxins in their flesh than non-predatory fish, since their food already has toxins concentrated in its flesh.

So if you choose to consume fish, always beware of consuming fish meat from large, predatory fish. Oh, and did you know that the tuna in your cupboard may have come from a fish that weighed over 1000 pounds? Bon appetite!

➤ **Shellfish:** Some believe that shellfish such as crab must be fine to eat, since it "very low in fat." True, crab meat is relatively low in fat, compared to fish, beef or chicken.

But perhaps we should compare it to some plant foods. Ounce for ounce king crab meat has four times the fat of spinach and lentils, and nearly eight times the fat of sweet potatoes. Low fat? Not exactly.

And remember, crab fat is unhealthy, inflammation-causing animal fat, whereas the fat in the veggies is health promoting.

Among shellfish, shrimp is particularly problematic to health. Wild-caught is not as bad as farm-raised, but 90% of the shrimp in stores and restaurants is the latter. Also, 90% of shrimp sold in the U.S. is imported from China and elsewhere. Very little of it is inspected, and it has been known to contain antibiotic drugs, carcinogenic xenoestrogens, and banned chemicals and toxins.

One more point regarding supposed "low fat" shellfish: Who eats crab or lobster without added fat? It is always cooked and served with butter, fried, in an oily gumbo, etc. And of course it has animal protein, inflammatory arachidonic acid and industrial toxins. No, shellfish is not healthy food for humans.

Chicken

➢ **Chicken a healthy meat?:** Many believe red meat to be bad for your health, and chicken to be good. We hear over and over health professionals promoting the consumption of chicken, especially chicken breast meat. But in the extensive investigating I have done I have been surprised to learn that, contrary to these popular claims, **the serious research studies consistently conclude that consuming chicken and other poultry comes with serious health consequences – worse than red meat and even fish for many specific diseases.**

Chicken has a lot of fat and cholesterol, and of course animal protein. It also often contains many toxins, as well dangerous bacteria. And turkey and other poultry are similarly problematic.

➢ **Chicken and obesity:** Chicken consumption has been shown to be responsible for causing obesity more than the consumption of other meat. This has been traced to an obesity causing virus, which is contracted from chicken meat.[116]

➢ **Chicken and bladder infections:** The raw chicken you purchase at the store is normally "bathed" in E. coli bacteria, which comes from chicken feces, traces of which remain on the chicken even though it looks so pretty wrapped in cellophane in your fridge. **Bladder infections have been traced to this chicken-sourced E. coli.** The number of such infections in women may run into the millions every year. But the infection doesn't result from eating the bacteria. It's from handling the raw chicken, as when putting it away after shopping or preparing it for cooking. The bacteria stays on the hands and the

---

[116] Greger, Infectobesity: Adenovirus 36 and Childhood Obesity
http://nutritionfacts.org/video/infectobesity-adenovirus-36-and-childhood-obesity/

woman then infects herself when she uses the toilet.[117]

> **Chicken and antibiotics:** Chickens are typically fed antibiotics to help them stay healthy and gain weight. But the heavy use of antibiotics in this way tends to breed antibiotic resistant strains of bacteria, including E. coli and salmonella. When people then get infected with these bacteria, standard antibiotics used to treat the resulting diseases, such as bladder infections and salmonella, may be ineffective.

> **Chicken and hormones:** It is illegal in chicken and egg farming to give the chickens hormones. So one needn't fear artificial hormones in chicken meat. However, there is still a hormone-poultry consumption connection related to health. Actually, this connection relates to all meat consumption, including fish.

The Harvard Nurses Study found that women who ate meat (including fish and chicken) had a more difficult time getting pregnant than those who did not eat meat. It appears that any type of meat has this effect. But poultry had the greatest impact on female fertility. **One serving of chicken a day (e.g. half a chicken breast) caused the women in the study to experience a 50% greater risk of infertility compared with those who didn't eat meat.**

Why would this be? It is thought that animal protein causes the IGF-1 growth hormone levels in a woman's body to rise, triggering a disruption in the normal ovulation cycle. Apparently chicken protein causes this effect more than protein from other animals. High IGF-1 levels also has been shown to encourage cancer to develop. Plant protein, on the other hand, does not have this effect.[118]

> **Chicken and arsenic:** Chickens grown in factory farms get a lot of parasites, since they are all crammed into one giant pen

---

[117] Greger, Avoiding Chicken to Avoid Bladder Infections
http://nutritionfacts.org/video/avoiding-chicken-to-avoid-bladder-infections/
[118] Greger, Meat Hormones and Female Infertility
http://nutritionfacts.org/video/meat-hormones-female-infertility/

together. These parasites keep the chickens from being healthy and gaining weight. So in some factory farms the chickens are fed arsenic-laced drugs. These drugs kill the parasites, and thus the chicken gains weight quickly. But some of the arsenic remains in the meat when it is sold in the market.[119]

Actually, the arsenic they feed to the chickens, and which is in the raw chicken meat, is organic arsenic, which is apparently not too dangerous. Thus the chicken producers can claim no one will be harmed. But when you cook the chicken, the organic arsenic converts to the inorganic form, the one which causes cancer, and for which there is no safe level. If you eat cooked chicken from a factory farm, there's a good chance you are eating dangerous inorganic arsenic.

➢ **Chicken and breast cancer:** One group of researchers followed 4000 women with breast cancer for seven years. Many died before the study ended. The researchers analyzed the study subjects' diets to see if dietary choices had an impact on who lived and who died. They found that the 25% of the women who ate the most saturated fat were 41% more likely to die of their cancer than the 25% of the women who ate the least.

So, what are the foods with the most saturated fat? The top four are, in this order, cheese, wheat flour desserts (cakes, cookies and doughnuts), ice cream, and chicken. And high temperature cooking methods such as grilling and frying makes chicken even more carcinogenic.

Hmmm. So, there is good evidence that eating fried chicken contributes to breast cancer deaths. But that being the case, why would it be that the breast cancer advocacy group Susan G. Komen for the Cure[120] teamed up with KFC in a national

---

[119] Greger, How Many Cancers Have Been Caused by Arsenic-Laced Chicken http://nutritionfacts.org/video/how-many-cancers-have-been-caused-by-arsenic-laced-chicken/
[120] The Komen website says: "At Susan G. Komen, our mission is pretty simple: to save lives and end breast cancer forever... We educate, support research, offer grants that provide financial and emotional assistance and advocate for better breast cancer policy."

"Buckets for the Cure" campaign?

During the campaign, KFC donated 50 cents to Komen for each pink bucket of chicken sold, up to $8 million. Maybe the campaign should have been called, "Buckets for a Cause" instead, since there is good evidence fried chicken causes breast cancer deaths. "Each bucket makes a difference" indeed. You can't make this stuff up, folks.[121]

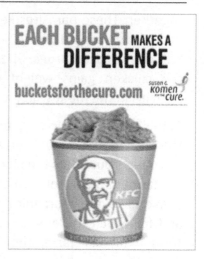

➤ **Chicken and salmonella:** Salmonella causes serious disease, the debilitating effects of which can last for years; it can be fatal. Yet these bacteria are present in most chicken sold in our stores, because the chicken meat is contaminated with chicken feces. **You don't even have to eat the chicken to get contaminated and get sick.** Simply having it in your kitchen almost guarantees your floor, countertops, sink, dish sponge, cupboard knobs, fridge handles, etc. will get the germs on them.[122]

➤ **Chicken feed:** Factory farm chickens are commonly fed "feather meal," which is composed of recycled chicken feathers and other chicken body parts which aren't otherwise sellable. **So they have made cannibals out of chickens.** Certainly not their natural diet!

Chicken feathers were tested to find out what chickens are being fed. Several substances were found in the feathers which chickens are not supposed to eat. These include several types of antibiotics, including some which had been banned years ago. They also contained several other drugs including Prozac,

---

[121] Greger, <u>Breast Cancer Survival, Butterfat, and Chicken</u>
http://nutritionfacts.org/video/breast-cancer-survival-butterfat-and-chicken/
[122] Greger, <u>Chicken Salmonella Thanks to Meat Industry Lawsuit</u>
http://nutritionfacts.org/video/chicken-salmonella-thanks-to-meat-industry-lawsuit/

antihistamines, fungicides, and caffeine. The antihistamines are needed to combat the respiratory problems associated with crowded living conditions of factory farms, and the caffeine is given to the birds so that they stay more alert and presumably eat more.[123] And I suppose it would be depressing to live one's life in a factory farm environment, so the Prozac is quite understandable.

The point, of course, is that if it is in the feathers, it is most likely in the meat, and in the body of any who eat the meat.

➤ **"Free range" chickens:** See section on **Eggs** above for more insights into what the "free range" label might mean for the quality of the chicken meat.

Red meat

➤ **"Lean" meat:** As stated above, all meat, poultry, and fish has a lot of fat. Don't be taken in by advertisers who

> *All meat is high in fat, including "lean" cuts.*

promise their product is "low in fat," or a "lean cut." It's a lie. Or at least a stretching of the truth by using fuzzy terminology. And when doctors or dieticians say you should eat "lean cuts of meat," don't be deceived. There is no such thing in absolute terms, only in relative terms. Compared to fatty cuts, lean cuts are leaner, true. But compared to a whole plant food meal, not at all! And besides, when one considers the research studies which show so clearly the dangers of animal protein, a 3 ounce "lean" steak just may be more harmful to your health than a 3 ounce fatty steak, because the former contains more animal protein, which as we saw above is especially harmful to health.

Furthermore, high quantities of fatty meat, i.e. any kind of animal flesh, is not what our digestive systems were designed to deal with. See **Chapter 12** for the clear evidence of this from a physiological perspective.

---

[123] Greger, Illegal Drugs in Chicken Feathers
http://nutritionfacts.org/video/illegal-drugs-in-chicken-feathers/

➢ **Meat and acid:** Eating meat and dairy products lowers the pH of the body, making it more acidic. This is hard on the kidneys, and can contribute to osteoporosis. Most importantly, an acidic environment in the body encourages cancer growth.[124] Whole plant foods do an excellent job of balancing the body's pH to its optimal level.

➢ **Meat and inflammation:** All meat and dairy contains arachidonic acid (AA). Our bodies need AA in order to produce inflammation when and where appropriate, such as for wound healing or to deal with certain diseases. But our bodies produce all the AA we need. So we don't need to supplement with AA from outside sources such as meat and dairy. And in fact eating meat and dairy increases the level of AA in our bodies, which is one reason these foods promote unhealthy levels of inflammation. Inflammation in artery walls leads to heart disease and stroke.

Studies support the idea that eating meat can trigger arthritis, a disease caused by inflammation, and switching to a plant based diet can be curative.[125] Another study concluded that "a high fat (i.e. meat, including poultry, fish, and dairy) diet may contribute to chronic inflammatory diseases of the airway and lung."[126]

It is debatable whether meat-induced inflammation is primarily produced as a result of the animal fat, the animal protein, or the AA, or a combination of all of these (as well as certain toxins, covered below). But it really doesn't matter. The logical response to this information is the same no matter what the specific cause of the inflammation is: **to avoid excess inflammation and the chronic diseases it causes, avoid meat and dairy.**

---

[124] Ian Forrest Robey, *Nutrition and Metabolism,* Examining the relationship between diet-induced acidosis and cancer http://www.nutritionandmetabolism.com/content/9/1/72

[125] Greger, Diet & Rheumatoid Arthritis http://nutritionfacts.org/video/diet-rheumatoid-arthritis/

[126] SK Rosenkranz, *European Journal of Applied Physiology,* Effects of a high-fat meal on pulmonary function in healthy subjects http://www.ncbi.nlm.nih.gov/pubmed/20165863

➢ **Animal protein and endothelial cells:** You have about 60,000 miles of blood vessels in your body. The smallest capillaries are so small that the blood cells have to slip through single file. The inner surface of every blood vessel is lined with a single layer of cells called the endothelium. This single organ, your vascular system, has a total surface area of about 700 square meters, the size of a tennis court and a basketball court put together! So one might expect that it would be rather important that we keep it healthy.

And indeed it is. For eons no one knew about the endothelium, and no one cared. Yet their proper function is indeed extremely important to vascular health.

In former generations, thanks to dietary customs, and the relative high cost of meat, the masses lived primarily on a whole food plant based diet, and their endothelial cells were healthy and happy. The only exceptions were the rich, who could afford a deadly diet of meat two or three times a day.

But in Western societies all that has changed. Now the masses can afford a rich diet – they can eat like kings! And get the chronic diseases of kings, too.

You see, **the animal protein found in meat and dairy damages the fragile endothelial cells so that they can't function properly.** One result is plaque in arteries and veins.

> Reducing red meat proteins in your diet and replacing them with vegetable and soy proteins [in whole plant foods] will help the endothelium. Animal proteins contain mixtures of amino acids that produce more of the amino acid methionine, which is the precursor for homocysteine, which can damage the endothelium. Vegetable proteins are healthier because they contain no saturated fat and less methionine.[127]

When the endothelium it is healthy and functioning properly it produces nitric oxide, a gas which keeps the inner surface of your blood vessels slippery. This enables the blood to flow

---

[127] Joan Beal, Endothelial Health http://www.ccsvi.org/index.php/helping-myself/endothelial-health

freely, as it should.

But eating animal protein, sugar, oil and fat, causes inflammation, as well as substances toxic to the endothelium. Together these conditions caused plaque to form. Plaque is little sores along the lining of your blood vessels. They are filled with fat, cholesterol, calcium, and other stuff found in the blood. If the endothelium isn't damaged too much, it will keep this plaque in place, and it may never bother you.

However, as the endothelial cells are continuously assaulted by animal protein and other elements of the SAD, the plaque will build up, narrowing the path through which blood may pass. Eventually the result is partial blockages. But if left unchecked these partial blockages can lead to angina (chest pain near the heart), macular degeneration, erectile dysfunction, and other problems.

If nothing is done to improve the diet, eventually some plaque will likely break loose, and cause a complete blockage of the blood vessel, possibly resulting in a heart attack or stroke. **Dairy and meat consumption thus leads to these and many other serious, painful, costly, and sometimes life threatening conditions.**[128]

Dr. Caldwell Esselstyn has done significant research in this area, and has shown that when heart patients with advanced disease stop eating animal protein, and start eating a whole food plant based diet, their endotheliums recover, their heart disease symptoms are greatly reduced or completely disappear, and **in some cases their disease actually reverses**.[129]

---

[128] Esselstyn, The Collapse of Cardiology: A Time to Rejoice? http://www.dresselstyn.com/site/study-12/
[129] Esselstyn, Resolving the Coronary Artery Disease Epidemic through Plant-Based Nutrition http://www.dresselstyn.com/site/study03/

In fact, since the endothelial cells can become damaged in any blood vessels in your body, there are quite a few diseases which can be triggered by this damage. These include (but are not limited to)

- Diabetes
- Atherosclerosis (hardening of the arteries)
- Heart disease and Stroke
- Hypertension
- Multiple sclerosis
- Lupus
- Scleroderma (hardening of the skin)
- Rheumatoid arthritis
- ALS (amyotrophic lateral sclerosis, Lou Gehrig's disease)
- Parkinson's
- Hypercoagulation of blood, thrombosis, clotting disorders
- Kidney disease, renal failure
- Metabolic syndrome[130]
- Sleep apnea (as a cause of endothelial dysfunction)
- Glaucoma[131]
- Macular degeneration[132]

---

[130] Metabolic syndrome is a group of risk factors which include high blood pressure, high blood sugar, unhealthy cholesterol levels, and abdominal fat. Any of these risk factors can be dangerous, but when a person has all of them they are at serious risk of disability and death from chronic disease. For example, a person with metabolic syndrome has double the risk of vascular and heart disease, which can lead to heart attacks and strokes; their risk of diabetes is five times greater than for those without metabolic syndrome. For more specifics, see WebMD: http://www.webmd.com/heart/metabolic-syndrome/metabolic-syndrome-what-is-it

[131] Joan Beal, Endothelial Health http://www.ccsvi.org/index.php/helping-myself/endothelial-health

[132] Macular Degeneration Foundation, Adult Macular Degeneration http:// www.eyesight.org/Macular_Degeneration/Adult_MD/adult_md.html

- Erectile dysfunction[133]
- Dementia/Alzheimer's[134,135]
- Back pain[136]
- Hypertension (high blood pressure)[137]

Wow. All those diseases? Yes, all those and more!

Why so many diseases? Because your blood vessels are the lifeline for all of your organs. If they get stopped up by plaque, the organ they are servicing ceases to function optimally. If enough of them get clogged, disease results. The common ones we are familiar with are heart disease and stroke. But many more have been identified, as the above list indicates.

For example, many who have been diagnosed with Alzheimer's in their old age, when they die and their brains are autopsied, are found to have suffered from countless microinfarcts, or mini-strokes. These are often not even noticed by the sufferer when they occur, but with each one some small portion of their brain dies off, and brain function is lost. The cumulative effect is a disease which, for all practical purposes, is Alzheimer's (though there are other causes of Alzheimer's symptoms as well).

A probable example of this effect from dietary meat surfaced in The Adventist Health Study conducted in Loma Linda, California: The matched subjects who ate meat (including poultry and fish) were more than twice as likely to become demented as their vegetarian counterparts...

---

[133] Greger, Pills vs. Diet for Erectile Dysfunction
http://nutritionfacts.org/2014/05/20/pills-vs-diet-for-erectile-dysfunction/
[134] 60 Minutes, 90+ (minute 20.)
https://www.youtube.com/watch?v=nAfmRQbrqKE
[135] Greger, Preventing Alzheimer's with Lifestyle Changes
http://nutritionfacts.org/video/preventing-alzheimers-with-lifestyle-changes/
[136] Greger, Back in Circulation: Sciatica and Cholesterol
http://nutritionfacts.org/video/back-in-circulation-sciatica-and-cholesterol/
[137] Canadian Institutes of Health Research Multidisciplinary Research Group on Hypertension, American Journal of Hypertension, Beyond blood pressure: the endothelium and atherosclerosis progression
http://www.ncbi.nlm.nih.gov/pubmed/12383592

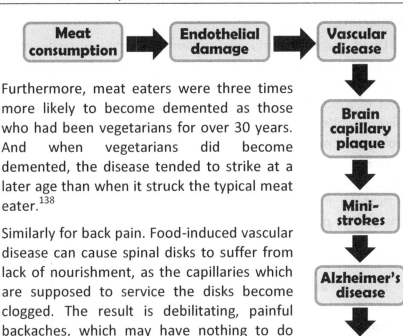

Furthermore, meat eaters were three times more likely to become demented as those who had been vegetarians for over 30 years. And when vegetarians did become demented, the disease tended to strike at a later age than when it struck the typical meat eater.[138]

Similarly for back pain. Food-induced vascular disease can cause spinal disks to suffer from lack of nourishment, as the capillaries which are supposed to service the disks become clogged. The result is debilitating, painful backaches, which may have nothing to do with taking a fall or lifting heavy objects.

Hypertension is often a very correctible symptom of diet-caused endothelial impairment. Many with high blood pressure find their condition resolve upon switching to a whole food plant based diet.[139] "But my hypertension is hereditary. It's been in my family for generations." Well, maybe your diet has, too. But you can change that!

Another thing to keep in mind is that if any of your blood vessels show evidence of endothelial damage, it is likely that all of them are damaged to some degree. This is why one vascular disease, such as back pain or erectile dysfunction, is a warning sign that more serious disease is on the horizon.

For more discussion of the endothelium, see **Chapter 7** under

---

[138] P. Giem, et al, *Neuroepidemiology* 1993, The Incidence of Dementia and Intake of Animal Products: Preliminary Findings from the Adventist Health Study http://www.karger.com/Article/Abstract/110296

[139] McDougall, High Blood Pressure (Hypertension) https://www.drmcdougall.com/health/education/health-science/hot-topics/medical-topics/hypertension/

Animal fats.

➢ **Dead meat bacteria endotoxemia:** Another reason meat (including chicken, fish, etc.) causes inflammation is that it contains a lot of bacteria, and bacteria contains toxins. (The raw meat of a Burger King quarter pounder has about 100 million bacteria cells.) **Some of these toxins are not destroyed by cooking, no matter how long or at what temperature the meat is cooked.** Nor are they destroyed by stomach acid. They pass directly into the blood from the stomach and small intestine, causing an inflammatory response in the body as the body struggles to deal with them. And researchers suggest (it would be impossible to prove) that this leads to heart disease, stroke, and diabetes, all inflammation diseases.[140]

➢ **Fake meat burgers:** If you avoid meat you also avoid consuming unknown animal products and other ingredients in restaurant burgers. In one study, pathologists from the Cleveland Clinic analyzed the meat content in burgers from 8 fast food restaurants. They found there was from 2.1% to 14.8% meat. The rest was blood vessels, nerves, cartilage, bacteria, parasites, and ammonia.[141]

➢ **Beef and hormones:** Though it is illegal in the U.S. to use hormones in chicken farming, it is legal to use them in the raising of beef and milk. The hormones which may be used in beef production include estradiol, progesterone, testosterone, melengesterol acetate, trenbolone acetate, and zeranol.[142] These hormones are often present in the meat when it is purchased and consumed.

Of course many claim these hormones are safe to consume, but typically those who make such claims are those who have a financial reason to defend their use. And anyone who

---

[140] Greger, Dead Meat Bacteria Endotoxemia
http://nutritionfacts.org/video/dead-meat-bacteria-endotoxemia/
[141] Greger, What's in a Burger? http://nutritionfacts.org/video/whats-in-a-burger/
[142] Weiert Velle, The Use of Hormones in Animal Production
http://www.fao.org/docrep/004/X6533E/X6533E01.htm

understands the profound effects hormones can have on the body will know that the burden of proof must lie with those who would make the claim of safety. Yet they don't present such proof, they just give unfounded assurances.

And there is evidence of the hormones' toxicity. When Japan began importing large amounts of hormone laden beef from the U.S., cases of breast, ovarian, and endometrial cancers increased in the country dramatically. Correlation doesn't prove causality, but it does raise strong suspicions. U.S. beef has 600 times the estrogen of Japanese-raised beef, and excess estrogen is a known risk factor for these cancers.[143]

Another interesting fact: Athletes eating meat from animals which were injected with steroids can test positive in drug screening.

➤ **Meat glue:** The enzyme transglutaminase, which is toxic to breathe, was originally derived from guinea pig livers, but now is derived from the blood of pigs and cows. It is mixed with smaller pieces or trimmings of beef, pork, poultry, or fish to glue the bits together and produce larger pieces which can then be sold at a higher price as steaks or roasts. So far that sounds kind of gross, but the main problem with this practice is that **fecal bacteria on the outside of meat can end up inside a glued-together steak, making it harder to kill the bacteria when cooking.**[144] Yup, pretty gross for sure.

➤ **Poultry litter cattle feed:** The term "poultry litter" refers to the straw bedding, spilled poultry feed, feathers, feces, and other debris which is swept up from the poultry factory farm floor.

---

[143] Greger, Anabolic Steroids in Meat http://nutritionfacts.org/video/anabolic-steroids-in-meat/

[144] Greger, Is Meat Glue Safe? http://nutritionfacts.org/video/is-meat-glue-safe/

Heme Iron

Another concern with diets that are rich in meat and offal is an excess intake of heme iron, found exclusively in animal tissue. As iron is a pro-oxidant and excess iron cannot be excreted from the body, excessive absorption of iron can contribute to progressive inflammatory and degenerative diseases. It has been shown in controlled feeding experiments that the absorption of heme iron is considerably less regulated than that of non-heme iron [which plant foods provide], and therefore a high intake can lead to excess iron absorption.

Recent meta-analyses of prospective cohort studies found that an increment of 1 mg/day of heme iron was associated with an 11%, 16% and 27% increased risk of colorectal cancer, type II diabetes and coronary heart disease respectively. When taking into consideration the fact that diets very rich in meat and offal can supply well over 10 mg of heme iron per day, these findings cast considerable doubt on the long-term safety of such diets. Heme iron intake has also been associated with oxidative stress and an increased risk of stroke, gestational diabetes, gallstones and cancers of the prostate, lung, stomach, esophagus, endometrium and kidneys. [See article for referenced documentation.]
— McDougall Newsletter, August 2013

For most people, taking extra iron [i.e. supplements] is a bad idea. And in fact [excess iron] may be one reason there are higher cancer rates among meat eaters, because they get heme iron, or blood iron, which our bodies are unable to down-regulate the absorption of.
— Dr. Michael Greger

Safe disposal of this material is costly, as is cattle feed. And it happens that cattle can digest poultry litter and convert it into meat. So poultry litter is often used as cattle feed. That hamburger you ate last night may well have contained meat from a cow that was fed chicken feces, etc.

Additionally, the chicken feed in the poultry litter may have contained beef byproducts. It is illegal to make cannibals out of cows, feeding them beef byproducts, because of the danger of mad cow disease. However, cattle are commonly fed poultry litter which contains spilled poultry feed which may contain beef byproducts. There is a simple way to avoid the dangers (and yuck factor) posed by this ridiculous situation.

➢ **Pork:** Pork carries the same dangers as do other meats, if not worse, due to the increased parasite infection danger. God knew what He was doing when He forbade the Israelites from eating it. Type "pork" in the www.nutritionfacts.org search box for the yucky facts about this yummy food.

➢ **Wild meat:** Wild meat, such as deer and duck, is probably the least unhealthy form of meat to eat. Generally wild animals live on a more natural diet than domestic ones do, and no one is sticking them with hormone shots or intentionally feeding them poisons.

However, that doesn't mean wild meat is toxin free. It can still have some toxins concentrated in the flesh from the chemicals in their environment (crop pesticide over-spray, for example). Significant lead exposure can be obtained from eating wild meat, as buckshot and shattered bullet fragments leave traces behind.[145] Dead meat bacteria endotoxemia would be just as much a problem in the consumption of wild meat as domestic. And your body will still struggle to deal with dangerous levels of inflammation caused by excessive arachidonic acid and animal fat and protein.

---

[145] Greger, Filled Full of Lead http://nutritionfacts.org/video/filled-full-of-lead/

Processed meat

➢ **The most dangerous meat:** Processed and cured meats include hot dogs, sausage, bologna, salami, ham, bacon, etc. (For convenience, we will refer to all processed and cured meats as processed meats.) These are the most dangerous meats to eat, posing the greatest health risks. Consumption of these products is significantly associated with the following cancers: bladder, endometrial, prostate, thyroid, throat, esophageal, stomach, colon, rectal, lung, pancreatic, testicular, kidney, leukemia[146], and breast[147]. Not to mention the other health risks associated with meat consumption.

The primary reason processed meats cause cancer is the presence of nitrates and/or nitrites, which have been added to the meat to keep its color pink and to keep it from spoiling. These chemicals do not harm us directly. Rather, nitrates convert to nitrites, and in the absence of vitamin C, nitrites convert to *nitrosamines*. This can happen in the meat before you even eat it. **It is the nitrosamines which are carcinogenic.**

Nitrites also occur in many vegetables, and in fact are nutritious phytochemicals in that context. They don't convert to nitrosamines in plant foods, so are not dangerous.[148] Eating vitamin C with your bacon or hot dogs does not solve the problem, since the meat probably already contains nitrosamines, which the vitamin C will not protect you from.

➢ **Processed meat compared to cigarettes:** The nitrosamines in cigarette smoke are known to cause kidney cancer. Yet as smoking continues to decrease in the U.S., cases of kidney

---

[146] Greger, Bacon and Botulism http://nutritionfacts.org/video/bacon-and-botulism/
[147] Camille Pouchieu, et al, *International Journal of Epidemiology*, Prospective association between red and processed meat intakes and breast cancer risk: modulation by an antioxidant supplementation in the SU.VI.MAX randomized controlled trial http://ije.oxfordjournals.org/content/early/2014/07/03/ije.dyu134.short
[148] Greger, Are Nitrates Pollutants or Nutrients? http://nutritionfacts.org/video/are-nitrates-pollutants-or-nutrients/

cancer continue to rise, and now there are about 13,000 deaths from this disease per year.

Meat also has nitrosamines, and processed meat has high levels of the stuff. One hotdog has the same amount of cancer-causing nitrosamines as five cigarettes! (Of course, hotdogs are eaten, not smoked. Whether this substance is more lethal when absorbed through the stomach or the lungs, I don't know, but either way, cancer is in the picture.) Thus it is thought that processed meat consumption explains at least part of the continued rise in kidney cancer.[149]

➢ **Second-hand bacon fume carcinogens:** Most of us love the smell of frying bacon. But with that lovely odor comes a "quite significant" amount of "nitrosopyrrolidine, one of the more potent nitrosamines," which we learned earlier are dangerous carcinogens. When breathed, particles of this stuff are deposited deep in the lungs, where they can cause cancers to develop.[150] One wonders how many "mysterious" cases of "non-smoker's lung cancer" have been caused by this danger.

If you must have bacon, it is recommended that you fry it outside whenever possible, as this decreases the toxic exposure considerably. And when frying bacon indoors, or any meat for that matter, be sure to use the exhaust fan above the stove.

Frying, grilling, barbecuing, smoking and broiling other meats has a similar toxic effect. Unsurprisingly, it has been observed that cooks tend to have an abnormally high rate of respiratory cancers. Also, pregnant women breathing these fumes (as well as eating such meat) has been demonstrated to result in poorer fetal development.[151]

➢ **Hot dogs and infant brain tumors:** Are there other risks to

---

[149] Greger, Can Diet Protect Against Kidney Cancer?
http://nutritionfacts.org/video/can-diet-protect-against-kidney-cancer/
[150] Greger, Carcinogens in the smell of frying bacon
http://nutritionfacts.org/video/carcinogens-in-the-smell-of-frying-bacon/
[151] Greger, Meat Fumes: Dietary Secondhand Smoke
http://nutritionfacts.org/video/meat-fumes-dietary-secondhand-smoke/

the baby in utero when mom eats processed meat? One study concluded that

> A substantial risk of paediatric brain tumour appears to be associated with relatively high levels of maternal cured meat consumption during pregnancy.[152]

➤ **Hot dogs and leukemia:** A study found that children eating 12 hot dogs per month were over nine times as likely to get leukemia as those who didn't eat hot dogs.[153]

➤ **What's in a hot dog?:** Hot dogs were analyzed to determine what they contained. Ingredients included bone, blood vessels, nerves, cartilage, skin, corn syrup, sodium nitrate and nitrite (carcinogenic, promotes heart disease, diabetes), sodium erythorbate (can cause headaches, nausea, etc.), heterocylic amines (carcinogenic when the meat is cooked). The meat content was less than 10%.[154]

Children eating 12 hot dogs per month were found to be over nine times as likely to get leukemia as those who didn't eat hot dogs.

➤ **Ditch the dogs and prevent death:** A large European study of over 448,000 subjects estimated that if everyone's processed meat consumption were reduced to ½ hot dog per day, the improvement in public health would result in 3% fewer deaths

---

[152] JM Pogoda, S. Preston-Martin, Maternal cured meat consumption during pregnancy and risk of paediatric brain tumour in offspring: potentially harmful levels of intake Public Health Nutrition http://www.ncbi.nlm.nih.gov/pubmed/11299090

[153] Dr. John M. Peters, et al, *Cancer Causes and Control,* Processed meats and risk of childhood leukemia http://link.springer.com/article/10.1007/BF01830266#page-2

[154] Greger, What is Really in Hot Dogs? http://nutritionfacts.org/video/what-is-really-in-hot-dogs-2/

from all causes.[155]

An American study of over 600,000 subjects determined that 20% of all heart disease deaths in women could be averted if on average they would cut their processed meat intake down to about ½ strip of bacon per day.[156,157] Hmmm. I wonder what would happen everyone's consumption were zero.

➤ **Processed meat euphemisms:** Beware of new slick terminology which the food industry will come up with from time to time to make their products not seem so objectionable. For example, the current term preferred by the processed meat industry for their products is "convenience meats." Diseases caused by processed meats are definitely not convenient.

➤ **Meat as a spice:** Dr. Daphne Miller traveled the world visiting traditional cultures where the people live long lives remarkably free of typical Western chronic diseases. Her goal was to research their diets and recipes in preparation for writing a book. Like the Blue Zone researchers (**Chapter 3**), she found that these healthy populations did consume meat, but almost everywhere it was used quite sparingly. When a dish did contain meat, it was usually served as a flavoring for the plant foods which comprised the main part of the meal. Her advice: "Use meat as a spice."

---

[155] Sabine Rohrmann, et al, Meat consumption and mortality - results from the European Prospective Investigation into Cancer and Nutrition
http://www.biomedcentral.com/1741-7015/11/63
[156] Rashmi Sinha, Ph.D., et al, Meat Intake and Mortality: A Prospective Study of Over Half a Million People
http://archinte.jamanetwork.com/article.aspx?articleid=414881
[157] Greger, From Table to Able: Combating Disabling Diseases with Food
http://nutritionfacts.org/video/from-table-to-able/

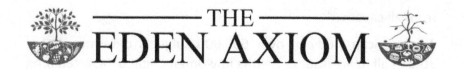
Chapter 7:

Foods Which Promote Disease:

Oils, Fats and Sugar

The matter of edible oils is a complex subject. As with other topics in this book, I do not claim to be an expert on this one. But I have done some study, and do understand some of the basics, which I will try to explain in this chapter. I suggest you read carefully, as understanding these things can help you make wise choices for a truly healthy diet.

There is much controversy about which oils and fats are good for health and which ones are bad. One nutritionist put it this way: oils in their natural state are good; damaged oils (by high heat, chemicals and other processing) are bad. Others stress that omega-3 oils are good but omega-6 oils are bad. Some say olive oil is good, but other oils should be avoided. And still others say all foods with added oils are bad, and even plant foods with naturally high concentrations of oils (like nuts and avocados) should be avoided. We'll see if we can make some sense of all this in this chapter.

Sugars and other sweeteners are another important subject related to diet and health. We will look at the evidence that these substances promote chronic disease.

Omega oils

➢ **Omega-6 and omega-3 fatty acids:** Most edible oils provide one or both of two major nutrients: omega-6 fatty acids and omega-3 fatty acids. (Think of "fatty acids" as just another term for "oils.") **Both are needed for good health.** Omega-6 fatty acids support the inflammatory system of the body. Omega-3 fatty acids support the anti-inflammatory system of the body.

Both types of oils and both systems are needed, because sometimes your body needs an inflammatory response, such as when it needs to respond to trauma, a germ, or a toxin, and sometimes it needs an anti-inflammatory response, such as when the trauma, germ, or toxin has been dealt with and it is time for the inflammation to stop.

So the problem isn't that omega-6 oils are bad in and of themselves. The real problem with them is threefold.

The first is where they come from. Are they a constituent of a whole food you are eating? Or are they from an added oil, likely damaged from processing and rancid?

The second problem is the quantity consumed. When added to foods, these oils are consumed in much higher quantities than they occur in whole plant foods.

And third, the relative quantities of omega-6 and -3 oils consumed. If you consume them out of balance toward the 6s, which is universal in Western diets, your body is likely in a constant state of inflammation. This tends to encourage chronic inflammatory diseases: heart disease, stroke, diabetes, cancer, Alzheimer's, etc.

From 1909 to the present, in the U.S. there has been a steady rise in the consumption of omega-6 oils, which correlates with the rise in inflammatory diseases over the same period. That correlation alone doesn't prove causation, but there are many studies which show convincingly that this imbalance is a significant contributor to these diseases.

➢ **Polyunsaturated Fatty Acids:** PUFAs are basically the unsaturated oils commonly added to foods, such as soybean, canola (rapeseed), corn, safflower seed, cotton seed, and sunflower seed. These oils consist primarily of omega-6 fatty acids, and so are the primary force behind the imbalance of omega-6 to omega-3 consumption in the SAD.

Before the 1900s many PUFAs were never consumed as added oils, because the technology didn't exist to extract them. So when they were introduced they were a new "food" which became a part of our everyday diet. Yet they are a food the human body was never designed to consume.

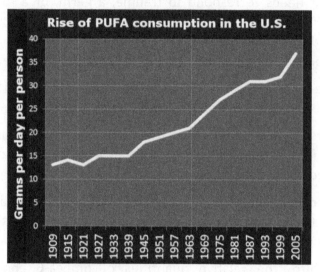

There was much money to be made from the sale of PUFAs, so food companies not only manufactured the oils, but also lies about how healthy these new oils were to eat. For example, they claimed that margarine, manufactured from PUFAs and high in trans fat, was healthier than butter. Even medical students were taught that they should recommend margarine to their patients, and that is exactly what doctors did for many years. The reality is that, though butter is bad for one's health, margarine is worse!

But as the above chart shows, the public believed the lies. In reality PUFAs have promoted an epidemic of chronic disease and caused untold suffering.

➢ **Omega-6/omega-3 ratios – the dangers of getting them wrong:** Many authorities say **the optimal intake ratio of these fatty acids is 1/1.** That is, we should eat the same amount of 6s as we do 3s. The SAD provides a ratio of about 16/1. That means most Americans eat 16 times as much omega-6 oils as omega-3 oils. (Some say the ratio is actually more like between 20/ and 50/1.) A scientific paper summarized the findings of several studies:

> In the secondary prevention of cardiovascular disease, a ratio of 4/1 was associated with a 70% decrease in total mortality. A ratio of 2.5/1 reduced rectal cell proliferation in patients with colorectal cancer, whereas a ratio of 4/1 with the same amount of omega-3...had no effect. The lower omega-6/omega-3 ratio in women with breast cancer was associated with decreased risk. A ratio of 2-3/1 suppressed inflammation in patients with rheumatoid arthritis, and a ratio of 5/1 had a beneficial effect on patients with asthma, whereas a ratio of 10/1 had adverse consequences.[158]

Notice that the lower the ratio, the more the benefit for all diseases researched. Hence the often heard recommendation to increase your intake of omega-3 oils.

People on the SAD ingest anywhere from 16 to 50 times as much inflammatory omega-6 oils as omega-3 oils.

But is it really realistic to correct the imbalance only by increasing omega-3 oil consumption? Why do we much more seldom hear recommendations that we decrease omega-6 oil consumption? The "increase omega-3 oils" mantra implies that the amount of omega-6 oils commonly consumed does not in and of itself pose health risks. This is at best naïve and at worst deceptive. Actually, at worst it is deadly.

Making a concerted effort to cut omega-6 oils from the diet will have a significant impact on the 6/3 ratio we are consuming, thus reducing the likelihood of developing inflammatory disease, while at the same time contributing toward healing from these diseases if we already have them.

➢ **Omega-6 in meat:** Leaves tend to contain more omega-3 oils, while grains tend to contain more omega-6 oils. When

---

[158] A.P. Simopoulos, The importance of the ratio of omega-6/omega-3 essential fatty acids http://www.ncbi.nlm.nih.gov/pubmed/12442909

cattle eat their natural diet of grass, they get omega-3 oils from the grass, and their meat has a larger proportion of omega-3 oils in it than does the meat from cows whose diet consists of grains such as corn. In the U.S., in the last months prior to slaughter cattle are typically fed a diet consisting primarily of corn. The Union of Concerned Scientists found that steak from grass fed cattle had almost twice the omega-3 fatty acids as steak from corn fed cattle.[159]

Other animals grown for meat, including chickens, are the same. Though seeds naturally make up a portion of a chicken's diet, when given a chance they will also eat various leaves, bugs, etc. But in a factory farm chickens are primarily fed grain. And thus their flesh and their eggs are abnormally high in omega-6 oils.

So this unnatural diet fed to the animals we consume partially explains the 6/3 imbalance in the SAD, and the chronic inflammation and resulting chronic disease suffered by meat eaters. And this is why, if you feel you must eat animal products, you should insist on grass fed "free range" or "pastured" meat, eggs and dairy.

➢ **Fish oil studies:** Often oily fish consumption and/or omega-3 fish or krill oil supplements are prescribed to help correct the omega-6/omega-3 imbalance and improve heart health. In the past there have been studies which indicated that omega-3 oil supplementation was beneficial to heart health. However, other studies contradicted those findings. A meta-analysis[160] of several studies published in the Journal of the American Medical Association found that *fish oil supplementation is not actually associated with decreased cardiovascular disease, heart*

---

[159] *Union of Concerned Scientists,* Pasture-Based Operations FAQ
http://www.ucsusa.org/food_and_agriculture/solutions/advance-sustainable-agriculture/greener-pastures-faqs.html#.VLRUJ3tICWQ
[160] A meta-analysis is a study which compiles the data from several previously published studies which examined a similar topic. It is thought that this approach has a good chance of producing more reliable results than any one study can.

disease, and all-cause mortality.[161] Another study showed that even for heart patients, there is no benefit.[162]

➤ **Fish oil toxins:** If you still think you should take fish oil supplements, consider that fish oil can contain many toxins. You should never take these supplements if you are not sure they are high quality, purified from heavy metals, PCBs, etc. Note that PCBs are found in some fish oil supplements at higher levels than in any food – over 1400 times as much plant foods! And even some brands claiming to be toxin free have been shown to be contaminated.[163]

Many consider krill oil to be superior because krill are lower on the food chain, and thus have fewer concentrated toxins in their bodies.

Omega-3 oil supplements derived from algae have become popular with vegans, who try to avoid all animal products. They also have the advantage of, reportedly, being free of the toxins associated with fish oil.

However, eating any oil supplement violates the whole food principle. Thus we should immediately be suspicious that oil supplements may damage the body in some way. We should also expect that whatever benefit the oil supplement is supposed to confer, we can get that benefit from a whole plant food diet. Even if no evidence is known to prove that a given oil supplement is harmful, before considering taking it we should 1) insist on solid evidence that it is helpful, and 2) know for a fact that a better, whole plant food alternative has not been discovered.

As we shall see below, the facts show that for good health no one should be taking omega-3 oil supplements; they are in fact unnecessary. It is better to take all that money you have been

---

[161] Greger, Is Fish Oil Just Snake Oil? http://nutritionfacts.org/video/is-fish-oil-just-snake-oil/
[162] *Ibid.*
[163] Greger, Is Distilled Fish Oil Toxin-Free? http://nutritionfacts.org/video/is-distilled-fish-oil-toxin-free/

spending on omega-3 supplements and instead buy healthy plant foods which will supply all of your omega-3 needs.

➢ **Omega-3 needs supplied by plant foods:** Though plant foods often don't contain high amounts of omega-3 oils per se, they do contain α-linolenic acid, ALA, which you own body converts to the omega-3 oils you need.

> Omega-3 fatty acids are derived from linolenic acid. The principal omega-3 is alpha-linolenic acid (ALA), which is then converted into eicosapentaenoic acid (EPA) and docosahexaenonic acid (DHA) by the body. *This makes ALA the only essential omega-3 fatty acid.* ALA can be found in many vegetables, beans, nuts, seeds, and fruits. [Emphasis added.][164]

Drs. Esselstyn and McDougall agree. They also maintain that we can get all the omega-3s we need from whole foods. **Whole plant foods contain omega-3s and/or the ALA ("parent" or precursor) oils which the body converts into omega-3s as needed.** Additionally, this way of eating is free of all added omega-6 oils, which helps bring the 6/3 ratio to where it should be. So omega-3 supplementation is unnecessary, not to mention a waste of money.

➢ **Inadequate research:** To my knowledge the research studies done to assess the benefits of omega-3s, whether sourced from pills or oily fish, have always compared people on the SAD eating extra omega-3s with people on the SAD not eating extra omega-3s. And of course all people on the SAD are getting an overdose of inflammatory omega-6s.

I know of no study comparing people on a whole food plant based diet with those taking extra omega-3s on various diets. Thus there is apparently no reliable evidence that the dubious study-supported omega-3 supplementation recommendations, which most doctors and nutritionists promote, can be applicable to anyone except those on the SAD – and that it really applies to those on the SAD is even doubtful.

---

[164] *Physicians Committee for Responsible Medicine,* Essential Fatty Acids
http://www.pcrm.org/health/health-topics/essential-fatty-acids

Avoid added oils

It is best to avoid eating any foods with added oils. Added oils have been shown to damage blood vessels, leading to vascular diseases such as heart disease, stroke, macular degeneration, dementia, etc. Added dietary oils also slow down the movement of blood in the circulatory system, an unhealthy condition.

➤ **Oil is empty fat calories:** Oil, any kind of oil, has nine calories per gram, which is equivalent to **120 calories in every tablespoon!** (That's as many calories as a medium sized sweet potato or a pound of broccoli. You have to walk about a mile to burn 100 calories!)

These are almost completely non-nutritive calories. When oil is added to food it does virtually nothing positive for the body of the one who eats it, but it does contribute to obesity and other chronic diseases. For most people, when they eat foods with added oils it causes weight gain, and it causes the weight to stay on.

Avoiding all oil is best, but it is most important to avoid omega-6 oils. These are oils that are liquid even when kept in the fridge, which is all plant-sourced oils except olive, coconut, and palm.

➤ **Olive oil:** Olive oil is almost universally touted as a healthy oil. Some seem to think that they can make a salad or other dish more healthy by drizzling some olive oil on it. Absolutely not so! Though probably less damaging to health than the liquid (when cold) oils (see above), **olive oil has been shown to promote heart disease, obesity and other health problems.**[165] Dr. McDougall notes:

> Serial angiograms of people's heart arteries show that all three types of fat—saturated (animal) fat, monounsaturated (olive oil), and polyunsaturated (omega-3 and -6 oils)—were associated with significant increases in new atherosclerotic lesions over one year of study. Only by decreasing the entire fat intake, including poly- and

---

[165] *Pritikin Longevity Center*, Olive Oil Nutrition – What's Wrong With Olive Oil? https://www.pritikin.com/your-health/healthy-living/eating-right/1103-whats-wrong-with-olive-oil.html#.VHNqZ8kXLPw

monounsaturated-oils, did the lesions stop growing.[166]

"Virgin" or "extra virgin" olive oil is little better; it still has this effect.

Dr. Michael Klaper notes that

The Greeks, by the way, are the fattest country in Europe. They have the highest rate of obesity of all the European nations. And when (researchers) looked at (Greek) women who were obese, they did fat biopsies of the actual fat in their fat stores, 55% of the fat came from olive oil. It sticks to you.[167]

Olive oil has been shown to promote heart disease, obesity and other health problems.

Note that the omega-6 to omega-3 ratio in olive oil is in the neighborhood of 14/1, far from the ideal intake we should be getting of 1/1. Thus consumption of olive oil only hinders your efforts to achieve a healthy balance of omega oils.[168]

The bottom line is that the evidence indicates that consumption of any added oil is damaging to health. Oil is not whole food, and so immediately we should consider it suspect. And the known science regarding the consumption of olive and other edible oils again gives evidence that the whole food principle of the Eden Axiom is valid.

➢ **Oils damaged in processing:** Not only are omega-6 oils bad because they provide an overdose of omega-6 fatty acids, but also because of the way they are processed. High temperatures are typically used in the refining process, which causes the molecules to break down. **This heat and molecular breakdown makes the oil rancid.** The bad, rancid odor is removed with

---

[166] McDougall, NEJM Study Promotes Olive Oil and Dismisses Low-fat Diet
https://www.drmcdougall.com/misc/2013other/news/oil.htm
[167] Dr. Michael Klaper, M.D., *VegSource* 2012, Olive Oil Is Not Healthy
https://www.youtube.com/watch?v=OGGQxJLuVjg
[168] *Ibid.*

further heating and/or chemical treatments. So the nice looking and not-bad-smelling cooking oil you use in cakes, cookies, frying and on salads may actually be rancid. **And the molecule fragments of this rancid oil are toxic to the body**, providing free radicals which degrade your DNA, further encouraging disease to develop.

The Best By date on oils have been shown to be quite inaccurate, so if you do consume these oils you are taking your chances from that standpoint as well.[169]

The worst oils to consume are PUFA oils such as corn oil, sunflower oil, soybean oil, canola oil, etc. If you feel you absolutely have to use them, always choose virgin, extra virgin, and cold pressed. This means the processing was done at lower temperatures, and should mean the fatty acids are not broken down as much into toxic substances. And, if you do use these oils, do not heat them very hot, such as in frying, as this produces free radicals and other toxic compounds, including toxic fumes. And remember that any added oils, whether heated or not, are toxic to your blood vessels and promote weight gain.

➤ **Fries and chips:** Usually French fries, fried chicken, tater tots, fried okra, all sorts of chips, etc. are deep fried in severely damaged toxic omega-6 oils. **Thus when you eat these foods you are consuming large quantities of inflammation-causing disease-promoting substances.**

Of course your body has ways of protecting itself from these toxins to some degree, which explains why one can eat these foods for years without apparent harm. But they do put unnecessary stress on the body, cause inflammation, degrade the endothelium (lining) of your veins, arteries, and capillaries, and will often eventually lead to obesity, heart disease, diabetes, cancer, and other diseases.

Instead of fried choose baked chips, which supposedly contain

---

[169] Greger, True Shelf Life of Cooking Oils http://nutritionfacts.org/video/the-true-shelf-life-of-cooking-oils/

less oils. Or better, make your own: put corn tortillas (check ingredients lists and try to get a brand without chemical additives – maybe not possible) on a cookie sheet and bake at the lowest temp possible for a few minutes till crisp. Or better still, make your own tortillas with Masa Harina corn flour. The only ingredients are the flour and water – and some seasoning if desired. Easy and delicious!

➢ **Margarine:** Margarine and "spread" are fake food. They have been described as "edible plastic." Well, at least the second part of that description may be accurate. Though I don't advocate consumption of dairy products, real butter is way safer than margarine or "spread." Coconut oil is even better – delicious spread on toast. Or try to learn to enjoy foods without butter or oil – the healthiest alternative.

Oils in cooking and oil substitutes

➢ **Animal oils and frying:** The science is clear that eating animal products and fried foods promotes chronic disease, not good health. But if you do choose to fry, and don't have coconut or palm oil, I believe the best alternative is free-range, grass-fed lard or butter, as it is less dangerous than using an omega-6 oil. But it is much better to just learn to live without frying at all.

➢ **Oils for cooking:** When considering cooking with oil, keep these things in mind:

Frying with oil not only produces toxic substances, it also destroys much of the nutrition of the food. Frying meat will produce toxic substances in the meat. And if that weren't bad enough, frying releases toxic gasses into the air which are carcinogenic when breathed, much like second-hand tobacco smoke.

If you do choose to use oil in cooking (not frying), the best oils to use are coconut and palm. (There is controversy about this claim; some would suggest other oils.) Generally these can only be used for cooking and baking (not for salad dressing, for example), since they are solid at room temperature.

There are many substitutes you can try for oil in cooking. For example, for stir frying veggies you can use water or vegetable broth. Just add it little by little as needed. For baking, unsweetened applesauce often is a good substitute (most healthful is homemade applesauce with the apple skins, thoroughly pureed in a blender). Check online for other possibilities.[170]

➤ **Salad dressing:** As indicated earlier, if you absolutely have to have a liquid at room temperature oil, such as on a salad, choose extra virgin cold pressed olive oil. But finding non-oil alternatives is better. I like salsa on salad, or thick lentil stew, or both (really, it is good!). Some like vinegar straight. Or a little lemon juice. Lots of no-oil salad dressing recipes are available on the web. It might be hard to change your habit and tastes in this area, but if you do you will soon be used to the new normal and glad you made the switch, knowing that it will have a positive impact on your long term health.

Animal fats

It is best to avoid animal fat altogether. Animal fat is primarily made up of saturated fat. Saturated fats can often be recognized by the fact that they are solid at room temperature.

➤ **Saturated fat and the endothelium:** In the last chapter, in the **Red meat** section, we discussed how animal protein can damage the endothelium, the fragile layer of cells lining the inside of every blood vessel in your body. Saturated fat has been shown repeatedly in studies to damage the endothelium as well.

Dr. Joel Fuhrman explains the function of the endothelium:

> The endothelium is a specialized layer of cells that forms the inner lining of all blood vessels. Endothelial cells produce nitric oxide and other substances that regulate blood pressure, maintain balance between pro-thrombotic (blood clotting) and anti-thrombotic

---

[170] For example, this web page has some good suggestions:
http://www.fitday.com/fitness-articles/nutrition/healthy-eating/healthy-substitutes-for-oil.html

mechanisms, and act as a selective barrier between the blood and surrounding tissues. The functions of the endothelium are crucial; endothelial dysfunction is an early event in atherosclerotic plaque development and cardiovascular disease.[171]

When the endothelium is functioning properly, it is able to cause the blood vessels to relax and expand as needed to maintain proper blood pressure, and keep the blood moving as it should.

> *Eating a meal containing animal fat or added oil impairs the proper function of the endothelium, which can lead to vascular disease.*

When the endothelium's function is impaired, blood vessels will not be able to do this, and this is an unhealthy condition, leading to vascular disease.

The Brachial Artery Tourniquet (BART) test is a harmless, non-invasive test which can measure the ability of blood vessels to adjust properly to changing conditions. If they don't respond properly, this indicates the endothelium is impaired. Thus the BART test is a good way to determine the effect of various foods on endothelial function.

In his book, "Prevent and Reverse Heart Disease," Dr. Esselstyn described how this test was used by Dr. Robert Vogel, of the University of Maryland School of Medicine, to compare the effects of two types of breakfasts: high fat and non fat:

> One group of students then ate a fast-food breakfast that contained 900 calories and 50 grams of fat. A second group ate 900-calorie breakfasts containing no fat at all. After they ate, Dr. Vogel again constricted their brachial arteries for five minutes and watched to see the result. It was dramatic. Among those who consumed no fat there was simply no problem: their arteries bounced back to normal just as they had in the pre-breakfast test. But the arteries of those who had eaten the fat-laden fast food took far longer to respond.

---

[171] Dr. Joel Fuhrman, M.D., It's Just One Meal. How Bad Could It Be? http://www.drfuhrman.com/library/Its_just_one_meal.aspx

> Why? The answer lies in the effect of fat on the endothelium's ability to produce nitric oxide. Dr. Vogel closely monitored endothelial function of subjects and found that two hours after eating a fatty meal there was a significant drop. It took nearly six hours, in fact, for endothelial function to get back to normal.
>
> If a single meal can have such an impact on vascular health, imagine the damage done by three meals a day, seven days a week, 365 days a year – for decades.[172]

Thus this test revealed evidence that a high fat meal impairs the production of nitric oxide by the endothelium. And this is significant, because of the important role this nitric oxide plays in arterial health. Dr. Esselstyn goes on to list some of the important things nitric oxide does to keep our blood vessels functioning well:

- It relaxes blood vessels, selectively boosting blood flow to the organs that need it.

- It prevents white blood cells and platelets from becoming sticky, and thus starting the buildup of vascular plaque.

- It keeps the smooth muscle cells of arteries from growing into plaques.

- It may even help to diminish vascular plaques once they are in place.[173]

While a high fat diet, which includes animal products and added oils, impairs nitric oxide production, a diet which avoids those extra fats and instead emphasizes dark green leafy vegetables and other whole plant foods actively promotes a healthy endothelium, able to produce all the nitric oxide needed.

Dr. Esselstyn has found that when his patients are on such a diet, not infrequently their previously plaque-encrusted arteries begin to clear. Reversal of heart disease, true healing, actually happens, and many who were expected by their cardiologists to die of heart disease within months instead live for 10, 15, even

---

[172] Esselstyn, 2007, "Prevent And Reverse Heart Disease", Penguin Group, New York, p.39
[173] *Ibid.* pp. 41-42

20 years or longer. See the **Appendix** for the address of Dr. Esselstyn's website, where you will find the many papers he has published documenting his remarkable work.

The BART test has also been done to evaluate the effect of various added oils. The effect is the same. All added dietary oils impair endothelial function, and thus contribute to vascular disease.

So the next time you consider eating some eggs, sausage, a burger, a piece of fried chicken, pizza or cheesecake, think about your fragile endothelium and how it will be impacted by that meal. Think about your loved ones, about the high cost of healthcare, and about your responsibility before God to be a good steward of all He has blessed you with. **I think you will find that knowing a few of these interesting and important facts about human physiology, as well as seriously considering the spiritual implications of your efforts to maintain good health – or otherwise – really can help you have the willpower to make healthy, God honoring dietary choices!**

➢ **Saturated fat increases cholesterol and inflammation:** Saturated fat also causes cholesterol and inflammation levels to rise in your body.[174] This also can lead to damage to the arterial walls, and thus many vascular diseases including heart disease and stroke.

This inflammation associated with saturated fats affects the lining of the colon as well. This causes the condition called "leaky gut,"[175] which can lead to many autoimmune diseases, including

---

[174] Greger, Trans Fat, Saturated Fat, and Cholesterol: Tolerable Upper Intake of Zero http://nutritionfacts.org/video/trans-fat-saturated-fat-and-cholesterol-tolerable-upper-intake-of-zero/
[175] Greger, The Leaky Gut Theory of Why Animal Products Cause Inflammation http://nutritionfacts.org/video/the-leaky-gut-theory-of-why-animal-products-cause-inflammation/

arthritis, lupus,[176] Crohn's disease,[177] colitis, multiple sclerosis, and others.[178] And of course often the best cure for such conditions is a whole food plant based diet.[179]

All meats and dairy (except fat-free dairy) have a lot of saturated fat, even "lean" cuts. This includes fish and fowl, even chicken breast. Lots of saturated fat.

There is also some controversy here. Some believe animal fat to be healthy, if it's not "damaged" fat, that is through cooking at high temperatures (frying, char broiling), refining, or from animals fed a unnatural diets and/or hormones, drugs, etc. But it is clear that the weight of evidence indicates that the fat definitely does promote chronic diseases such as vascular disease, diabetes, and cancer.

➤ **Dietary fat causes diabetes:** Diabetes has for a long time been recognized as a diet-caused disease. This being the case, why is it that it has most commonly been treated primarily with drugs? Diabetics routinely receive advice regarding making dietary changes to slow the progression of their disease. But typically those diet changes don't stop or reverse the disease, and eventually drugs and/or insulin injections are required to control blood sugar levels. But even with those measures, the disease continues to progress, and many diabetics suffer severe complications such as amputations, kidney disease, high blood pressure, heart disease, stroke, and others. The drugs and insulin cannot cure diabetes.

In fact, the American Diabetes Association website has this

---

[176] McDougall, Mayra: Almost Lost to Lupus
https://www.drmcdougall.com/health/education/health-science/stars/stars-written/mayra/
[177] *WebMD*, Leaky Gut Syndrome: What Is It?
http://www.webmd.com/digestive-disorders/features/leaky-gut-syndrome
[178] McDougall, Diet: Only Hope for Arthritis
https://www.drmcdougall.com/health/education/health-science/featured-articles/articles/diet-only-hope-for-arthritis/
[179] McDougall, Ten Cases of Severe, mostly Rheumatoid, Arthritis Cured by the McDougall Diet
https://www.drmcdougall.com/misc/2014nl/may/tencases.htm

statement, which I presume is meant to encourage diabetics:

> Diabetes increases your risk for many serious health problems. The good news? With the correct treatment and recommended lifestyle changes, many people with diabetes are able to prevent or delay the onset of complications.[180]

The best encouragement they can give is that with "correct treatment" (i.e. drugs, insulin) **and** implementing their recommended lifestyle changes, "many" are able to prevent or delay complications from occurring. They imply that drugs will be needed, and of course that is true, if diabetics follow their lifestyle recommendations.

If I were a diabetic, I would not consider this to be encouraging, or "good news."

But wait a minute. If diabetes is a disease caused by diet, shouldn't it be also curable by diet? Not just complications delayed?

We know there are diets which do not cause diabetes. Many large populations of people have lived with no apparent problem with diabetes. So doesn't it make sense that a diabetic should eat like those populations which have no diabetes?

Dr. Neal Barnard, M.D., has been successfully treating diabetics for years. He explains type 2 diabetes[181] this way:[182] Cells need glucose for energy. There are little doors in the cells through

---

[180] American Diabetes Association, Complications
http://www.diabetes.org/living-with-diabetes/complications/
[181] Type 1 diabetes, often called childhood onset diabetes, is due to the inability of the pancreas to produce insulin. Most of the information in this book regarding diabetes relates specifically to type 2 diabetes, described in this section. Type 1 diabetes cannot be cured with diet, but it is important to note that it may be prevented by a low fat whole plant food diet. In fact, milk and meat consumption by small children is specifically indicated as a cause of this terrible disease. This study report is representative of the evidence for this: Sandro Muntoni et al, *The American Journal of Clinical Nutrition,* Nutritional factors and worldwide incidence of childhood type 1 diabetes
http://ajcn.nutrition.org/content/71/6/1525.abstract
[182] Barnard, *TED Talk,* Tackling diabetes with a bold new dietary approach
http://www.youtube.com/watch?v=ktQzM2IA-qU

which the glucose can enter. But the doors are locked. Insulin is the key which unlocks the doors, allowing the glucose to enter. This is why when you eat starches and sugars your blood insulin levels rise as your pancreas responds to the presence of glucose.

Fat from meat and added dietary oils, however, will clog the keyholes as if someone had stuffed chewing gum in them, so the insulin can't unlock the doors, and the glucose can't enter. If this is the situation, does it seem that the best solution to this problem is to increase the amount of insulin? If you have a keyhole clogged with chewing gum, will throwing a bunch more keys at it solve the problem? No. The best solution is to remove the chewing gum from the keyhole, clear out the extra fat from the cells. Then the key will be able to do its work.

So how does one clear the fat from the cells? You can probably guess.

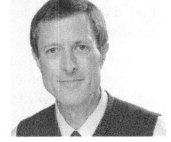

Dr. Barnard found that a whole food plant based diet, which has no meat or animal products (thus no animal fat), and no added vegetable oils or sugar, effectively clears the fat from the cell keyholes, curing diabetics of this supposedly incurable disease in 14 weeks, making them asymptomatic. And they continue to be healthy and free of the symptoms of diabetes as long as they maintain this diet.

Aside from the "clogged keyhole" analogy, another reason the available insulin is unable to get glucose into the cells is that they are already full. The cell shuts the doors and puts out a "no vacancy" sign. Taking insulin injections overrides the "no vacancy" sign, rudely forcing the glucose into the cell anyway. Thus insulin injections often cause weight gain, already a serious problem for many diabetics.

But why are the cells full of glucose? Because of a high-sugar and refined flour diet. That is why cutting out those partial foods from the diet completely, along with getting adequate exercise to help burn up the extra glucose, are also very important lifestyle measures to take.

Dr. Barnard and Dr. McDougall have been very successful at guiding their diabetic patients into a dietary program which, for many, effectively cures their diabetes.

How does the remarkable success of the protocol prescribed by these doctors compare to the results of the recommendations of the American Diabetes Association? Regarding meat, the ADA recommends the patient "choose the leanest options," which, they say, include T-bone steaks, sirloin, etc. They also approve of the consumption of chicken, and recommend at least two fish meals per week. So you can probably predict what the outcome of following this diet will be for the diabetic patient.

Your prediction was correct. Unlike the patients of Drs. McDougall and Barnard, diabetics on the ADA diet do not see their disease cured. In fact **typically their condition continues to deteriorate**.

So, you diabetics reading this now know what you can do to address your disease. And for those of us who don't have diabetes, we know what to do to avoid ever getting it!

➢ **Dietary fat and menstruation:** High levels of dietary fat, such as that which is obtained from eating meat, dairy, and foods with added vegetable oils, can significantly exacerbate the pain women experience during menstruation. Eliminating this dietary fat reduces the amount of estrogen in the blood, which reduces the severity of monthly hormone shifts which many women experience. This has been found to reduce cramping, PMS, and unhealthy food cravings. Even a single high fat meal during the month can be sufficient to increase the estrogen level in the body, bringing on the uncomfortable symptoms.[183]

---

[183] Barnard, Chocolate, Cheese, Meat, and Sugar – Physically Addictive (minute 27:40) https://www.youtube.com/watch?v=5VWi6dXCT7I

Trans fat

➤ **What is trans fat?:** In trans fat, "trans" refers to a certain configuration of the molecules (most fats in our body are the "cis" configuration rather than the "trans" configuration).

> The vast majority of trans fats in our food are manufactured by adding hydrogen bonds to unsaturated fats. This makes the fat more stable, so it doesn't spoil as quickly. These fats are usually referred to as "hydrogenated fats" or "partially hydrogenated fats". "Fully hydrogenated fats" should not contain significant amounts of trans fats. The evidence is reasonably clear that this type of fat contributes to heart disease.[184]

Trans fats occur in nature, but only in animal products. Whole plant foods do not contain them. The process of manufacturing trans fat artificially was developed in 1901, and in 1911 Proctor and Gamble began selling Crisco shortening. Hydrogenated trans fats then began to replace lard, beef tallow and butterfat in cooking.

Cooks and food manufacturers like the properties of trans fat. They can improve the taste of food and extend shelf life. But in 1988 trans fat was linked to heart disease, and more studies followed. Now the science on its dangers to health is so solid and well known that almost everyone in the West knows they shouldn't eat it.

➤ **Foods containing trans fat:** Frying foods at high temperatures will make the oil more toxic to consume, and some claim it may produce trans fat even in non-trans fat oils. And of course trans fat-containing hydrogenated oils are still sometimes used in frying. Other foods commonly containing trans fat include pie crust, margarine and spread, cake mixes and frostings, pancake and waffle mix, ice cream, coffee creamers, microwave popcorn butter flavoring, cookies, biscuits and sweet rolls, crackers, frozen dinners, rice noodles, and many other foods.

---

[184] Laura Dolson, *About Health,* Trans Fat
http://lowcarbdiets.about.com/od/glossary/g/transfat.htm

➢ **No safe limit:** Dr. Greger wrote this about trans fat:

> The most prestigious scientific body in the United States, the National Academies of Science (NAS), concluded that the only safe intake of trans fats is zero. In their report condemning trans fats, they couldn't even assign a Tolerable Upper Daily Limit of intake because [the NAS report concluded,] **"any incremental increase in trans fatty acid intake increases coronary heart disease risk."** [Emphasis added.][185]

Compare this to mercury, arsenic, lead, aluminum, etc., which do have "safe" levels, according to the FDA.

➢ **Trans fat and food labeling:** Food labeling laws state that any amount of trans fat over .5 gram per serving must be indicated on the label. If it has less than .5 gram per serving the label can say "0 trans fat." **So if you eat several servings of "0 trans fat" processed foods in a given day, you can actually be ingesting a significant amount.** And no amount is safe. Another good reason to avoid eating packaged foods.

➢ **Trans fat and meat:** All meat (including poultry, fish, eggs) and dairy contains some level of trans fat. But since it isn't "added" by the producer, the label will not state that it contains trans fat, or the amount per serving. But one 3 oz. serving of beef has .9 gram trans fat, one cup of milk .2 gram trans fat.

➢ **Trans fat and logic:** Proposition A: No amount of trans fat is safe to consume. Proposition B: All meat and dairy contains some level of trans fat. If both A and B are true, then the logical conclusion would be... I'll let you figure it out.

Note that some experts in this area consider artificially produced trans fats to be dangerous, but insist that naturally occurring trans fats in meat and dairy are harmless, and maybe even healthy. However, apparently this remains to be proven.

Fats/oils in whole plant foods

Fats and oils which occur in whole plant foods, when consumed

---

[185] Greger, Trans Fat in Animal Fat http://nutritionfacts.org/2014/02/27/trans-fat-in-animal-fat/

in their natural state, inside the whole food, rather than separated from it, promote good health in healthy people. God put oils in food because they are part of the complete nutrient complex that our bodies need to live and stay healthy.

However, thanks to years of consuming a toxic diet, many people are not healthy. Dr. Esselstyn believes heart disease patients should not eat avocados, nuts or seeds, because he sees evidence that these foods' high fat content can impair cardiovascular health and prevent healing. Some studies, however, indicate nuts are beneficial to heart health.

> Based on the data from the Nurses' Health Study, we estimated that substitution of the fat from 1 ounce of nuts for equivalent energy from carbohydrate in an average diet was associated with a 30% reduction in CHD risk and the substitution of nut fat for saturated fat was associated with 45% reduction in risk. [186]

It may well be that the above is true for those who do not yet have heart disease, while those with heart disease should stay away from nuts (and avocados), as Dr. Esselstyn recommends. Certainly Dr. Esselstyn's impressive results should compel the prudent heart patient to take his advice seriously.

Dr. McDougall recommends that those who wish to lose weight eat a starch based whole food diet without avocados and nuts, since these are the highest calorie foods.

Coconut and palm oil

Many consider coconut and perhaps even palm oil to be healthy alternatives to the PUFA oils like corn, soy and safflower. But, as stressed earlier, it is best to avoid consuming any added oils, as there is good evidence that any added dietary oil, no matter what kind, is damaging to the body. Even coconut and palm oil are implicated in this.

---

[186] F.B. Hu, M.J. Stampfer, Department of Nutrition, Harvard School of Public Health, *Current Atherosclerosis Reports,* Nut consumption and risk of coronary heart disease: a review of epidemiologic evidence 1999 http://www.ncbi.nlm.nih.gov/pubmed/11122711

Fat in the Okinawan diet

The Japanese people living on the island of Okinawa have a reputation for being the longest living on the planet. They have the most centenarians of any population, and live to an average age of 81.2 years.

One study compared age-adjusted mortality of Okinawans versus Americans and found that, during 1995, an average Okinawan was 8 times less likely to die from coronary heart disease, 7 times less likely to die from prostate cancer, 6.5 times less likely to die from breast cancer, and 2.5 times less likely to die from colon cancer than an average American of the same age (Wilcox, et al, Caloric Restriction, the Traditional Okinawan Diet, and Healthy Aging).

Sweet potatoes have traditionally been an Okinawan staple. Little meat is eaten. A low amount of dietary fat is considered to be a key to the Okinawans' remarkable good health.

% of calories obtained from dietary fat

Traditional Okinawa diet 6

Whole food plant based diet .... < 10

USDA recommendation .... 20 - 35

American Heart Assoc. recommendation*....25 - 35

Standard American Diet .... ~ 37

*This is the figure for fats from "foods like fish, nuts, and vegetable oils." Percent of calories from saturated fats should be <7%, and from trans fats <1%, they say. As we will see later, this diet leads to worsening of heart disease.

Dr. McDougall cites a study in which several dietary oils were tested to see which ones caused the most increase in triglycerides and blood clotting. The oils tested were canola, olive, sunflower, palm, and butter. All were found to have a similar effect of increasing both triglycerides and blood clotting.[187]

➢ **Coconut oil – Alzheimer's and dementia:** These mental diseases (actually, Alzheimer's is a type of dementia) have various causes, but one condition responsible for them is described as "diabetes of the brain."[188] The evidence indicates this form of diabetes is also caused by an unhealthy diet rich in animal products.[189,190] As a result of this diet, the brain cells get to the point that they can't imbibe glucose for energy as they should, so are starved for energy, and start to malfunction. So the best strategy for preventing and treating these conditions is a whole food plant based diet.

A possible complementary treatment of Alzheimer's and dementia involves coconut oil. Though consuming even coconut oil apparently damages blood vessels, the effects of Alzheimer's and dementia are so devastating that the risks of this treatment may be worth the possible benefit.

Here's how it is said to work: Besides glucose, brain cells can also burn ketone bodies. Coconut oil is 60% medium-chain triglycerides (MCTs), the highest concentration of any food. The liver converts MCTs into ketone bodies, which travel to the brain and help out brain cells which aren't able to take in glucose. Thus some Alzheimer's and dementia patients have experienced

---

[187] McDougall, Vegetable Fat as Medicine
https://www.drmcdougall.com/health/education/health-science/featured-articles/articles/vegetable-fat-as-medicine/

[188] Jessica Griggs, New Scientist, Are Alzheimer's and diabetes the same disease? http://www.newscientist.com/article/mg22029453.400-are-alzheimers-and-diabetes-the-same-disease.html#.VHN438kXLPw

[189] McDougall, Alzheimer's Disease Can Be Safely Prevented and Treated Now
http://www.nealhendrickson.com/mcdougall/2004nl/040600pualzheimer.htm

[190] Greger, Preventing Alzheimer's With Lifestyle Changes
http://nutritionfacts.org/video/preventing-alzheimers-with-lifestyle-changes/

improvement of symptoms if they eat 4-9 tbsp. coconut oil/day.[191]

I suggested an acquaintance at our church give her dementia-plagued husband coconut oil, and some weeks later she contacted me, excited to share about how he was improving.

If someone consumes coconut oil to treat Alzheimer's or dementia they should evaluate the results after a week or two. If they see no improvement, they would do well to consider stopping the treatment to reduce the chance of the vascular damage which consuming large amounts of oil can cause.

> **Coconut oil – healthy food or no?:** There are many books and websites dedicated to spreading the news that coconut oil is very healthy, a nutritious food and natural remedy for many maladies. But most of this appears to be pop science, based on anecdotal evidence and the desire to sell product. According to many health authorities, the hard scientific evidence for these claims is not compelling – at least not yet. WebMD reports:

> There is very limited evidence on disease outcomes [from the use of coconut oil], says Dariush Mozaffarian, MD, DrPH, of Harvard Medical School and Harvard School of Public Health. "All that has been studied well is the impact of coconut oil on cholesterol levels and the findings are intriguing but we still don't know if it is harmful or beneficial," Mozaffarian says.[192]

Of course, WebMD and Dr. Mozaffarian are not free from bias either; I don't know if they are intending to promote a particular agenda regarding the use of coconut oil. M.D.s are often reluctant to consider that a dietary intervention can really make a significant difference in factors such as cholesterol levels. More in **Chapter 15: Doctors' knowledge is limited** regarding this.

Dr. Greger reports that reliable studies indicate coconut oil

---

[191] Dr. Mary Newport, M.D., Medium Chain Triglycerides and Ketones: An Alternative Fuel for Alzheimer's
http://www.youtube.com/watch?v=feyydeMFWy4
[192] Kathleen M. Zelman, M.P.H., R.D., L.D., The Truth About Coconut Oil
http://www.webmd.com/diet/features/coconut-oil-and-health

consumption raises blood cholesterol somewhat, likely due to the high saturated fat content. However, unlike saturated fat-loaded dairy and meat consumption, coconut oil does not cause a rise in inflammation in the body. Dr. Greger doesn't report on any studies directly linking coconut oil consumption to vascular or any other disease, however.[193,194]

Eating any oil will damage artery endothelium, thereby increasing risk of heart attack, as discussed above. Dr. Matthew Lederman, M.D., an associate of Dr. Esselstyn, also makes the logical connection that since other oils, especially those containing saturated fat, have been proven to cause inflammation, raise cholesterol, and promote vascular disease, it follows that coconut oil does, too. Thus he cautions strongly against its consumption.[195]

There is at least one study which suggests that coconut oil may be helpful in *preventing* cardiovascular disease.

> This review highlights the mechanism through which saturated fatty acids contribute to CV [cardiovascular] disease (CVD), how oils and fats contribute to the risk of CVD, and the existing views on VCO [virgin coconut oil] and **how its cardioprotective effects may make this a possible dietary intervention** in isolation or in combination with exercise **to help reduce the burden of CVDs.** [Emphasis added.][196]

Additionally, Dr. Mary Enig, Ph.D. did considerable research in an effort to exonerate coconut oil and show it is safe and healthful. She cites many studies which she says prove this to be the case. (I would be interested in her take on the BART test results, but

---

[193] Greger, Does Coconut Oil Clog Arteries?
http://nutritionfacts.org/video/does-coconut-oil-clog-arteries/
[194] Note that Dr. Greger doesn't really answer the question in the title of this video, since the studies he cites only indicate a rise in cholesterol, not artery clogging. Though the one is usually assumed to cause the other, many now doubt this is necessarily so.
[195] Matthew Lederman, M.D., Is Coconut Oil Healthy or Hazardous?
http://nutritionstudies.org/coconut-oil-healthy-hazardous/
[196] A.S. Babu, et al, *Postgraduate Medicine*, Virgin coconut oil and its potential cardioprotective effects 2014 http://www.ncbi.nlm.nih.gov/pubmed/25387216

alas, she died in 2014; I don't know if she ever published any comments on that subject.) If you want to look into this further, I encourage you to study her paper and check out her sources carefully: <u>Health and Nutritional Benefits from Coconut Oil: An Important Functional Food for the 21st Century</u>.[197]

So you can take this information and come to your own conclusions regarding whether or not you should consume coconut and/or palm oil as a part of your whole food plant based diet.

I, for one, can't discount the research and opinions of Drs. Esselstyn, Campbell, McDougall and Greger, who all agree that it is best to avoid coconut and palm oil. I admit it was hard for me to come to this position, as I had previously bought into the notion, promoted by Drs. Enig, Mercola, and others, that these oils are a great addition to a healthy diet.

Oils in the Heart Attack Proof diet

NO OIL! Not even olive oil, which goes against a lot of other advice out there about so-called good fats. The reality is that oils are extremely low in terms of nutritive value. They contain no fiber, no minerals and are 100% fat calories. Both the mono unsaturated and saturated fat contained in oils is harmful to the endothelium, the innermost lining of the artery, and that injury is the gateway to vascular disease. It doesn't matter whether it's olive oil, corn oil, coconut oil, canola oil, or any other kind. Avoid ALL oil.   *— Dr. Caldwell Esselstyn*

---

[197] Dr. Mary Enig, Ph.D., *The Westin A. Price Foundation* 1996, <u>Health and Nutritional Benefits from Coconut Oil: An Important Functional Food for the 21st Century</u> http://www.westonaprice.org/health-topics/a-new-look-at-coconut-oil/

If you have a history of heart or other vascular disease, I urge you to follow Dr. Esselstyn's advice and avoid all oils altogether, including coconut and palm oil (not to mention all animal products, sugar, and white flour), as that is the protocol which has produced such dramatic positive results for his patients.

Keep in mind, also, that consuming coconut and palm oil violates the whole food principle, so the likely fact that it is unhealthy is not surprising.

To be honest, however, I will admit that in our household we do use coconut oil very sparingly. In the context of our otherwise extremely healthy diet, we don't expect to experience any adverse effects from this.

One thing to bear in mind is that the issue of whether or not to consume coconut oil is relatively trivial compared to the consumption of meat, eggs, dairy, other oils, sugar, and refined flours. If you continue to eat these things, whether or not you choose to eat coconut oil is probably immaterial; it will likely have little additional adverse impact on your health compared to those other substances.

Sugar and other sweeteners

God created our bodies to consume starch, from our tongues to our colons. So naturally we crave sweets. And that is fine if the sweets are found in their natural environment, in whole fruits and veggies. But when the sweet component, the sugar, is extracted from the plant, concentrated, and then consumed, it becomes, in a word, *toxic*.

This was rarely a problem in the past, as the human technology to produce a lot of sugar cheaply in most parts of the world did not exist. (Bees were the most efficient at this task, of course.) But now sugar is cheap and plentiful, as are numerous artificial sweeteners. The natural craving for sweets, combined with their easy availability, shameless and irresponsible advertising, and unbridled consumption has contributed to untold and unprecedented human suffering due to chronic disease.

➢ **Sugar consumption – Historical perspective:** It is estimated that in 1776 Americans consumed about four pounds of sugar per year. By 1850 it was 20 lbs., and by 1994 it was up to 120 lbs. Today one estimate has it at about 160 lbs. of added sugar consumed by each person each year. That's right, on average **each American consumes about 7 oz. of sugar every day, which is 50 tsp.** You heard right, fifty teaspoons, which is the amount of sugar in about 5 cans of Coke. And that's 40 times as much as the average American consumed at our country's founding!

Is it any wonder we have a plague of chronic diseases which our forefathers never, or only extremely rarely, suffered from? Though consumption of sugar isn't solely responsible for all of these diseases, it surely is a main reason for the epidemic.

Sugar makes a greater contribution to our diets, measured in calories, than does meat or bread or any other single commodity.[198] Many diseases, unknown in previous eras, are now commonplace thanks to our addiction to sugar.

➢ **Sugar promotes disease:** Sugar promotes inflammation in the body; encourages diabetes; feeds cancer cells, promoting their growth and proliferation; damages the endothelium of your blood vessels, increasing risk of cardiovascular and other vascular diseases; contributes to obesity; promotes tooth decay; and is responsible for many other serious diseases.[199]

George A. Bray of the Pennington Biomedical Research Center, Louisiana State University, wrote,

> Most meta-analyses have shown that the risk of obesity, diabetes, cardiovascular disease, and metabolic syndrome are related to consumption of beverages sweetened with sugar or high-fructose corn syrup. Calorically sweetened beverage intake has also been related to the risk of nonalcoholic fatty liver disease, and, in men, gout. Calorically sweetened beverages contribute to obesity through their caloric load,…. By worsening blood lipids, contributing to

---

[198] Greger, How Much Added Sugar Is Too Much?
http://nutritionfacts.org/video/how-much-added-sugar-is-too-much/
[199] Dr. Robert H. Lustig, M.D., Sugar: The Bitter Truth
https://www.youtube.com/watch?v=dBnniua6-oM

obesity, diabetes, fatty liver, and gout, fructose in the amounts currently consumed is hazardous to the health of some people.[200]

"Some people"?!! Well, technically that's true. It is only hazardous to those who consume it.

The best advice anyone can give regarding sugar is to **try to avoid eating anything to which it has been added.** Of course it isn't practical or perhaps even possible to avoid all added sugar. And it is unlikely that a little sugar in your food or drink from time to time will cause a problem. But being conscious of how severely sugar can damage your body should go a long way in helping you to minimize the amount you consume.

➤ **Sugar and cancer:** Cancers are constantly trying to take root and grow in our bodies. Our immune system is usually able to keep them under control. But certain factors can encourage cancer to grow out of control, causing disease. One of those factors is high sugar intake. Much research has proven that cancer cells feed on sugar. For example, this from University of Copenhagen researchers:

> The process of glycosylation, where sugar molecules are attached to proteins, has long been of interest to scientists, particularly because certain sugar molecules are present in very high numbers in cancer cells. It now turns out that these sugar molecules are not only present but actually aid the growth of the malignant cells. In the long term this discovery is an important step towards a cure that can stop the growth of cancer cells.[201]

This is representative of many other studies confirming that added dietary sugar both helps get cancer started and helps enable it to sicken and kill.

This being the case, why is it that cancer patients *are not* routinely counseled to avoid dietary sugar? Why is it that

---

[200] George A. Bray, *Advances in Nutrition,* Energy and Fructose From Beverages Sweetened With Sugar or High-Fructose Corn Syrup Pose a Health Risk for Some People http://advances.nutrition.org/content/4/2/220.abstract
[201] University of Copenhagen, *Science Daily* 2013, Specific sugar molecule causes growth of cancer cells
http://www.sciencedaily.com/releases/2013/09/130916103646.htm

cancer patients undergoing chemotherapy, especially children, are routinely given cancer-promoting candy by their caregivers?

This grieves my heart greatly. It should grieve us all.

➤ **Sugar and diabetes:** High consumption of added sugar is known to contribute to the onset of type 2 diabetes. And diabetes is the third major chronic disease killer, accounting for 3.8 million deaths worldwide in 2006 alone. Add to that the many tens of thousands of amputations due to the disease each year, and the magnitude of this disaster begins to be realized. And it is only compounded by the fact that for most victims it is entirely preventable via lifestyle choices.

Dr. Robert Lustig, a pediatric endocrinologist and sugar researcher, says sugar isn't *empty* calories, as is often said, but rather *toxic* calories. He says his studies show that 29% of the type 2 diabetes cases worldwide are due solely to the daily consumption of the amount of added sugar found in a single can of soda. In other words, suppose you drink one can of soda per day. If you stopped that habit and didn't replace that sugar in your diet, your risk of getting diabetes would be cut by 29% based on that single dietary choice. It is such effects of sugar on the body which, in Dr. Lustig's view, earns sugar the designation *toxic*. [202,203]

Unfortunately, from what I have seen of Dr. Lustig's work, it appears that he doesn't recognize the important role dietary fat plays in causing and exacerbating diabetes. The evidence I have seen suggests that not only a diet very low in added sugar, but also a diet very low in animal fat, i.e. a largely whole food plant based diet, is necessary to really be sure you will not get diabetes, and to be cured of this terrible disease if you already do have it.

---

[202] Lustig, <u>Sugar: The Bitter Truth</u>
<u>https://www.youtube.com/watch?v=dBnniua6-oM</u>
[203] Lustig, <u>Sugar: The Elephant In The Kitchen</u>
<u>https://www.youtube.com/watch?v=gmC4Rm5cpOI</u>

➢ **Sugar and acne:** Acne is largely a diet-induced disease. Adolescents in Western countries commonly suffer from this disease at rates of 79-95%. In many underdeveloped nations, however, the rate is closer to 0%![204] High sugar consumption is a significant contributor to this problem.[205]

➢ **Disguised sugar in product labels:** Learn to recognize disguised sugar on product labels. Some of the ways food companies try to hide the fact that their products contain lots of sugar is to call it euphemistic names such as agave nectar, brown rice syrup, high fructose corn syrup or HFCS, dextrose, evaporated cane juice, glucose, lactose, malt syrup, molasses, sucrose, honey, etc. All of these are essentially just sugar, and all damage the body like plain old sugar.

A list of ingredients may begin well, making you feel good that the first ingredient is something "healthy," such as wheat flour. But then the next two or more ingredients may be sugar under various names. This of course is done in an attempt to hide the fact that sugar makes up a considerable proportion of the product, and may in fact be the main ingredient.

Note the ingredients label below: wheat flour, which contains a bunch of added-in artificial pretend nutrients, followed by no less than *six* forms of sugar, and several types of added oil. What's left is a long list of chemicals and partial foods. Whatever this product is, my friend, it is toxic and should not be consumed by anyone who cares about their health.

By the way, one of the side benefits of eating whole food plant based is that you don't have to take a course on food labels to really understand what it is you are eating. Most of the best, most nutritious foods are those with no ingredients label!

---

[204] McDougall, Acne Has Nothing to Do with Diet – Wrong!
http://www.nealhendrickson.com/mcdougall/031100puacne.htm
[205] Ayren Jackson-Cannady, *WebMD*, 10 Lifestyle Steps to Help Your Acne,
http://www.webmd.com/skin-problems-and-treatments/acne/features/lifestyle

INGREDIENTS: ENRICHED FLOUR (WHEAT FLOUR, NIACIN, REDUCED IRON, THIAMIN MONONITRATE [VITAMIN B$_1$], RIBOFLAVIN [VITAMIN B$_2$], FOLIC ACID), CORN SYRUP, SUGAR, SOYBEAN AND PALM OIL (WITH TBHQ FOR FRESHNESS), CORN SYRUP SOLIDS, DEXTROSE, HIGH FRUCTOSE CORN SYRUP, FRUCTOSE, GLYCERIN, CONTAINS 2% OR LESS OF COCOA (PROCESSED WITH ALKALI), POLYDEXTROSE, MODIFIED CORN STARCH, SALT, DRIED CREAM, CALCIUM CARBONATE, CORNSTARCH, LEAVENING (BAKING SODA, SODIUM ACID PYROPHOSPHATE, MONOCALCIUM PHOSPHATE, CALCIUM SULFATE), DISTILLED MONOGLYCERIDES, HYDROGENATED PALM KERNEL OIL, SODIUM STEAROYL LACTYLATE, GELATIN, COLOR ADDED, SOY LECITHIN, DATEM, NATURAL AND ARTIFICIAL FLAVOR, VANILLA EXTRACT, CARNAUBA WAX, XANTHAN GUM, VITAMIN A PALMITATE, YELLOW #5 LAKE, RED #40 LAKE, CARAMEL COLOR, NIACINAMIDE, BLUE #2 LAKE, REDUCED IRON, YELLOW #6 LAKE, PYRIDOXINE HYDROCHLORIDE (VITAMIN B$_6$), RIBO-FLAVIN (VITAMIN B$_2$), THIAMIN HYDROCHLORIDE (VITAMIN B$_1$), CITRIC ACID, FOLIC ACID, RED #40, YELLOW #5, YELLOW #6, BLUE #2, BLUE #1.

➢ **Honey:** As indicated above, basically honey has the same negative effects on your body as added sugar.

What?!! Honey isn't good for you? Sounds like health food heresy.

But think about it. What is honey? It is processed, concentrated flower nectar, that is, mostly processed sugar. Processed not by people, but by some really cleverly designed and hard working bees. But it is still a processed, non-whole food sugar product, with only very minute trace amounts of anything that might be healthy for us – not enough to normally be of much value.

Of course, after the bees get done with it a lot of honey gets a good dose of processing at the hands of man as well, which certainly doesn't improve its nutritional value.

Honey has been known to infect babies with botulism.[206] Some beekeepers give their bees antibiotics, and hives may be contaminated with pesticides. These substances can end up in the honey. Aside from the botulism, exposure to such contaminants from eating honey will probably never be proven to cause harm in humans, however. It is the sugar content and what that does to the body which is most concerning.

---

[206] *WebMD,* Honey http://www.webmd.com/vitamins-supplements/ingredientmono-738-HONEY.aspx?activeIngredientId=738&activeIngredientName=HONEY

Now I know some will protest that they only eat local raw honey, and only to help them with their allergies. Fine. No doubt that would be safer than taking allergy medications. The practice probably won't cause problems if you are otherwise healthy and the quantity of honey is small.

I do consider honey to be more "natural" than refined sugar, and if one has to choose between the two, honey is of course better. I trust bees more than sugar factories for sure. But for good health it is best to try to break the sugar addiction and learn to require less sweet in your diet. Whole foods are always best.

➢ **Sugar is addictive:** Sugar is addictive in the same way many illicit drugs are addictive. It stimulates similar parts of the brain that other addictive substances do to deliver pleasure to the user.[207] Some people are more prone to this addiction, and thus it can be much harder for such people to give up sugar than it is for others who are not prone to have this addiction (just as is the case with addictions to tobacco, alcohol, gambling, etc.). So if you find it "impossible" to get off sugar, recognize that it is an addiction. You are being controlled by it, in a sense. And recognizing it for what it is will help you to take it seriously.

Don't resign yourself to being addicted. Don't give up and give in! Take charge of your life. Or better, give Jesus control. Does He want you addicted to sugar? No, of course not. Ask Him for help. If you are serious, He will help you.

Also, ask a loved one to help you make right choices. Or talk it over with your family and decide together to make a healthy change which will free you from the bondage of sugar addiction. Explain the problems with sugar consumption carefully and clearly to your children. Have them read this section of the book and ask them what they think your family should do. This is a great opportunity to prepare them to face more serious addiction issues in the future. Get them involved in planning a strategy for beating this problem.

---

[207] Kris Gunnars, How Sugar Hijacks Your Brain and Makes You Addicted
http://authoritynutrition.com/how-sugar-makes-you-addicted/

If you can't quit cold turkey, make a concerted effort to do it gradually. For example, if you drink two cans of soda per day, determine to only drink one per day for a week, then just one every other day, etc. If you usually eat a bowl of ice cream before bed, force yourself to grab a coffee mug this time, and dish out a smaller serving. After a few days, start taking just one spoonful per day. **And when the ice cream is gone, don't buy any more.** (Hint: Eat a big meal before going grocery shopping, and stay in the produce department – don't even *think* about doing window shopping in the ice cream section.)

At first, your sugar craving may demand you give in. Ask God to help you be strong in your resolve to break this addiction, and remember that the cravings will fade away as you develop new habits and your body gets used to the new healthy normal.

If you have a lot of tension and stress in your life, if you are going through a hard season emotionally, this may make breaking the sugar addiction nearly impossible. Seek help from God and those who love you. Make peace with those around you, and with your circumstances. When your emotional stability is restored, you will be able to tackle this addiction.

➢ **Moderation can be dangerous:** But surely consuming a little added sugar is okay, right? Moderation is the key, is it not?

Sugar consumed in the quantity typical of the SAD is clearly disease-promoting. Consuming no added dietary sugar is health-promoting. Exactly how much sugar you can consume and remain free of sugar-induced disease is not known.

It is doubtful that eating a little added sugar, such as one cookie a day, or one teaspoon in your morning coffee, in the context of an otherwise whole food plant based diet, would cause problems.

However, we must remember the addictive power of sugar. The more you consume the more you crave. That small daily serving of sugar may lead to "just one more cookie," and going down that slippery slope has resulted in disaster for millions. So consider making an effort to avoid added sugar whenever possible. Eat whole fruits to satisfy your sugar craving.

"Moderation" is a nice concept, but if a substance has been proven to be toxic, and on top of that it is addictive, is it really wise to consume it, even in moderation?

Is it okay to just do just one line of cocaine a day, since "moderation" is good? No, we would say that person is an addict. We would say he should try to quit completely.

Consuming sugar is more culturally acceptable than consuming cocaine, but it is not inaccurate to say that sugar harms, and kills, many more people than cocaine ever will.

> *Who would know-ingly and willing-ly, on a regular basis, eat food heavily laced with a known toxin? Only an addict.*

> **Learning to live without sugar:**
Part of adjusting to a whole food plant based diet is learning to enjoy foods that aren't made extra sweet with added sugar or other sweeteners. **If you wean yourself off sugar, before long you will find that you really can enjoy foods even when they don't contain added sugar.** Your taste buds will become more sensitive to the actual taste of the food, since the sugar isn't overpowering.

Keep learning more about how sugar damages the body, becoming increasingly convinced about how dangerous it is. Read the articles and watch the videos referenced in this section, for example. This will help you have the willpower to "just say no," because after all, **who would knowingly and willingly, on a regular basis, eat food heavily laced with a known toxin? Only an addict.**

> **The best natural sweetener:** If you feel you must use a sweetener, such as in making some yummy whole plant food cookies, **the best natural sweetener to use is date sugar.** It is simply ground-up dates, so it is a whole food.[208] Though dates

---

[208] Greger, The Healthiest Sweetener http://nutritionfacts.org/video/the-healthiest-sweetener/

are 80% sugar, they don't spike the blood sugar nearly as much as other sugary sweeteners do. And you can make your own date sugar for your recipe by putting some pitted dates in the blender with some of the wet ingredients (like applesauce) and blending well. Many great truly healthy cookie recipes are available on the Internet.[209]

Molasses is also a somewhat nutritive sweetener, so that would be a second choice if you must sweeten something.

But of course date sugar and molasses aren't so great for sweetening tea or coffee. Try to learn to enjoy your tea or coffee without sugar. But if you can't, and don't want to give up your daily fix, read on...

➢ **The least dangerous artificial sweetener:** The least dangerous artificial sweetener seems to be erythritol, which so far has no known health problems associated with it. Xylitol and sorbitol can have a laxative effect on some people, otherwise they seem to be relatively benign. (Chewing xylitol gum, sweetened with xylitol only, may be good for your teeth as some say it protects them from cavities). Data on whether Stevia/ Truvia is safe is not yet clear. All other artificial sweeteners (Saccharin/Sweet n Low, Sucralose/Splenda, Aspartame/Equal, Sugar Twin, Sweet One) have been found to cause certain serious health problems.[210]

I'll say it again: It's best to just wean yourself off the need for added sweeteners as much as possible. Grab an apple or some raisins instead of that cookie or piece of cake. Put raisins, banana or berries on your oatmeal instead of sugar. If you can't drink your coffee unsweetened and/or without adding milk or cream, you should seriously consider trying to break the coffee habit.

---

[209] For example, see this page for some ideas:
http://wholefoodvegan.com/tag/whole-foods-plant-based-dessert/
[210] Greger, A Harmless Artificial Sweetener http://nutritionfacts.org/video/a-harmless-artificial-sweetener/

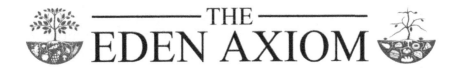

THE
EDEN AXIOM

Chapter 8:

Drinks

In the last chapter we saw the injurious impact the wrong kind of beverage can have on our health. Think about the various things you typically drink throughout the day. How do those beverages measure up when we consider the Eden Axiom? What sort of beverages did God provide for Adam and Eve in Eden?

➤ **What should you drink?:** One nutrition expert said he is often asked if a person were to make only one change in their diet to benefit their health, what should it be? His answer is to stop drinking sweet drinks, whether sugar free or whatever. Consuming sugar is of course harmful. Artificial sweeteners are chemicals which our bodies are not designed to tolerate well. Moreover, studies have found that people who switch to artificially-sweetened sodas actually gain weight as a result (maybe because they feel they can compensate by eating more junk food). Thus this doctor recommends only drinking water and herbal or green tea (unsweetened).

Sounds a bit restrictive, doesn't it? But, sadly, all other beverages are problematic from a health standpoint. And no wonder, considering how far so many depart from the whole food principle.

➤ **Tap water:** Generally tap water is not recommended for drinking. Municipal water systems are good at delivering water which doesn't contain harmful bacteria, but otherwise it isn't good. It typically has many dissolved solids in it, minerals which may or may not be healthful. But worse is the chlorine and (usually) fluoride which tap water contains. Often it also contains traces of pharmaceutical drugs. You do not want to be drinking these harmful chemicals. More on this in **Chapter 15: Toxins in water**.

➢ **Spring water:** Many consider truly contaminant-free river or spring water to be the best water to drink, as it contains healthy minerals. However, such water is hard to find, and it is expensive to have water tested, including bottled spring water, to verify that it is safe. For example, even the snow on the slopes of Mount Shasta, a pristine environment if ever there was one, have been found to have levels of aluminum many times higher than the safe upper limit, and it seems likely that that aluminum would end up in any springs and rivers near the foot of the mountain.[211]

➢ **Distilled water:** We can assume that the water in Eden which Adam and Eve drank came from springs and/or the rivers mentioned in Genesis 2, and that it had minerals (there was no rain at that time so presumably no distilled drinking water available). So we would expect that mineralized water would be the most healthy.

However, some claim that the minerals in water can't be used by the body since they aren't organic, that is, bound up in plant tissue. Some even say that these minerals cause harm, and that distilled water promotes good health.[212,213] Others of course dispute these claims.[214]

➢ **Drink lots of water:** Drink lots of water each day. How

------

[211] It is proposed by some that this aluminum comes from the exhaust of jet liners flying overhead.

[212] Vivian Goldschmidt, M.A. (nutritional science), The Benefits of Drinking Distilled Water http://www.waterwise.com/productcart/pc/PDFs/vivian-goldschmidt-the-benefits-of-drinking-distilled-water.pdf

[213] George Malkmus, The Best Water to Drink http://www.myhdiet.com/healthnews/best-water-drink/

[214] Zoltan P. Rona, M.D., M.Sc., Early Death Comes From Drinking Distilled Water http://purewater101.com/wp-content/uploads/2013/07/Early-Death-Comes-From-Drinking-Distilled-Water-Zoltan-P.-Rona-MD-MSc.pdf

much? Divide your weight in pounds in half. Drink that many ounces each day, more if you spend a lot of time in the heat and sweat a lot. For example, if you weigh 128 lbs., drink at least ½ gallon, which is eight 8 oz. glasses. Water is a critical nutrient. Don't neglect it!

See **Toxins in water** in **Chapter 15** for ideas on how to provide your family with healthy drinking water.

➢ **Tea – preparation:** Tea drinking is one of the very few healthful dietary habits which don't involve truly whole food. Drinking tea has many reported health benefits. Principal among these is the high antioxidant content of tea.

> *Tea drinking is one of the very few healthful dietary habits which don't involve truly whole food.*

Non-herbal tea tends to contain relatively high levels of fluoride, which is a toxic substance best avoided. So some suggest that it is best to steep black, white, or green tea for in hot water for no longer than four minutes. Herbal teas have very little fluoride.

➢ **Green and white tea:** These teas have been tested and found to have high levels of antioxidants, and to be protective from cancer.[215,216] There are other health benefits as well, and research suggests that drinking seven cups a day may be ideal. Dr. Greger recommends not exceeding 10 cups a day due to the fluoride exposure.[217]

➢ **Hibiscus tea:** Dr. Greger compared 282 beverages and found that the one with the most cancer-fighting antioxidants is

---

[215] Greger, Cancer Interrupted Green Tea
http://nutritionfacts.org/video/cancer-interrupted-green-tea/
[216] Greger, Antimutagenic Activity of Green Versus White Tea http://nutritionfacts.org/video/antimutagenic-activity-of-green-versus-white-tea/
[217] Greger, Overdosing on Tea http://nutritionfacts.org/video/overdosing-on-tea/

hibiscus tea.[218,219] You can put four teabags in a ½ gallon of drinking water (or 8 in a gallon, or adjust to taste) and keep it in the fridge. Check the herbal tea label. Be sure hibiscus is the first ingredient. Celestial Seasonings Red Zinger is a popular one. You can get hibiscus tea more cheaply in bulk, by the pound, if you drink a lot of it. And of course you can drink green tea this way as well.

One caution: Hibiscus tea is acidic, and can be a bit hard on tooth enamel. So it is best to not drink it while eating a meal. When done with your tea, drink some water and swish to rinse off your teeth.

➢ **Coffee:** Many studies have been done on coffee which indicate it is healthful, while others indicate it should be avoided. There is some evidence that heart patients should consider abstaining from coffee. The researchers in one small study found that "caffeinated coffee induces significant endothelial dysfunction."[220] For this reason Dr. Esselstyn has added coffee to his "do not consume" list for heart patients.

Coffee also tends to raise cholesterol (unless a paper filter is used in brewing) and blood pressure. It can cause the lower esophageal sphincter to not function as it should, leading to reflux, heartburn and damage to the esophagus. And these effects are entirely apart from the effect of the caffeine.[221]

Again, many studies tout the benefits of coffee consumption, and many of those findings may in fact be true. But as with many things, one must decide whether the benefits outweigh the potential harm.

---

[218] Greger, Herbal Tea Update: Hibiscus http://nutritionfacts.org/video/herbal-tea-update-hibiscus/
[219] Greger, How Much Hibiscus Tea Is Too Much? http://nutritionfacts.org/video/how-much-hibiscus-tea-is-too-much/
[220] Dominic Marro, R.D., C.D.N., Caffeine and Your Arteries http://www.wholefoodplantbasedrd.com/2013/11/caffeine-and-your-arteries/
[221] McDougall Coffee – Pleasure and Pain https://www.drmcdougall.com/misc/2004nl/040700pucoffee.htm

Health concerns of coffee consumption

Coffee contains several hundred different substances (in addition to well-known caffeine) and many of these have powerful pharmacological effects on the human body....

Coffee causes the blood vessels to constrict and the heart to beat stronger, resulting in an elevated blood pressure for most people. Within minutes of drinking this concoction of invigorating chemicals, the systolic blood pressure (top number) can rise 5 to 15 mmHg and the diastolic (bottom number), 5 to 10 mmHg.[2] One 5-ounce (150 ml) cup of regular coffee contains 150 mg of caffeine – a substance known to raise blood pressure. However, decaffeinated coffee also increases blood pressure; therefore, ingredients found in the coffee bean other than caffeine also have pressure-raising effects....

Irregular heart beats (arrhythmias), nervous tremor, headaches, anxiety, teeth-grinding, jaw-clenching, insomnia, frequent urination, elevated eye pressure (glaucoma), diarrhea, osteoporosis and periodontal diseases may be other reasons to add to your list for quitting. When the fear of future health problems, like heart attacks, and the suffering from anxiety, indigestion, and the urge to urinate every few minutes becomes sufficiently troubling, you then may decide life would be better without this upsetting drug.

— Dr. John McDougall

➢ **Alcohol:** Alcohol can be considered a drug and a toxin in the human body. With that said, the body has the ability to detoxify moderate amounts of alcohol (in the liver) without ill effects.

Some studies suggest that consumption of 4-6 oz. of red wine/ day has been found to be healthy for the heart. Some studies have found no health benefits to drinking white wine or other alcoholic drinks. One study of older people, however, found that those who lived the longest were more likely those who drank 1- two drinks per day of any type of alcohol – there was no statistical difference between them, and more than two drinks was not found to be helpful.[222]

In fact, more than two drinks per day increases the chance of chronic disease. Think about what alcohol is. It is *alcohol!* And what is alcohol used for? To kill germs. Surgical instruments are sterilized with it. So what happens when you drink alcohol and it gets to your colon, which is full of bacteria needed for proper digestion, proper immune function, etc.? It kills off some of that good bacteria. If you drink alcohol, just drink a little!

If you are on a whole food plant based diet you shouldn't need the possible extra heart protection afforded by red wine or other alcohol, since you are not damaging your heart or blood vessels in the first place by eating meat, dairy, sugar, oils, or white flour. So I don't believe there is any health reason to consume it.

Of course if one uses alcohol, it should always be done with caution. Some people can easily become addicted, so generally, unless you already know you have no problem controlling your alcohol intake, it is best to avoid it.

---

[222] *60 Minutes* 90+ https://www.youtube.com/watch?v=nAfmRQbrqKE

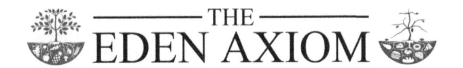

THE EDEN AXIOM

Chapter 9:

Exercise, Sleep, Stress

and Relationships

As explained in **Chapters 2** and **4**, the Eden Axiom includes the principle of a physically active lifestyle; this can be seen in Genesis 1-3. As with issues relating to diet, the best science we have clearly supports this principle as well. But since this principle generally isn't particularly controversial, I will not spend many pages on it nor take the trouble to marshal a lot of authoritative proof for my assertions.

The issues of sleep, stress and relationships are also very critical to good health, so we will deal with those briefly in this chapter as well.

Exercise

➢ **An active lifestyle:** The evidence indicates that a consistently active lifestyle, where you are moving about frequently throughout the day, is more healthful than adding a time of exercise on to a relatively sedentary daily routine. **The more you can be active throughout the day, the better**.

If your daily routine is not very active, you can consciously modify your behavior in positive ways. For instance, if you have to be out running errands for the morning, deliberately park a block away, or at the far end of the parking lot, from each appointment or store; walk up and down stairs instead of taking the elevator; etc. If you have to sit most of the day, be sure to get up every 30 to 60 minutes and walk around a bit, walk up and down some stairs, do some pushups or sit-ups, etc. Put your computer printer across the room or in a different room from your desk, so that you are forced to get up whenever you need to retrieve a document, add paper, etc.

If you can't manage or modify your daily routine to allow you to log at least 10,000 pedometer steps, it is wise to make it a priority to fit a concentrated sustained time of exercise into your day as well.

> **Sitting disease:** This is a newly recognized issue which health researchers are just starting to be concerned about. A study was published in 2010 by the American Cancer Society examining the health impact of daily physical activity. Statistics were kept on over 123,000 people from 1993 to 2006. The researchers noted how long each study participant spent each day sitting – whether working at a desk, driving, sitting at home watching T.V., etc. They also noted which ones lived till the end of the study and which ones died.

For people who sit most of the day, their risk of heart attack is about the same as smoking.
— Martha Grogan, cardiologist, Mayo Clinic

The results? They calculated that **women who sat an average of over six hours per day were 94% more likely to die than women who sat less than three hours.** For men the figure was 48%. And even if those who sat a lot got a lot of exercise otherwise, their risk was still great.[223]

Wow. I don't know about you, but that motivates me to think

---

[223] *Juststand.org,* Sitting Disease Infographic http://www.juststand.org/tabid/674/language/en-US/default.aspx. Of course a study like this can't control for many possible additional factors which may have influenced the outcome. But the large number of study subjects increases the reliability of the figures.

seriously about finding ways to spend more time standing and walking, and less time sitting. If you have to spend a lot of time at a desk, you might want to find a way to raise up your desk surface, computer, monitor, etc. so that you can stand while working. (I did this and am typing this while standing!)

➢ **The best exercise**: If your daily routine doesn't allow sufficient activity, what is the best form of exercise? Participating in sports is great. For most of us brisk walking or jogging are probably the best and most practical exercises. Swimming is excellent, but it requires a body of water, which is not available to most, and pool swimming is usually not ideal, thanks to the chlorine exposure (see **Chapter 15: Toxins in water: Chorine in swimming pools**).

Many fitness authorities recommend rebounding (jumping on a mini-trampoline), either as a supplement to other forms of exercise you participate in or as a primary activity, because of the unique health benefits it provides. See more on this in **Chapter 15: A few more facts and tips: Rebounding**.

➢ **Exercise duration:** If you are unable to be active throughout the day, an absolute minimum of 30 minutes 3 days per week of exertion equivalent to brisk walking or jogging is essential for good health. **Sixty minutes six days per week is ideal.** You should break a sweat! If you are out of shape, start out slowly (e.g. 15 minutes 3x/week) and gradually work your way up to your goal. And spend a little time stretching before and after you exercise.

➢ **Exercise intensity: If your goal is good health, don't exercise too hard.** Sustained strenuous workouts provide no health benefit over moderate ones, and they can be damaging to the heart and joints.[224]

It's fine if you like to run fast 10k races and marathons, play long intense basketball or soccer games, etc. But realize that the

---

[224] Dr. James O'Keefe, M.D., <u>Run for your life! At a comfortable pace, and not too far</u> https://www.youtube.com/watch?v=Y6U728AZnV0

extreme intensity and duration of these activities aren't more effective at helping your body to be healthier than consistent, moderate exercise. Instead they are actually subjecting your body to risks, as with many other active sports (skiing, mountain climbing, football, moto cross, etc.).

Thus taking a brisk walk, at a pace which gets your heart going a bit faster than normal, causing you to break a sweat, is really ideal. Any other exercise which approximates this level of intensity is adequate for maintaining good health. Remember the Blue Zone people. Their only exercise is a good amount of moderate physical activity throughout the day as they walk where they need to go, herd their sheep, fish, work around the house, etc. This appears to be the most health-promoting exercise habit.

➢ **Exercise motivation:** If you have a hard time being motivated to be more active, **get yourself a pedometer**, or if you keep your smart phone or iPod Touch attached to your person all the time, download a pedometer app. Research found that people who started using a pedometer began walking an average of 2000 more steps per day – about a mile – than they had previously. **Shoot for 10,000 steps total per day**.

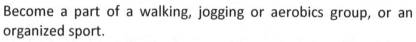

For most people, exercising socially helps them maintain motivation. Become a part of a walking, jogging or aerobics group, or an organized sport.

Another good motivator is to **keep learning about the benefits of an active lifestyle**, and the dangers of the alternative.

➢ **Weight training:** Don't just walk or jog. **Good bone health requires some weight training**. As your muscles pull on your bones, they are stimulated to stay strong by building mass. This reduces the chance of fractures, and provides a hedge against osteoporosis later in life. More on osteoporosis later.

Push ups, sit-ups, and lifting weights are all good. It is not necessary to lift heavy weights. Unless you are a young man and/or particularly strong already, you might want to start with 3 or 5 pound dumbbells and work your way up to perhaps 10 pounds or more as it is comfortable.

➤ **Impact of exercise vs. impact of diet on cholesterol:** Often exercise is prescribed for those with high cholesterol, since studies show it can help lower cholesterol, and thus, it is thought, prevent heart disease.

However, I did not find exercise to be helpful. My total cholesterol was around 300 while I was running regularly and eating probably less than an average amount of meat, fried food, and sweets. For a time I was on the cholesterol lowering drug fenofibrate,[225] which had lowered my cholesterol to 227. Whenever I got off that drug, my cholesterol level went back up to 300. But after only 3 months on a plant based diet, and no cholesterol lowering meds and exercising much less than previously, it was down to 223. After 18 months on the diet my total cholesterol was down to 182. That's a drop of almost 40%! **So for me, exercise didn't seem to have much effect on my cholesterol levels, while the effect of this diet was huge.**

Avoiding dietary cholesterol, i.e. animal products, as well as other foods which tend to cause inflammation such as oils, sugar, and other processed foods, allows the body to achieve healthy normal cholesterol levels. Even though some would say 182 is still somewhat high, I am confident that it is a normal level for my body, and it was achievable only while eating a healthy whole food plant based diet. I don't believe I have any risk of cardiovascular disease, because I only eat foods which promote a healthy endothelium, none which promote plaque and clogged arteries. No amount of exercise can give you that level of protection from chronic disease.

---

[225] Fenofibrate, though probably safer than statins, does have adverse side effects, and has never been shown to prevent heart disease or lower mortality. I did not know these things while I was taking it. More on this in **Chapter 15: Cholesterol.**

➢ **Impact of exercise vs. impact of diet on vascular health:** When I was young I wrongly assumed that regular intense workouts would help keep my arteries clear of disease causing plaque. It made sense to me. A rapidly moving stream doesn't get clogged up with silt. But our arteries are not streams, and arterial plaque is not silt. Jim Fixx's experience, as well as scientific studies, demonstrate that my theory was incorrect.

➢ **The case of Jim Fixx:** Jim Fixx is the famous author of "The Complete Book of Running," which contributed to the running craze of the 1970s and 80s. When I took running class for P.E. in college, each day the coach would read a snippet out of this book and discuss it before we hit the track.

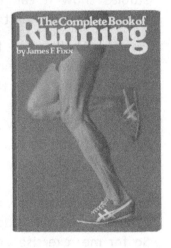

Fixx was in great shape in some respects due to his daily workouts, but he had an unhealthy diet. It is very likely that healthy eating could have compensated for his family history of heart disease (which killed his father at 43), and kept him going strong into old age.

In spite of warnings by some that he should eat better, he refused, believing he could enjoy a diet high in animal products processed foods, and still be healthy thanks to his regular workouts.[226]

But it was not to be. One day when he was 52 years old Mr. Fixx went out on his daily run. He never came back. His body was found by the side of the road. He had died of a heart attack. Autopsy revealed that three of his coronary arteries were clogged by from 70 to 95%.

Plant foods do not cause vascular blockages; in fact they actively prevent them. Animal   products   and   other

---

[226] John Robbins, <u>What Should We Learn From The Deaths Of Fitness Icons?</u>
<u>http://www.huffingtonpost.com/john-robbins/what-should-we-learn-from_b_815943.html</u>

inflammation-causing substances, such as sugar and oils, do cause plaque and blockages. **And no amount of exercise can compensate for this effect.**

Sitting and osteoporosis

People who spend a lot of time sitting have a higher risk of osteoporosis than do those who are more active. Any weight-bearing exercise and activities that promote balance and good posture are beneficial for your bones, but walking, running, jumping, dancing and weightlifting seem particularly helpful.

— Mayo Clinic

➤ **Exercise and osteoporosis:** There is a common misconception that the key to fighting osteoporosis is getting enough calcium. And if that doesn't work, there are drugs which supposedly help. But this approach is ill-informed and dangerous, because it tends to perpetuate and exacerbate the problem – and the drugs can have dangerous side effects.

To ensure healthy bones into old age, the best prescription is a whole food plant based diet, supplemented by a physically active lifestyle. The plants, plus sunshine (for vitamin D), provide all the nutrients you need for healthy bones. And the active lifestyle, which includes lifting some small weights, ensures your body is using those nutrients to optimize bone health. This is because when your muscles work, tugging on your bones, the bones are stimulated to build mass and stay strong.

Population studies in many cultures around the world confirm this, as does the known science. Osteoporosis is rare or unknown in many cultures where their diet is mainly plants, where they consume no dairy or calcium supplements, but where they are physically active, out in the sun, working in the fields, lifting loads, carrying babies, pounding rice, walking long distances, etc.

Calcium supplements and consuming dairy do not prevent osteoporosis! A few years ago, the USDA increased their recommended daily amount of milk consumption from two glasses to three, but the epidemic of osteoporosis just continues to get worse, while dairy sales continue to hum along. For more discussion about osteoporosis, see **Chapter 15: Nutrients and supplements: Calcium**.

Sleep

> *Then Jesus said,*
> *"Let's go off by*
> *ourselves to a*
> *quiet place and*
> *rest awhile."*
> *Mark 6:31*

Getting adequate quality and quantity of sleep is critical to good health.

➤ **Sleep debt:** Many of us, perhaps most, fail to get adequate sleep. We rack up sleep debt, and rarely if ever get caught up as we pile up successive nights of going to bed too late and/or getting up too early.

And it doesn't work to accumulate sleep debt during the week, expecting to "pay it back" on the weekend. Getting extra sleep on the weekend is better than getting too little sleep every night of the week, but for optimal health the sleeping routine, the times of rising and retiring, should be as consistent as possible.

➤ **Health risks of poor sleep:** Many diseases and other problems have been linked to not getting enough sleep – or too much – including obesity, high blood pressure, diabetes, negative mood and behavior, depression, and decreased productivity.

Dr. Mercola notes:

> There's compelling research indicating that sleeping less than six hours may increase your insulin resistance and risk of diabetes. And recent studies show that less than five hours of sleep at night can double your risk of being diagnosed with angina, coronary heart

disease, heart attack or stroke. Interestingly enough, the same appears to be true when you sleep more than nine hours per night.[227]

And Dr. Rubin Naiman adds:

The American Cancer Society did a study of a million American adults, and short sleepers showed a dramatic increase in risk of cancers across the board. So we know that there is a mountain of data showing if you don't sleep enough, you're going to get yourself sick...[228]

This is largely do to the effect lack of adequate sleep has in depressing the immune system.

People who don't get enough sleep end up performing poorly at school and work. And of course many fatal accidents are caused by drowsy driving. The Centers for Disease Control reports

(T)he National Highway Traffic Safety Administration estimates that 2.5% of fatal crashes and 2% of injury crashes involve drowsy driving. These estimates are probably conservative, though, and up to 5,000 or 6,000 fatal crashes each year may be caused by drowsy drivers.

Among nearly 150,000 adults aged at least 18 years or older in 19 states and the District of Columbia, 4.2% reported that they had fallen asleep while driving at least once in the previous 30 days. Individuals who snored or usually slept 6 or fewer hours per day were more likely to report this behavior.[229]

➢ **How much to sleep:** Here is what sleep expert Dr. Rubin Naiman has to say about this:

I think asking "how many of hours of sleep should I get?" is like asking, "Doctor, how many calories should I eat?" Of course the answer to that depends on who that person is. It's so individual. It also depends on the quality of those calories. Again, a lot of people are knocking themselves out night after night after night with sleeping pills. They may be getting seven to eight hours, but is it sleep? It looks like sleep. It might feel like sleep, but you know what, it's not really sleep. That's part of the question too—the

---

[227] *Ibid.*

[228] *Ibid.*

[229] Centers for Disease Control, <u>Drowsy Driving: Asleep at the Wheel</u> http://www.cdc.gov/Features/dsDrowsyDriving/index.html

quality of it."[230]

And Dr. Mercola comments:

> The general consensus seems to be that most people need somewhere between six and eight hours of sleep each night.[231]

➢ **Too much sleep:** Too much sleep can contribute to health problems, including depression, according to Dr. McDougall:

> Oversleeping leads to troubles as irritating as insomnia and as serious as suicidal depression. Studies have shown that there is a "depressogenic" substance that is produced during sleep... Even people without diagnosed depression improve their moods by not oversleeping.[232]

➢ **When to sleep:** Some sleep experts say it is important to get to bed early in the evening so that you can get as many hours of sleep as possible before midnight. Apparently this is because normally it is during the first part of your night's sleep that you sleep most deeply. It is at that time that your body gets the highest quality restorative rest.

➢ **Sleeping paralyzed:** While you sleep, your body is dealing with many of the stresses dealt it during the day, both physical and mental. There is a period of your sleep in which you are basically paralyzed. That is when the most rest and healing is taking place. And for children, that is when physical growth happens. **If you don't reach that level of sleep, your health will suffer**, according to Dr. Stasha Gominak, a neurologist and headache doctor.[233]

Dr. Gominak found that many of her patients' headache and other symptoms disappeared when they got their sleep

---

[230] Mercola, <u>Sleeping Less than 6 Hours Can Double Your Risk of Heart Attack</u> http://articles.mercola.com/sites/articles/archive/2012/04/09/dr-rubin-naiman-on-how-much-sleep-do-you-need.aspx

[231] *Ibid.*

[232] McDougall, <u>Sleep Like a Baby – Lessons from My Grandson on How to Cure Insomnia</u> https://www.drmcdougall.com/misc/2005nl/050100puinsomnia.htm

[233] Dr. Stasha Gominak, <u>Vitamin D, Sleep Apnea, Headache, Migraine, Depression</u> https://www.youtube.com/watch?v=GHCD3fONV1k&list=PL8725D4BAB54B0A71

problems resolved. And often one of the keys to that was getting them to adequate blood levels of vitamin D. If you are interested in this subject, please watch her referenced lecture.

➢ **Insomnia and sleeping pills:** I suffer from insomnia from time to time. In the past I have taken sleeping pills. Lunesta and Ambien work great for me! But I don't take them anymore. The possible side effects are just too dangerous to take the risk.

Now, if I can't sleep, I do what many sleep experts suggest: If you try to go to sleep for 20 minutes or so, but still feel wide awake, get up, go into another room, and read for a few minutes till you feel more drowsy. Don't turn on the T.V. or computer or other device! The bright light and brain stimulation of the screen will likely wake you up more. Just read your Bible or other book or a magazine. But the subject matter should be something calming.

➢ **Preparing for sleep:** Often problems with insomnia can be addressed by correctly preparing yourself for sleep. Allow me to share five important lifestyle factors which affect how quickly we get to sleep, and how well we sleep.

1. Our bodies' *wake sleep cycle* is largely regulated by the amount of light that enters the eyes. The norm is for the amount of light to be reduced in the hour or more before one goes to bed. This signals to your body that bedtime is coming. Thus if your body sees clearly that it is nighttime, when you actually go to bed, you fall asleep fairly quickly. Of course modern life with artificial lighting being everywhere 24/7 really messes up our bodies' normal rhythm, and for many, insomnia results. So it is a good practice to dim the lights in the hour or so leading up to bedtime.

    The light entering your eyes while you are sleeping can cause problems as well. Thus many sleep experts recommend being sure your bedroom is totally dark – use heavy drapes, no nightlight, no glowing clock, etc. If that is not possible, you might try wearing a blindfold while you sleep.

2. Your visual and mental stimulation during the time before

bed is another important factor. If immediately before bed you are surfing the net, or you watch a T.V. program or movie, especially one with a lot of action, tension and shocking images, or read a book of that type, your mind is not prepared for sleep, and insomnia may result.

3. Strenuous exercise in the late afternoon or evening can keep your body from allowing you to get to sleep. Try to exercise earlier in the day.

4. Eating less than 2½ hours before bed can also be a problem.[234] If you are digesting food, your body's energy is focused on that process, and it may have a harder time allowing you to fall asleep. It is best to finish your evening meal no later than 7pm whenever possible. And avoid snacking after dinner is over, unless you find it does not hinder your sleep.

5. Maintaining good relationships with God and others around you, and successfully managing other potential stressors in your life, will help you to fall asleep more quickly and sleep more soundly.

Some can sleep well even if they ignore the above suggestions. But for the rest of us who do struggle with insomnia, if you establish this kind of routine, soon your body will become accustomed to it, and it will know when it is time to sleep. It may or may not work for you. But it is worth a try.

If getting into the habit of properly preparing for sleep helps you get to sleep sooner and sleep better, it can have a profound effect on your overall health, your mood, your performance at work, your studies, and it can make you a safer driver.

Stress and right relationships

We saw in **Chapter 2** how the low-stress environment of Eden was transformed into a very high stress situation when

---

[234] Note also that going to bed less than 2½ hours after eating a meal tends to cause weight gain.

relationships were destroyed. Stress and relationships are very closely related.

So the principle of stress which we get from The Eden Axiom is that for optimal health, the stress in one's life should be minimal. And such a condition requires harmonious relationships with one another and with God. And of course we find that the research on this subject, as well as practical experience, supports this principle.[235]

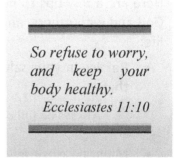

So refuse to worry, and keep your body healthy.
Ecclesiastes 11:10

Some stress, however, is appropriate in our lives; it is proper and healthy. For example, the stress you feel when driving in traffic can increase your alertness and keep you driving safely. The stress you experience thinking about how certain poor lifestyle choices can harm a person's health will drive you to embrace healthy habits. The stress which comes about when you offend a loved one eats at you till you make things right and are reconciled. The stress you feel when you sin drives you to repent and confess to God, who is always faithful and just to forgive. This is good stress. It is temporary. It gets you through a situation, and then is relieved, and you have peace.

But most of us have too much chronic stress. We neglect to do the things we should do when we should do them. We worry about health problems or money or the direction our country is heading. We go through long periods living in tension with those around us and with God.

When stress is not dealt with properly, not resolved, and turns to worry and anxiety, things are getting out of hand. Chronic stress will hinder your body's ability to fight off disease and stay healthy. Having a lot of chronic stress in your life will undo many

---

[235] *WebMD,* Stress Management - Effects of Stress
http://www.webmd.com/balance/stress-management/stress-management-effects-of-stress

of the other positive lifestyle measures you are taking to achieve good health and long life.

Here are a few tips to help you improve your relationships with God and with others, and decrease the amount of stress in your life:

- Rejoice in your salvation. Nothing else matters as much as that.

Always be full of joy in the Lord. I say it again—rejoice!
Philippians 4:4

- Maintain close fellowship with God. Be honest about your sin, confess it to Him, and take joy in His forgiveness. It's real, and it's forever!

If we claim we have no sin, we are only fooling ourselves and not living in the truth. But if we confess our sins to him, he is faithful and just to forgive us our sins and to cleanse us from all wickedness.
1 John 1:8-9

- Maintain harmonious relationships with those around you.

So now I am giving you a new commandment: Love each other. Just as I have loved you, you should love each other.
John 13:34

- Forgive others. "Unforgiveness is the poison you eat hoping the other person will die." It is poison. It will kill you, physically **and** spiritually.

Make allowance for each other's faults, and forgive anyone who offends you. Remember, the Lord forgave you, so you must forgive others.
Colossians 3:13

- Take life seriously, but remember Who is in charge. Rest in Him, His sovereignty, His love, His grace.

Let my soul be at rest again, for the LORD has been good to me.
Psalm 116:7

- Don't take yourself too seriously. Learn to laugh at yourself. Take time to laugh every day. Be happy.

A cheerful heart is good medicine, but a broken spirit saps a person's strength.
Proverbs 17:22

- Keep things in perspective. Someone cut you off on the highway, or your team or candidate lost. So what? How important is that, really, in light of the wonderful things God is doing in your life today, and in light of eternity?

No eye has seen, no ear has heard, and no mind has imagined what God has prepared for those who love him.
1 Corinthians 2:9

- When tempted to feel stressed about some injustice, rest in knowing that God will make all things right. That's not your job.

Don't say, "I will get even for this wrong." Wait for the Lord to handle the matter.   Proverbs 20:22

- Don't act like an unbeliever by worrying about how you will be provided for. God knows your needs and will provide for you.

"So don't worry about these things, saying, 'What will we eat? What will we drink? What will we wear?' These things dominate the thoughts of unbelievers, but your heavenly Father already knows all your needs."
Matthew 6:31-32

- Are you God's child? God is a loving Father who takes care of His children. He will always provide good things for us, exactly the things we really need.

Even strong young lions sometimes go hungry, but those who trust in the LORD will lack no good thing.
Psalm 34:10

- Rest in God's will for you. His will is that you be thankful for even the hard things life throws at you. If you are joyful and prayerful, you can be thankful.

[16]Always be joyful. [17]Never stop praying. [18]Be thankful in all circumstances, for this is God's will for you who belong to Christ Jesus.   1 Thessalonians 5:16-18

- Know that whatever is stressing you right now, God is working through it to accomplish the greatest good for you and others around you. Rest in His sovereignty in your life.

And we know that God causes everything to work together for the good of those who love God and are called according to his purpose for them.   Romans 8:28

- The antidote to worry is prayer. Pray and have peace.

Don't worry about anything; instead, pray about everything. Tell God what you need, and thank him for all he has done. Then you will experience God's peace, which exceeds anything we can understand. His peace will guard your hearts and minds as you live in Christ Jesus.   Philippians 4:6-7

- Make the decision to reduce stress from your life by paying attention to and acting on the above.

So refuse to worry, and keep your body healthy.
                                                      Ecclesiastes 11:10

A formula for health

Here is a suggested formula to calculate your "health sum":

Discerning Diet + Excellent Exercise + Sufficient Sleep

+ Slight Stress + Right Relationships = Highest Health

All of these elements are important. Don't depend on exercise alone, or any other single factor or combination of four or fewer factors to keep you healthy.

At the end of the book we will revisit this formula and discuss it a little more.

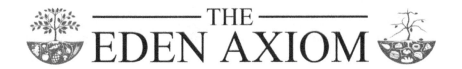

THE EDEN AXIOM

Part 3: The Response

Chapter 10:

"Brothers, What Shall We Do?"

After the Apostle Peter's convincing and convicting sermon recorded in Acts 2, the Bible says that the Jews who were listening were "cut to the heart." The powerful message they had heard so convinced them that they had a need, that they asked Peter and the other apostles, "Brothers, what shall we do?"

It is my hope that having read this far you too are convinced by the message I have presented. Perhaps by now you have settled on a course of action. Or maybe you could use a concise summary, with some specifics on how you might respond.

We have learned that the right fuel for the body, that which will promote good health, is whole plant foods. And we have seen overwhelming evidence that partial foods, that is food extracts, as well as animal products and the toxins they contain, promote chronic diseases. We have explored briefly other topics which play a major role in good health, including exercise, sleep, stress, and relationships.

So you may be saying, "Okay, I got it. But help me here. In a nutshell, what exactly should I do in response to what I have learned?" Here are some important steps you might consider taking:

- Things to reduce in your diet:
  - o Meat, poultry, fish, eggs, dairy, and all other animal products
  - o Packaged, processed, or "enriched" foods – most foods with an ingredients label
  - o Sugar, including products with any form of sugar added (corn syrup, high fructose corn syrup, cane juice, etc.)
  - o Products containing white flour (bread, bagels, pancakes, doughnuts, tortillas, etc.)
  - o Foods with added oils (salad dressings, fried foods, chips, etc.)
  - o Foods with added artificial sweeteners, colors, nitrites, MSG, sodium benzoate or other chemicals
  - o Deep fried, char broiled, microwaved, or other foods cooked at very high temperatures (see **Chapter 15: Cooking**)
  - o Sodas, fruit juice, energy drinks, and other such beverages, regardless of how they are sweetened
  - o Coffee or tea if you must have cream and/or sugar added to it

Though some of the above foods contain some helpful nutrients. All of them have been found to cause disease, especially when eaten in excess. In other words, the harmful effects outweigh the positive, health promoting effects, so that they are net disease causers. Any amount you can reduce these items will be helpful. **You and your family will get the maximum benefit if you reduce them to zero**, or at least to near zero.

- Things to include in your diet:
  - o Whole plant foods: leafy and cruciferous veggies; other veggies including potatoes, sweet potatoes, carrots, squash, etc.; brown rice, oats and other whole grains; fruits, berries, beans, nuts and seeds
  - o Purified, filtered water, to total ½ oz. for each pound of body weight per day

- o (Optional) White tea, green tea, hibiscus or other herbal tea (but without sweetener or milk added)

- Get lots of midday sunshine to ensure adequate vitamin D. If you can't get much sunshine, consider taking a D3 supplement. If you avoid all meat and dairy, take a B12 supplement. See **Chapter 15: Nutrients and supplements** for more details on these topics.

- Be physically active throughout the day. If necessary, spend 30 to 60 minutes getting moderate exercise six days a week, or as much as you can get up to that amount. Find ways to spend less time sitting.

- Get about seven to eight hours of sleep per night, starting as early as possible. A few people may require as little as six hours per night.

- Be intentional about reducing stress, strengthening good relationships with family, friends and coworkers, keeping the right perspective regarding life's problems.

- Maintain a strong sense of purpose in your life, so that each day you look forward to accomplishing important things, things you are good at doing, which are in according with the gifts God has given you.

Baby steps

It may seem like it will be very hard to adopt such a lifestyle. I want to encourage you to try it. Try making baby steps. For example, try buying a non-dairy milk (e.g. soy or almond milk[236]) next time you go shopping, and drinking that instead of cow's milk. Try reducing the sugar in your coffee from two teaspoons

---

[236] Or better, make your own! Put ½ cup raw almonds in a blender along with 1 cup water. Blend on high for a few seconds. Add 2 more cups water and blend for a second or so. You may wish to add 1-3 dates and/or a bit of vanilla to enhance the flavor – and make it more likely your kids will like it. There will be small bits of nuts and dates in the milk. You can strain these out if you like and save to add to another recipe, or leave them in and just be sure to shake well before using.

to one. Then later to ½. Later to zero. Or better, kick the coffee habit. When you eat out, order meals with less meat in them. Ask to see the vegetarian menu. (Even if they don't have one, it is good to ask, as it will prompt the restaurant management to consider developing one.) When you shop, buy less meat, or no meat, and instead buy extra fruits, veggies, beans and nuts. Then when you make chili, use a vegan chili recipe instead of the one with ground meat in it. When you make soup or stew, use a veggie broth as the base and fill it full of beans and veggies instead of meat. When you want burgers, try a baked black bean burger recipe and use 100% whole grain bread for buns. There is no end to the great whole plant food alternative possibilities.

Work on the other areas little by little as well. Do it as a family and keep each other accountable, encouraging each other toward success. Remember why you are doing this!

Even if you only make very small changes, it still can have significant benefits. For example, if you bump up your veggie intake by adding one serving of dark green leafys per day, such as ½ cup of broccoli, you can cut your risk of heart disease, stroke, cancer, and other diseases significantly.[237]

As you move toward a whole food plant based diet, I would encourage you to make a good effort to ensure the transition goes smoothly. Please don't do it half-heartedly and then give up discouraged, because "it didn't work for me." Be radical now so you don't have to suffer the radical consequences later.

If you like a lot of variety in your meals, and taste and presentation is especially important to you, please look up plant based recipes on the Internet and/or get some good whole food cookbooks (see **Chapter 14: The palatability angle** for some suggestions). Also, there are many websites and videos online which are dedicated to helping people make the transition. For example, Dr. Greger has a good video in which he goes over many of the basic concepts you should know, and demonstrates

---

[237] Greger, <u>Stop Cancer Before It Starts</u> (minute 34:40)
https://www.youtube.com/watch?v=dYxpgwFip2M

some meal prep ideas (if you can endure his corny jokes).[238]

Feeling better – or not

For many people, once they get started on a whole food plant based diet, the thing t hat keeps them sticking with it is how great they feel. Weight comes off, they sleep better, aches and pains disappear. And if they were suffering from some chronic condition such as obesity, diabetes or cardiovascular disease, the improvement is often quite dramatic.

Some decide that they want to test the diet by making a total transition to whole plant foods all at once for three or four weeks or so, to see if it makes a difference in how they feel. After such a trial run, many feel so much better that they are firmly convinced that they made the right change, and they stick with it.

Some people experience a measure of discomfort during this transition, however, as their gut bacteria changes (see **Chapter 15: A few more facts and tips: Gut bacteria, good and bad**) and the rest of their body adjusts to the new normal. Such discomfort may not manifest for several months.

Dr. Michael Klaper describes the physiology of what seems to be happening in such cases.[239] Simply put, when the human body lives on a diet consisting mostly of meat and dairy for 30, 40, 50 years or longer, it finds strategies to adjust to this unnatural food and get the most nutrition out of what is being made available to it. A dramatic change to whole food plant based presents the body with a situation it is no longer prepared to deal with, even though originally it was created for this food.

Dr. Campbell puts it this way:

> According to some scientists our "chemosensory sensitivity" toward any particular food may vary depending on what we're used to

---

[238] Greger, <u>Maximum Nutrition: Transitioning Towards a Plant Based Diet</u>
<u>https://www.youtube.com/watch?v=Y9nNa81dSoY</u>
[239] Klaper, <u>Are Failed Vegans Addicts?</u>
<u>https://www.youtube.com/watch?v=0tJyb1wTxg4</u>

eating. In other words we are "programmed" by what we have eaten, and it may take a while to "reprogram" our bodies to some new tastes and our new diet.[240]

Look at what we have: We have the regular ingestion of a substance (meat), that when it's no longer ingested, the person experiences physical withdrawal symptoms. Is that not the definition of addiction?
— Dr. Michael Klaper

Thus a former SAD devotee eating exclusively plant foods may have low energy and may just not feel as well as they did when eating animal products. These are simply the withdrawal symptoms of an addict.

The solution, of course, is not to give up and continue consuming the "drug" as you have been. The solution is to stick with the plants, knowing the body will eventually adjust.

However, for some it may be necessary to continue to eat (or go back to eating) some animal products, but gradually phase them out of the diet over the course of several weeks or months. This will give the body time to make the adjustment and hopefully minimize the discomfort of the transition.

During the transition, oils, sugars, white flour and other partial (processed) foods should be phased out as quickly as possible as well, of course.

I have already shared about the improvement this diet made to my prostate health and my cholesterol numbers. My mother has adopted this diet and she says she has noticed a marked improvement in her overall health and how good she feels, including much less arthritis pain, and much more energy to be active each day. She is happy knowing she is giving her heart the

---

[240] Campbell, The China Project (booklet, p26), Paracelsian, Inc., Ithica, New York

best chance possible to keep going for many years. My wife has struggled with being heavier than she wanted to be for most of her life. Now, on a mostly whole plant diet, she eats as much as she wants, and is at a healthy, ideal size, "without even trying to lose weight," she says. And you have read the testimony of my brother-in-law in the forward to this book. None of us has suffered any of the ill effects of "withdrawal" which Dr. Klapper speaks of.

One of the greatest benefits of understanding the principles in this book, and of then responding by adopting a whole food plant based diet, as well as other positive lifestyle changes, is knowing you aren't a victim of your genes. You no longer have to wait in fear that chronic disease will strike and you can't do anything about it. Instead you have the confident assurance that you are doing something which really will make a positive difference in your health and longevity. And you know you are improving your stewardship of your body as you live a lifestyle more in line with God's original plan. **This new physical and spiritual outlook is truly significant and life-changing.**

How we manage a whole food plant based diet

Our kitchen is full of a variety of fresh fruits and veggies. We almost never buy meat or dairy products, and we purchase very few processed food items. When we shop we spend almost all of our time in the produce, frozen produce, and rice and beans sections of the market, and normally all we have in the house are plant foods.

Occasionally some social situation may demand that we prepare some food requiring butter and/or eggs. So we may have these on hand. But we prefer to look for a whole plant food alternative recipe we can try to meet the need.

We enjoy a variety of vegetable and bean soups, salads, baked veggies, fresh fruits, etc. For breakfast I eat a chunky smoothie each morning which contains a large variety of raw fruits, veggies, and seeds. I also have a bowl of oatmeal with berries and almond milk. Having a large, nutritious breakfast is a great way to start the day.

When we plan to have someone for a meal, we often look for a new whole plant food recipe to try. We recently served a delicious tomato sauce and eggplant casserole dish which was a big hit, even among the children who were visiting (who had seconds!). We usually serve a veggie salad and a fruit salad as well. And we keep some Italian salad dressing on hand for guests who want it.

We are not 100% meat free all the time. When someone has us for a meal, we eat what is served and don't worry about it – we're not paranoid about eating meat, of course, we just prefer not to if we have the choice (we still enjoy the taste!). If our hosts ask us ahead of time if we have any food issues, we briefly explain our diet, but we don't insist they adapt to what we prefer. Most who do ask us are happy to oblige, and some tell us they like the challenge of making a meat-free meal.

I realize that many may think eating this way would be impossible. But we and many others have proven that it is doable. If you are creative and determined, I'm sure you can succeed!

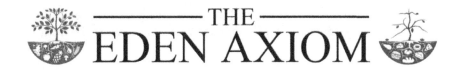

Chapter 11:

Diets: The Good, The Bad,

and the Dangerous

The term "diet" means different things to different people. For many it has negative connotations, reminding them of bad experiences as they have tried unsuccessfully to gain victory over weight issues. Often it refers to a temporary way of eating to accomplish a weight goal, as in "I'm on a diet."

In most places in this book where that word is used, that is not the meaning intended. A dictionary defines the word in this way:

> The usual food and drink consumed; a prescribed selection of foods.

This is usually what I mean by diet. It is not a temporary measure taken to lose weight. It is a sustained way of life, lived in the interests of good health.

In the context of the SAD, unnatural and dangerous disease promoting weight gain is inevitable for most people, as indicated by the fact that 2/3 of Americans are either overweight or obese.

Being fat is considered unattractive in our culture, and weight-loss hucksters take advantage of this, bilking vulnerable consumers out of billions of dollars for weight-loss diets, drugs and medical procedures which rarely really work in the long term, and can even be dangerous. Here are some interesting facts about this topic:

- $20 Billion – The annual revenue of the U.S. weight-loss industry, including diet books, diet drugs and weight-loss surgeries.

- 108 Million – The number of people on diets in the United States. Dieters typically make four to five attempts per year.

- 85 Percent – The percentage of customers consuming weight-loss products and services who are female.[241]

Perhaps the worst thing about all this is that the effort is focused on losing pounds and inches, not on good health. Yet many thin people die of chronic diseases. Losing weight while ignoring other important health issues is foolish.

I hope I have made it clear in this book that achieving good health, not reducing pounds or inches, should be the focus of our dietary choices. If weight loss is needed, we can expect that, barring some pre-existing medical complication, an ideal weight will gradually be achieved as we feed our bodies the fuel they were designed to run on, and work to improve other lifestyle areas such as stress and physical activity.

Note that, as mentioned earlier, if you are eating a whole food plant based diet, and you need to lose some weight for optimum health (see the section on **Obesity** in **Chapter 15**), it is best to avoid plant foods with high oil content, which means nuts and avocados. When you achieve your ideal weight, then you may wish to try adding some of these foods to your diet and see how your body reacts.

If you have read the whole book up to this point, you have all the info you need to make healthy food choices. But if you prefer to have more specific guidance, there is a lot more help available. Some will require the purchase of a book. But tons of specific information is available for free on the Internet as well.

---

[241] *ABC News* May 8, 2012, <u>100 Million Dieters, $20 Billion: The Weight-Loss Industry by the Numbers</u> http://abcnews.go.com/Health/100-million-dieters-20-billion-weight-loss-industry/story?id=16297197

Diets to consider

➤ Dr. Esselstyn's "heart attack proof" diet

I have mentioned previously Dr. Caldwell Esselstyn of the Cleveland Clinic. He has done significant work in the area of lifestyle medicine. He has developed what he claims is a "heart attack proof diet." It is heavy on leafy veggies like kale, collards, and chard. These and other veggies promote healthy artery linings (endothelium) and thus protect against heart disease. His diet, designed to save the lives of cardiac patients with severe disease, also includes all the other whole plant food items I have been promoting in this book, except oily ones like avocados and nuts. And he is very strict about avoiding foods which damage the endothelium, such as meat, dairy, sugar and oils.

Many of Dr. Esselstyn's patients had been told by their cardiologists, after many drugs, surgeries, stents, etc., that there was nothing else medical science could do for them. Some were told they only had months to live. But Dr. Esselstyn has found that nearly every one of those that followed his diet has seen their health improve, many making a dramatic recovery, including verifiable reversal of their disease. Others, who started on the diet but later reverted to the SAD ended up with more heart disease and suffering.

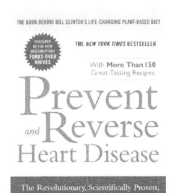

THE BOOK BEHIND BILL CLINTON'S LIFE-CHANGING PLANT-BASED DIET

THE *NEW YORK TIMES* BESTSELLER

With More Than 150 Great-Tasting Recipes

Prevent
and Reverse
Heart Disease

The Revolutionary, Scientifically Proven, Nutrition-Based *Cure*

Caldwell B. Esselstyn, Jr., M.D.
Foreword by T. Colin Campbell, Ph.D., author of *The China Study*

Look up Dr. Esselstyn on the Internet if you want to learn more (see **Appendix**). And remember, his diet is not only good for your heart, it will also help you avoid and heal from many other chronic diseases associated with diet, and has no negative side effects.

➤ Dr. McDougall's starch based diet

Dr. McDougall believes that starch, that is, carbohydrates from whole plant foods, is the backbone of a healthy diet. As evidence he cites the many civilizations throughout the ages which have lived and thrived on diets based on rice, corn, wheat, quinoa, potatoes, sweet potatoes, or other sources of starch. So he advocates getting most of your calories from these foods, and rounding out the diet with other veggies and fruits.

Dr. McDougall says it is okay to sprinkle a little sugar on food if it helps one stick with the diet, and not revert to eating animal products and oils. High quantities of sugar are indeed bad (sodas, cakes, candy, etc.), but a little used for flavor is not a problem, he says.

Dr. McDougall has proven his starch theory to be true as he has helped thousands of his patients recover from terrible chronic diseases and lose weight by being on his diet. He and his wife Mary have made a great contribution to the palatability of a plant based diet, developing and collecting hundreds of recipes, which they have published in books and online.

Dr. McDougall's website has years of searchable newsletters and articles which provide a treasure of helpful information, including referenced scientific studies and practical advice.

➢ Dr. Dean Ornish's dietary spectrum

Dr. Ornish's groundbreaking clinical research done in the 1980s yielded the first reliable scientific data proving that a whole food

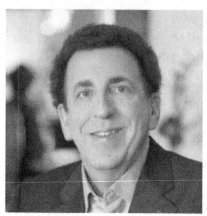

plant based diet could actually stop and reverse arterial plaque buildup and thus heart disease. He has shown that his diet is far superior to the American Heart Association diet for the prevention of heart disease.[242]

In Dr. Ornish's dietary "spect-rum" he categorizes foods into five groups, from most healthy

---

[242] Dr. Dean Ornish, M.D., *Preventive Medicine Research Institute,* Research Highlights http://www.pmri.org/research.html#heart-study

to least healthy. You can choose foods from any of the categories, but the ranking gives you a good idea of where you want your diet to be headed.

➤ The Physicians Committee for Responsible Medicine

This group, headed up by Dr. Neal Barnard, has a very good and simple-to-follow diet, summarized in their Power Plate graphic. If you eat approximately one quarter of your total food intake from each of these four whole plant food groups, you will get all the nutrition you need for optimal health.

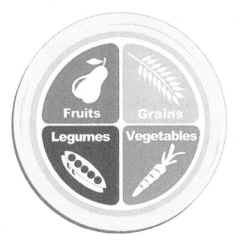

You can find out more about all of these diets by going to the links in the **Appendix**.

➤ Rev. George Malkmus' Hallelujah Diet

Rev. Malkmus was a successful pastor for many years. He claims to have been healed from a baseball-sized tumor in his colon by going on an all raw plant food diet. A key component of his healing diet was drinking a substantial amount of carrot juice. He also claims his vision improved substantially on this diet to the point where he no longer required glasses. That was nearly 40 years ago, and now at 81 he says he still has excellent vision.

Subsequently Rev. Malkmus did more research into diet and health and established a business/ministry called Hallelujah Acres (HA), which promotes the Hallelujah Diet (HD). This is a Christian-based outfit, and Rev. Malkmus uses Scripture liberally in his seminars. The diet prescribed by God in Eden is a key concept.

HA claims that thousands have been healed from serious chronic diseases by following their plan. Many of these, they say, were given no hope of healing by their doctors. Detractors from a more conventional medicine point of view, however, say these claims are unproven, and the diet is unbalanced and not healthful.

Rev. Malkmus contends that produce grown in our depleted soils has much fewer nutrients than the produce of Eden must have had. Therefore juicing vegetables, which concentrates the nutrients, is necessary and therapeutic, and able to heal in a powerful way.

HA sells certain supplements, cleanses, and juicing machines and other kitchen tools appropriate to the diet. Since they sell many of the same products they promote for good health, doubts arise as to their ability to remain objective and accurate. Many of their products are quite expensive, available cheaper elsewhere.

The diet consists of the barley greens, plus fruit, salads, and carrot juice, to total 85% of the food consumed. The remaining 15% may be cooked whole plant foods and grains. Some oils are allowed, but no salt, sugar, or white flour.

There are some features of the HD which are not normally necessary for good health, such as supplements and juicing. For most people all the ingredients they need to be on a healthy diet are available at the local supermarket. However, if even some of the many anecdotal claims to healing as a result of the HD are true, for some chronic diseases certain high quality supplements and especially juicing will likely be helpful.

And I do believe that many of the claims are true, as I have a personal friend whom I trust who used to be associated with HA, and he vouches for their legitimacy. Furthermore, partly as a result of learning of this diet I tried drinking carrot juice daily, and my vision improved substantially in just a few weeks. I have no other explanation except that the carotenoids in the juice have been doing their work.

It is good to note that if one learns and puts into practice the principles of this diet it is probably possible to get the same benefit without buying stuff from HA.

The HA website[243] has lots of helpful information. They really want to help people, but keep in mind the possible influence of their profit motive. Many videos are available on Youtube of Rev. Malkmus explaining his diet, as well as of their staff showing how to prepare various raw whole food meals.

Nutrient dense or calorie dense

As stated earlier, a person who is overweight or obese who wants to lose weight should not focus on their weight, but on their health, and eating foods which promote good health. As they do that, the weight issue will most likely take care of itself.

As I have read about the experiences of those who do focus on health, rather than weight, it has become clear to me that many are able to eat all they want, filling up every meal on whole plant foods, and still lose weight. A whole food plant based diet can thus be called **the "all you want to eat" diet**.

The exciting thing about this is that there is no more need to try and determine which slick diet ad is the best one to believe, to weigh out foods, to count calories, to strive for the recommended balance of good fats and bad fats and carbs and sugars, to buy expensive supplements, yada yada yada. Simplicity!

The all you want to eat diet is much simpler. One must simply be sure that whatever one eats are things "on the menu," that is, whole plant foods (except high-oil foods such as avocados and nuts). If one eats "off the menu" items, the "all you want to eat" approach will not likely result in losing weight.

This is because animal products, oils, foods with added sugars, refined flour, and other processed foods are dense with the calorie-laden macronutrients protein and fat. Calorie for calorie they have relatively few micronutrients such as vitamins, minerals and antioxidants, and no phytonutrients. Such foods tend to take up less room per calorie in your stomach. You eat at

---

[243] www.hacres.com

a relatively fast calorie-per-minute pace, and you get a full meal's worth of calories long before your stomach is full. Thus you will tend to eat too many calories before your stomach finally signals to your brain that it is time to stop eating.

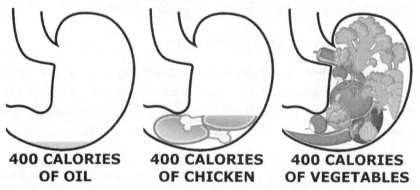

400 CALORIES OF OIL   **400 CALORIES OF CHICKEN**   **400 CALORIES OF VEGETABLES**

[Note: It is important to chew your food better than the above diagram might indicate!]

However, if your meal consists of less calorie-dense, more micronutrient-dense foods which tend to easily satisfy hunger, including starches like potatoes, sweet potatoes, squash, rice and oats, as well as other veggies, then you are eating at a much slower calorie-per-minute pace. Your stomach gets full before you have eaten too many calories. Your stomach then sends the signal to your brain that your are full, and you stop eating. Since you are full before you have consumed too many calories, you won't put on weight, and can even lose weight. You will also avoid the innumerable diseases associated with a eating those calorie dense foods.[244]

It should be kept in mind, however, that for weight loss, the kind of foods and the number of calories you eat are not the only factors which determine the potential for success. Emotional stress is a major factor for many people. A person may feel stressed about the whole area of "dieting" and weight loss. That stress can prevent weight loss from happening, even if very healthy foods, and very few calories, are eaten.

---

[244] McDougall, Successful Weight Loss Tips
http://www.nealhendrickson.com/mcdougall/021100puweight.htm

One explanation of this phenomenon is that stress is interpreted subconsciously by your body as indicating the food supply is limited. Your body responds by storing the energy you consume as a hedge against famine. Instead of burning the calories, they are socked away, stored as fat in your cells.

Emotional stress due to bad relationships with other people and with God can also play a role in keeping the weight on. Make sure your relationships with those around you are healthy. Stay close to God. Learn from His Word, the Bible. You need other mature believers to encourage you and build you up. Be the church with them as you learn together to walk in His grace and love. Relax in Him!

> *A person may feel stressed about the whole area of "dieting" and weight loss. That stress can prevent weight loss from happening.*

Your spiritual and relational vitality is a key to weight loss and good health. This allows a life free of unhealthy emotional stress, which liberates your body to respond well to the lifestyle changes you are making.

Don't focus on your weight or be stressed about losing weight. Focus on being a good steward of God's gifts, with the Holy Spirit's enablement. Be encouraged that you have the tools to improve your health by following Biblical principles. Make positive changes in your lifestyle. Expect healthy changes to happen. God willing, they will!

Diets to avoid

As mentioned earlier, having read and understood the material in this book so far, you have all the tools you need to evaluate which diets are helpful and which ones are to be avoided. Any diet which contradicts these principles may provide some limited benefit, but it is not going to be helpful in the long run, because it will contain elements which promote disease.

➢ **Low carb diets:** Low carb, high protein and fat (i.e. high meat and dairy product) diets have been promoted by various people since 1864. Most prominent among these are Atkins, South Beach, and Zone. These diets promise weight loss and improved blood lab numbers including cholesterol. Their authors claim high-carbohydrate foods promote unhealthy inflammation, and thus chronic disease. This is true if the carbohydrates come from refined sources, such as sugar and white flour. But high carb whole plant foods do not promote unhealthy inflammation.[245]

The Atkins foundation has funded a number of studies which purportedly prove their diet works not only for weight loss, but also for improving cholesterol, triglyceride and other lab numbers.

Independent studies, however, have found a different result, namely that when study subjects followed Atkins-type diets their LDL cholesterol levels rose and HDL fell. They suffered a number of other ill effects from the diet as well, including increased headaches, constipation, bad breath, and mortality.[246,247] A study of Swedish women reported the following conclusion:

> A diet characterized by low carbohydrate and high protein intake was associated with increased total and particularly cardiovascular mortality amongst women. Vigilance with respect to long-term adherence to such weight control regimes is advisable.[248]

A study was done measuring the effect of diet on blood flow

---

[245] McDougall, The Smoke and Mirrors behind *Wheat Belly* and *Grain Brain* https://www.drmcdougall.com/misc/2014nl/jan/smoke.htm

[246] McDougall, *McDougall Newsletter* November 2002, Atkins Diet Is As Good as Chemotherapy for Weight Loss http://www.nealhendrickson.com/mcdougall/021100puatkins.htm

[247] McDougall, *Newsletter September 2003*, Proof that the Atkins Diet Works Like Chemotherapy By Sickness-Induced Starvation https://www.drmcdougall.com/misc/2003nl/sep/030900puproofpositive.htm

[248] P. Lagiou, et al, *Journal of Internal Medicine*, Low carbohydrate–high protein diet and mortality in a cohort of Swedish women http://onlinelibrary.wiley.com/doi/10.1111/j.1365-2796.2007.01774.x/abstract;jsessionid=E66BD9DDC2E189C524A52273C70EC4CD.f04t02

through the heart. Study subjects who ate a vegetarian diet for one year had significantly greater blood flow. The blood flow was significantly reduced, however, in the group on low carb diets.[249]

Meanwhile, there are no studies to my knowledge which show any ill effects of a whole food plant based diet.

It is true that many people do lose weight on low carb diets, and some of their lab numbers may in fact improve somewhat. However these benefits appear to be short lived. It is fairly unusual, I understand, for anyone on a low carb diet to keep the weight off for more than a year.

> Over the long term, ... studies show that low-carb diets like Atkins are no more effective for weight loss than are standard weight-loss diets and that most people regain the weight they lost regardless of diet plan.[250]

Even Dr. Robert Atkins was not successful with his own diet; apparently he was overweight much of his life, and died in that state, with cardiovascular disease (though not directly because of it).[251]

Long term studies of the health outcomes of people on specific low carb diets have not been conducted. But other studies show

---

[249] Greger, Low Carb Diets and Coronary Blood Flow
http://nutritionfacts.org/video/low-carb-diets-and-coronary-blood-flow/
[250] Mayo Clinic Staff, Weight Loss: Results http://www.mayoclinic.org/healthy-living/weight-loss/in-depth/atkins-diet/art-20048485?pg=2
[251] Dr. Atkins had a heart condition for many years, but his physician claimed it was not a result of his diet. Dr. Atkins died in 2003 following a fall on the ice in which he sustained a head injury. There is some controversy surrounding his medical report which was released to the public. It shows that he was grossly overweight (258 lbs., 6 ft. tall; but his defenders claim that he gained 60 lbs. of water weight while in the hospital), had congestive heart failure, myocardial infarction (destruction of heart tissue resulting from obstruction of the blood supply to the heart muscle), and hypertension. Note that the company he left behind was worth over ½ billion dollars (they sell lots of books as well as Atkins approved products), so they stood to lose a lot of money due to negative publicity, and have done their best to defend their fallen founder and his diet.

a clear relationship between increased meat consumption coupled with reduced whole food carb consumption, and an increase in chronic disease and overall mortality.[252,253]

Some low carb diets such as Atkins stress the importance of taking nutritional supplements. Regarding supplements, Dr. Atkins wrote, "Don't even think of getting along without them!" Of course this is rather self-serving, since his foundation sells the supplements they insist are essential. But it is also evidence that they recognize their low carb diet is by nature deficient nutritionally. So how can it be the natural diet for humans to eat? A high carb whole food plant based diet contains all the nutrients a person needs, with the possible exception of B12 (due to the relatively sterile nature of the food we eat; see **Chapter 15: Nutrients and supplements**).

➢ **Paleo diets:** Paleo diets are similar to low carb diets, emphasizing meat consumption. Those who promote them claim their diet consists of the foods our supposed evolutionary ancestors ate, and thus they believe they are the foods our bodies evolved to live on. Paleo people believe grains and beans became part of the human diet relatively late in our history, and thus their consumption is not natural or normal for our physiology – and therefore must be unhealthy.

For those of us who believe the Bible's account of origins, we can easily see a major foundational flaw with this sort of approach. There are many historical and scientifically-based objections to the paleo diet philosophy as well, and the possibility that it can have any validity has been soundly

---

[252] Gary E. Fraser, *The American Journal of Clinical Nutrition,* Associations between diet and cancer, ischemic heart disease, and all-cause mortality in non-Hispanic white California Seventh-day Adventists
http://img2.tapuz.co.il/forums/1_161513157.pdf
[253] McDougall, The Smoke and Mirrors behind *Wheat Belly* and *Grain Brain*
https://www.drmcdougall.com/misc/2014nl/jan/smoke.htm

refuted.[254,255]

One of the major premises of the low carb/paleo argument is that high carb foods such as potatoes have high glycemic indexes, causing blood sugar spikes. This causes blood insulin levels to rise. Thus avoiding such foods, and instead eating lots of meat, will result in lower insulin levels and consequently better health. **Yet it has been demonstrated that meat consumption also raises insulin levels, and to a greater degree than carbs!**

Furthermore, those on diets emphasizing plant foods have been shown to have lower blood insulin levels than those who eat lots of meat. So if the promoters of such diets are indeed concerned about insulin, they really should change their message to emphasize a whole plant food diet.[256]

> *There's a little problem with this (paleo diet) story (about the diet our ancestors ate), which is that it is a total fairy tale, and it gets you eating a disease-inducing diet that's actually very harmful.*
> — *Janice Stanger, Ph.D.*
> *in Human Development and Aging*

If low carb and paleo diets are successful at all it is probably largely due to the restriction on sugar, white flour, other refined carbohydrates, and processed foods. Probably any diet which does that will have a measure of success. But if the claim is that

[254] McDougall, The Paleo Diet Is Uncivilized (And Unhealthy and Untrue)
https://www.drmcdougall.com/misc/2012nl/jun/paleo2.htm
[255] Christina Warinner, Debunking the Paleo Diet
http://tedxtalks.ted.com/video/Debunking-the-Paleo-Diet-Christ
[256] Greger, Paleo Diets May Negate Benefits of Exercise
http://nutritionfacts.org/video/paleo-diets-may-negate-benefits-of-exercise/

carbs from whole plant foods cause dangerous blood sugar spikes and disease-promoting inflammation, that is obviously false.[257]

➢ **The Mediterranean diet:** This diet has been touted by many health experts as a great way to promote good health, especially heart health. The Mayo Clinic website summarizes what this diet consists of:

- Eating primarily plant-based foods, such as fruits and vegetables, whole grains, legumes and nuts

- Replacing butter with healthy fats, such as olive oil

- Using herbs and spices instead of salt to flavor foods

- Limiting red meat to no more than a few times a month

- Eating fish and poultry at least twice a week

- Drinking red wine in moderation (optional)

The diet also recognizes the importance of being physically active, and enjoying meals with family and friends.[258]

Studies have been done which show this diet's health benefit over the SAD. No doubt this is due to the emphasis on plant foods and decreased meat and omega-6 oil consumption. But to suggest this proves one should be on this diet is like suggesting that it's healthier to get hit in the head by a baseball than a bowling ball. True, but it's a false dichotomy. As you know, having read this far, a third, better option exists. Which would be to just avoid the concussion entirely by skipping the fish, chicken and oil!

Whether you are a Mediterranean Presbyterian who likes to sprinkle it on your food, or a Mediterranean Baptist who likes to dunk your food in it, you can never make food healthier to eat by baptizing it in olive oil. Studies have shown that the fruits and

---

[257] McDougall, The Smoke and Mirrors behind *Wheat Belly* and *Grain Brain* https://www.drmcdougall.com/misc/2014nl/jan/smoke.htm
[258] *MayoClinic.com*, Mediterranean diet: A heart-healthy eating plan http://www.mayoclinic.org/healthy-living/nutrition-and-healthy-eating/in-depth/mediterranean-diet/art-20047801

veggies in the diet help to protect against some of the damage which tends to be inflicted on the body by eating olive oil. But how much better to skip the oil altogether! No matter what it is eaten with, olive oil has the same effect as other added oils, in that it slows down blood flow, increases inflammation, damages the endothelium, and causes weight gain. These are definitely not healthy effects.[259] Yet the Mayo Clinic calls olive oil a "healthy fat." Really?

To my knowledge there have been no studies comparing the health of people on the Mediterranean diet with that of those on a whole food plant based diet. But the numerous studies which show the chronic disease promoting effects of fish, chicken, and oils, including olive oil, probably make such studies unnecessary.

➤ **The American Heart Association diet:** The AHA has a recommended diet which they claim will protect against heart disease. Their web page on this diet starts out like this:

American Heart
Association

Learn and Live

> A healthy diet and lifestyle are your best weapons to fight cardiovascular disease.

Right on! So far they seem to have the right approach. We know that a whole food plant based diet is the most powerful weapon against cardiovascular disease. We have also learned that meat consumption causes heart disease. So does the AHA promote a truly heart healthy whole food plant based diet?

Later the AHA diet article gets somewhat more specific, giving recommendations regarding what should be eaten and what should be avoided. By this point in the book you should be able to accurately analyze these recommendations and pick out any problems yourself. But at the risk of telling you what should be obvious by now, I will spell out the problems I see; *[my comments in brackets]*.

---

[259] Jeff Novick, *Veg Source*, <u>Olive Oil is NOT Health Food but Sick Food</u>
https://www.youtube.com/watch?v=GfBKauKVi4M

As you make daily food choices, base your eating pattern on these recommendations:

- Choose lean meats and poultry without skin and prepare them without added saturated and trans fat.

[Amazing. They are actually telling people to consume meat, implying that consuming meat is good for heart health. We have seen that any sort of meat, lean or not, promotes the degradation of endothelial cells, and thus cardiovascular disease. Furthermore, the words "saturated and trans fat" are confusing; most people don't know what foods they are talking about. Of course these terms must be used to protect "corporate partners," those who pay the AHA to promote their products, such as The National Cattleman's Beef Association.]

- Eat fish at least twice a week. Recent research shows that eating oily fish containing omega-3 fatty acids (for example, salmon, trout and herring) may help lower your risk of death from coronary artery disease.

[Amazing again. They are actually telling people to consume fish, and that consuming fish is good for heart health. On the contrary, research shows that eating fish exposes the body to dangerous toxins and saturated fat, and promotes heart disease and other chronic conditions. The current research showing omega-3s being protective from heart disease is mixed, actually, some studies showing benefit, others not. And some show clear harm.[260] The case for fish consumption having a true net positive effect on coronary artery disease risk is at the very least uncertain, and certainly nonexistent for those on a heart healthy whole food plant based diet.]

- Select fat-free, 1 percent fat and low-fat dairy products.

[Amazing a third time. They are actually telling people to consume dairy, implying it is good for heart health. Assuming they know the facts regarding dairy and its negative effect on health, they are being quite patronizing in not laying out those facts, but instead assuming that since people won't be willing to give up dairy the best they can do is to tell them to consume dairy in a form which they believe to be the least harmful. Of

---

[260] Joseph Nordqvist, <u>Omega 3 fish oils linked to prostate cancer risk</u> http://www.medicalnewstoday.com/articles/263179.php

course, low- or nonfat means it's supercharged with animal protein (casein, a carcinogen), which certainly does not promote good health.]

- Cut back on foods containing partially hydrogenated vegetable oils to reduce trans fat in your diet.

[Good advice? Well, sorta. 1. Since any amount of these fats promotes heart disease, none at all should be consumed by anyone, especially those concerned about heart disease. So why do they use the words "cut back," and thus promote the false notion that consuming a little is good for your heart? Why are they so patronizing, assuming people can't handle the truth about the dangers of these fats? 2. The words "partially hydrogenated vegetable oils" are meaningless to most people, and so are worthless when not accompanied by an explanation. So to improve this point and make it truly helpful advice, a rewording such as this would be appropriate: "Do not consume any foods with partially hydrogenated vegetable oils, such as fried foods, frozen pizzas, cakes, cookies, margarine and spreads, pie, ready-to-use frosting and coffee creamers. Consuming these foods promotes heart disease." Few people will follow that advice, but at least they deserve the truth, so they can decide for themselves.]

- To lower cholesterol, reduce saturated fat to no more than 5 to 6 percent of total calories. For someone eating 2,000 calories a day, that's about 13 grams of saturated fat.

[Again, using a technical term, saturated fat, to confuse and soften a very serious message which has life and death implications. And again, using a mitigating term, "reduce," which gives a wrong impression about the dangers posed by this fat. Additionally, throwing around figures like 5-6%, 2000 calories, and 13 grams is worthless; does anyone really know how that translates to what one should actually eat or not eat? How much better if they had simply come right out and said, consistent with what the research demands, "For optimal heart health, do not eat any meat or dairy products." But then, that, again, would make their corporate sponsors angry, and we can't have that.]

- Cut back on beverages and foods with added sugars.

[If they really wanted to inform people about how to avoid heart disease (and other chronic conditions) they would say, "Don't consume any beverages or foods with added sugars." They must know the science supports such a dietary choice. Apparently they don't think that is practical or possible, or they assume no one would follow that advice anyway.]

- Choose and prepare foods with little or no salt. To lower blood pressure, aim to eat no more than 2,400 milligrams of sodium per day. Reducing daily intake to 1,500 mg is desirable because it can lower blood pressure even further.

[Actually, sodium intake affects the blood pressure of only a minority of people. Still, it is good to limit salt intake. But the best way to accomplish that is to stop eating animal products, which contain sodium naturally, and to which salt is usually added. Furthermore, blood pressure will be reduced much more effectively by a whole food plant based diet than by trying to reduce the sodium content of a diet containing meat.]

- If you drink alcohol, drink in moderation. That means one drink per day if you're a woman and two drinks per day if you're a man.

[Amen. They got one right! Interesting how they were able to spell out clearly what they mean in this case but were not able to do so with several of the other recommendations. Of course their clarity of message here might possibly have something to do with the fact that the AHA does not accept alcohol producers as corporate sponsors.[261]]

- Follow the American Heart Association recommendations when you eat out, and keep an eye on your portion sizes.

[These recommendations are for the most part unhelpful whether one eats out or at home! And again, nebulous, deceptive language: "Keep an eye on portion sizes" tells us that you can eat a little saturated fat and cholesterol-laden meat, sugary dessert, etc., and still have a healthy heart. The science says eating even what most would consider to be small

---

[261] *Integrity in Science,* Non-Profit Organizations Receiving Corporate Funding: American Heart Association
http://www.cspinet.org/integrity/nonprofits/american_heart_association.html

portions of such foods puts the heart at risk, especially for those who already have heart disease. See below.]

- Also, don't smoke tobacco — and avoid secondhand smoke.[262]

[Bingo. Two out of ten ain't bad. But why is it they have no trouble forbidding tobacco, yet they can't bring themselves to forbid meat, sugar, or oils? The science implicating these substances in heart disease is just as strong as that implicating tobacco. Of course the reason has to do with culture, money and politics, which constantly trump science when it comes to experts giving nutritional advice. And another would be, again, that no tobacco companies are accepted as AHA corporate sponsors.]

Note that this list of recommendations doesn't say anything about plant foods. These foods, especially vegetables, actively promote heart health, so it seems they should be emphasized heavily.

However, healthy foods are not completely neglected. Above this list on the AHA website it is stated that

> Eating a variety of fruits and vegetables *may* help you control your weight, cholesterol and your blood pressure. [Emphasis added.]

It *may not* help if the patient continues to eat a lot of animal products and processed foods. It *will certainly* help reduce these risk factors if these foods are drastically cut or eliminated entirely from the diet.

Thus, while *variety* is important, equally important is the sheer *quantity*, which when sufficient will displace the toxic foods which promote heart disease, and a reduction in weight, cholesterol, blood pressure and heart disease risk is guaranteed.

Regarding fruits and vegetables, the article continues:

> To get the nutrients you need, eat a dietary pattern that emphasizes:

---

[262] *The American Heart Association website,* The American Heart Association's Diet and Lifestyle Recommendations
http://www.heart.org/HEARTORG/GettingHealthy/NutritionCenter/HealthyDietGoals/The-American-Heart-Associations-Diet-and-Lifestyle-Recommendations_UCM_305855_Article.jsp

- fruits, vegetables,
- whole grains,
- low-fat dairy products,
- poultry, fish and nuts,
- while limiting red meat and sugary foods and beverages.

Again, you can detect the problems with the above, but at least they do suggest some healthy foods be emphasized.

It seems strange, however, that in the expanded list of recommendations analyzed above, which in the article follows this shorter list, they would repeat the recommendations related to dairy, fish, poultry, red meat, and sugar, but leave out those related to the good, truly healthy foods which do so much to promote heart heath.

So, what about the research data regarding the AHA diet? Since the "experts" recommend it, surely it has been proven to be helpful. Surely people on this diet don't have heart problems! Based on the above AHA recommendations, how effective do you think this diet really is?

Dr. McDougall describes a study which compared three groups of study subjects. One was on a very strict low fat diet. They were found to have a 6.6% chance of suffering a heart artery related event. The second group was eating the SAD, and their chance of an adverse cardiac-related event was 30.6%.

> There was also an intermediate group called "moderate treatment." They were on the American Heart Association Diet with 20% to 30% of the calories from fat and they were on cholesterol-lowering drugs. At the end of five years, 20.3% of these patients had cardiac events and after 2.6 years their scans showed worsening of their heart circulation. Thus, this approach, commonly prescribed by most practicing doctors, causes coronary artery disease to worsen, and more coronary events to occur.[263]

So it is safe to say that the AHA diet is another diet which is only appropriate for those who just want a slightly smaller chance of getting heart disease, or of their existing condition worsening. If

---

[263] McDougall, *McDougall Newsletter* June 2003, Cleaning Out Your Arteries https://www.drmcdougall.com/misc/2003nl/jun/030600puarteryclosure.htm

you want the best shot at avoiding heart disease altogether, the AHA diet is worthless.

➢ **Other diets:** Other diets to avoid would be ones which want to sell you some delicious shake or special supplements, or send you ready made meals, or any other diet which costs money. None of that is necessary, and it is not what is best for your health. **Remember, the most effective things you can do to achieve and maintain good health don't have to cost anything.** You are already buying food. It doesn't have to cost any more, and can certainly cost much less, to stop buying junk food and start buying healthful whole plant food.

When someone packages up some special program to sell it to you, there is a problem. The danger that the salesman's motives are tainted is high. He's looking for a way to get your money, and he will hawk his goods in such a way that it will keep you paying him as long as possible. This is true of food, supplements, drugs, and medical and alternative procedures.

That doesn't mean there is never any good in these things. Sometimes they are needed. And it doesn't mean that those selling these things always have selfish motives and only want your money. Many are sincerely convinced they are helping people with their products. **But beware that the profit motive will often cause people to shade the truth about how beneficial their product really is.** They may be reluctant to accept certain clear evidence which, if acted on in integrity, might undermine their livelihood.

So don't get sucked into some expensive and/or complicated diet scheme. All you need to do is learn and follow the simple diet principles we get from Genesis 1 and which the science supports, and take complete control of what you eat, so you don't have to pay anyone except your grocer or farmer's market.

If anyone tries to sell you on some diet, here are some questions you may want to ask them:

- **Has your diet been proven to prevent, stop and even reverse cardiovascular disease?**

- **Is your diet able to reverse and cure type 2 diabetes?**

- **Does your diet reduce the chance cancer will strike?**

- **Is your diet able to prevent and correct the problem of enlarged prostate (BPH) in men?**

- **Does your diet typically result in the normalization of blood pressure in people with hypertension, without the use of drugs?**

- **Is your diet able to cause symptoms of rheumatoid arthritis to resolve?**

- **Was your diet ever consumed by large, healthy populations of people for many generations?**

This last question would probably be answered in the affirmative by those promoting the paleo diet. However, they make many assumptions about the diet of ancient peoples which cannot be confirmed, and which are contradicted by many paleontologists. The historical record from the many great civilizations which were fueled by starch based diets is incontestable.

Some may point out that there is no known culture in history (or currently) which has lived exclusively on plant foods for several generations. Thus a whole food plant based diet doesn't pass the test. Technically this is true.

However, many healthy cultures have existed and continue to exist (though they are becoming more and more rare) which have diets consisting of over 90% whole plant foods. Meat plays a very minor role. The Blue Zone cultures are prime examples of this; typically they eat meat only five times per month. And furthermore, the meat they do consume is wild meat, and/or domestic meat which is raised on a natural diet and relatively free from toxins – a type of meat generally unavailable to most of us today.

So when we consider these facts from population data, and add to that what we know from scientific studies about the health damaging effects of animal products, all that evidence together argues rather convincingly that avoiding those foods altogether is in fact the best, most healthy course to take.

If our focus is on optimal all-around health, instead of just one or two factors such as weight or cholesterol numbers, the questions above are the ones we will ask when evaluating any diet. Questions regarding how much weight we can lose in a given period, or how much the cholesterol numbers are expected to drop, are not what our primary concern should be. These things are important, but they must not be the focus; optimal overall health is much more important. When we focus on the wrong things, bad diet choices are made, choices which are detrimental to good health.

I don't believe anyone can truthfully claim their diet has been proven to accomplish the above disease prevention and reversal miracles unless it is consistent with the whole plant food principle. And if a diet hasn't been proven to accomplish these things, but instead commonly allows these diseases to begin and to continue to progress, why in the world would anyone want to follow it?

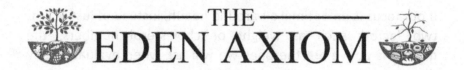

THE EDEN AXIOM

Part 4: More Data and Discussion

Chapter 12:

Human Physiology:

Herbivore or Carnivore?

"I'm a carnivore," a friend told me some time ago. "I eat meat and I'm not going to change that."

True, he was a carnivore in practice (actually an omnivore of sorts, since he did of course eat plant food as well). But was his carnivory a lifestyle forced on him by nature of his physical makeup, or was it just a choice he was making because he liked to eat meat? To put it another way, did God create us to eat meat (to be carnivores), did He create us to eat both meat and plants safely (omnivores), or did He create us to eat plants (herbivores), and just made it possible for us to tolerate some meat, giving us the freedom to do so if we so chose?

We can know two facts for certain regarding this question:

1. The first, most perfect environment God created for humans included a diet of whole plant foods only.

2. Eating meat, especially large quantities of meat, does injury to the human body, causing chronic deadly diseases; eating whole plant foods only promotes good health.

From these facts we can confidently conclude that God did not design us to eat large amounts of meat safely – or if He did so, the time when that was possible is long past.

But what about human physiology? If we compare it to that of carnivorous, omnivorous, and herbivorous animals, are our findings consistent with the above conclusion? The following points which may enlighten us regarding this question come from a lecture and related article by Dr. Milton Mills, M.D.[264,265]

➤ **Speed:** Carnivores tend to be fast runners, so that they can chase down prey. Herbivores tend to be slower; they don't need speed to chase down an apple or a carrot. Of course some herbivores, those who tend to be preyed upon by fast carnivores, are fast runners as well. But the point is that in order to obtain food, they don't need to be fast, and we find that humans fit into the slower herbivorous group. Factors which play into this aspect include the streamlined shape of carnivores' bodies, and the permanent "runner's crouch" structure of their frame. These features are lacking in herbivores.

➤ **Gestation period:** Carnivores tend to have relatively short gestation periods. This may be because the females need to hunt, and that would be difficult if they were pregnant for long periods, with huge bellies full of babies. Herbivores' gestation periods tend to be long. They can forage for their food just fine even when pregnant.

➤ **Birth weight:** At birth carnivore young tend to weigh less than 3% of their mother's body weight. Herbivore young tend to weigh 7-8% of their mother's body weight.

➤ **Facial bones and muscles:** There are distinct differences between the bone and muscle structure of carnivores' faces and that of herbivores. This has to do with optimal design for obtaining, chewing, and swallowing food.

➤ **Teeth:** The teeth of carnivores are designed for ripping,

---

[264] Dr. Milton Mills, M.D., Are We Designed To Eat Meat?
https://www.youtube.com/watch?v=Ee25u3YccHk
[265] Dr. Milton R. Mills, M.D., *Vegsource*, The Comparative Anatomy of Eating
www.vegsource.com/news/2009/11/the-comparative-anatomy-of-eating.html

tearing, and slicing. Carnivores don't tend to chew their food; they are incapable of chewing and grinding up their food the way herbivores do, because their lower jaw can only move up and down, not side to side. Instead, carnivores rip off pieces of meat and swallow them whole, in relatively large chunks. Herbivore teeth are designed for cropping and grinding food into very small pieces before swallowing.

➢ **Saliva:** Carnivores have no digestive enzymes in their saliva. Digestion doesn't begin till the meat enters the stomach. Herbivores have digestive enzymes in their saliva, which is mixed with the food during chewing, an important part of the digestive process.

➢ **Esophagus:** Carnivores have a relatively wide and distensible esophagus, adapted for swallowing large chunks of meat. Herbivores have a narrow, muscular esophagus, able to receive only small pieces of food which have been prepared by thorough grinding. Over 90% of people who choke to death choke on chunks of meat, which they were not designed to swallow. (Ever heard of the Heimlich maneuver being needed to dislodge a piece of spinach? By contrast, have you ever had to perform the Heimlich maneuver on your dog or your cat?)

➢ **Stomach size:** Carnivores tend to have very large stomachs, holding 60-70% of the total digestive tract capacity. The stomach can hold 30-40% of the animal's body weight. Thus a 300 lb. lion can consume 100 lbs. of flesh in a single meal. Herbivores have a much smaller stomach, which accounts for a much smaller percentage of the total capacity of the digestive tract. The herbivore stomach is designed for intermittent feeding, i.e. small, frequent meals, not infrequent gorging on large amounts of food. If humans were carnivores we would expect a 150 lb. person to be able to eat 50 lbs. of food in a single meal!

➢ **Stomach acid:** Carnivores have very strong, highly acidic digestive juices in the stomach, with a pH of 1-2. This enables them to digest not only meat protein, but also bones, hooves, etc., and helps destroy bacteria which is often present, especially if the meat is not fresh. Herbivore digestive juices are much less acidic, with a pH of 4-5. Strong acid is not necessary for dealing with plant foods.

> **Digestive ability:** In a carnivore's small intestine, protein and fat digestive enzymes predominate, and they have a poor ability to digest moderate to large carbohydrate meals. Herbivores can easily digest large carb meals, as their intestines are designed to do this, including handling the large amounts of fiber which comes with plant foods.

> **Small intestine:** Animal flesh is composed mostly of protein and fat. The cell walls are soft and extracting the nutrients from them is not difficult, requiring only a relatively short small intestine. Thus carnivore small intestines are only three to six times the animal's body length, measured from their head to the base of their tailbone. Herbivores, however, must be able to extract nutrients from plant cells. These also contain protein and fat, as well as carbohydrates and fiber. The plant cells are encased in a relatively tough fibrous cell wall. Thus the adequate digestion of plants requires thorough chewing, as well as a much longer small intestine, which averages 10 to 12 times the body length, again from head to tailbone.

> **Colon length and function:** The colon (large intestine) of carnivores and herbivores are similarly short and long, respectively. The carnivore colon has a smooth, non-pouched appearance, and its primary and perhaps only function is to convey waste out of the body. The herbivore colon, on the other hand, has a pouched appearance and has many complex functions, with the intestinal flora being especially important in processing the fiber, absorbing certain nutrients, and absorbing excess water back into the body.

> **Vascular health:** Carnivores such as dogs and cats can eat a diet of pure meat, and yet suffer no vascular damage, heart disease, etc. But when herbivores are fed high doses of meat they suffer serious vascular injury.

> **Bile:** Bile is a substance which functions like detergent, emulsifying fat and oils in the digestive tract. Carnivore bile is

very strong, able to emulsify fat very effectively. This protects them from gallstones. Herbivore bile is much weaker, since they encounter much less fat when eating their normal diet. When herbivores eat a lot of meat and/or plant-derived oils their bile is insufficiently strong to deal with the load of fat, and the result is often gallstones, which are usually composed primarily of cholesterol.

The above are just some of the points explained by Dr. Mills. Here are a few more interesting examples I have come across:

➢ **Vitamin C:** I don't know if this is true for all carnivores, but cats and dogs produce vitamin C in their bodies, so they don't need to get it from their diet. And of course the normal diet of cats and dogs does not include any vitamin C, since that vitamin is only found in plants. Humans, on the other hand, cannot produce vitamin C in their bodies, or produce very little, and so must obtain it from their diet, an indication they are herbivores.[266]

➢ **Arachidonic acid:** Dr. Greger explains how arachidonic acid provides a converse example. AA is necessary for a proper immune response. Cats do not produce AA in their bodies. They need to obtain it from their food. And of course AA is only found in flesh. Humans' bodies, however, produce their own AA, and need none from their diet.[267]

➢ **Taste buds:** Dr. McDougall points out that our tongues can taste bitter, sour, salt, and sweet. These are great for tasting plant foods. But we have no taste buds for protein. When was the last time you ate a piece of meat in its natural state, raw and unseasoned? Most of us recoil at the thought. Even cooked and unseasoned is not appetizing to us. Most of us have to add salt and/or other flavorings to make it tasty. Cats, and presumably

---

[266] *PetMD,* Cats Are Different: How a Cat's Nutritional Needs are Different from a Dog's
http://www.petmd.com/cat/nutrition/evr_ct_cat_nutritional_needs_different
[267] Greger, Chicken, Eggs, and Inflammation
http://nutritionfacts.org/video/chicken-eggs-and-inflammation/

other carnivores, however, do have amino acid tasting taste buds. When a cat eats raw meat it apparently tastes good to him.[268]

➤ **The bunny test:** This last example comes from a presentation by Dr. Neal Barnard, in which he gives some interesting illustrations which confirm humans do not instinctively seek to eat meat. Among them is what he calls the bunny test. When a child sees a bunny, what does he want to do with it? Touch it, pet it, hold it, snuggle it. He has no thought of hurting the bunny. What if he is very hungry? Does he have an instinct to rip the bunny apart and eat its flesh? Of course not.[269] But show him a strawberry and you will see a different reaction. Show a hungry cat a strawberry and his likely reaction will be similar to your reaction to a piece of raw meat. "No thanks."

We have compared herbivore physiology to that of carnivores. But what about **omnivores**? Do humans resemble them? No. Omnivores are basically built like carnivores, the main exception being their "hybrid" tooth and jaw structure which is designed for chewing plants as well as tearing meat. But their digestive systems have limited ability to digest plants, so they can only eat a limited variety of them.

In all of the above cited examples from the physiology of carnivores and herbivores, and many other such examples besides, humans fall squarely in the herbivore camp. Yes, we are capable of eating meat, and even apparently thriving on it for a time. But the way we are created gives clear indication that meat is not the most natural food for us. This is what we should expect considering the original diet God gave to humankind in the perfect environment of Eden. Thus the fact that eating meat causes myriad chronic diseases really is no surprise at all.

---

[268] McDougall, The Starch Solution (see minute 14:00)
https://www.youtube.com/watch?v=4XVf36nwraw
[269] Barnard, TED Talk, Tackling diabetes with a bold new dietary approach
(see minute 11:00) https://www.youtube.com/watch?v=ktQzM2IA-qU

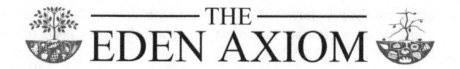

THE EDEN AXIOM

Chapter 13:

Theological Considerations

In **Chapter 2** we looked at the Scriptural basis for The Eden Axiom, and discussed some of the spiritual issues regarding our responsibility before God to exercise wise stewardship of our bodies. We briefly looked at several Bible passages which speak to this subject. Then in **Chapters 5-8** we learned some of the evidence that our food choices can promote good health, or conversely damage health and promote chronic disease. We saw that emphasizing whole plant foods in the diet, while decreasing non-plant foods and non-whole foods, is the most important change a person can make in their lifestyle if they value optimal health and wise body stewardship.

Based on what they see the Scriptures teaching, many Christians do come to believe that they should indeed make lifestyle changes to improve their health. But they often wonder just how the idea of a whole food plant based diet fits into the Biblical framework, especially in light of certain passages which may seem to contradict the whole food plant based dietary emphasis of this book.

So in this chapter we will turn again to the Scriptures, and look at more of the Biblical data which shows that this diet is indeed consistent with God's revelation, especially for us who live in modern times.

As we saw in the last chapter, physiologically a very strong case can be made that we were created to eat primarily plants. And this is consistent with the fact that the first perfect environment which God created for man and woman was a lush garden, complete with many whole plant foods which would supply all their nutritional needs. Animal products and partial foods were not part of the original menu ordained by God, and even in the newly fallen world man lived to great ages on this whole food plant based diet.

A modified diet

Then came the flood. When Noah and his family left the ark, God added a new food group to their menu: "every moving thing that lives" (Genesis 9:3; ESV), i.e. meat.

Though originally created to eat whole plant foods, in His wisdom and power God also made humans with the capacity to eat animals, and to derive sustenance from them.

In the generations following the flood a remarkable decrease in longevity occurred (Genesis 11). It might be tempting to blame this on the new diet, but it seems extremely unlikely that a simple addition of meat to the menu could have played a major role.

The primary reason for the decrease in post-flood lifespans is almost certainly genetic. The eight individuals who emerged from the ark constituted a "population bottleneck,"[270] a severe restriction on the diversity of the gene pool which would be inherited by future generations. There are good scientific reasons why this would result in accelerated aging and shorter lifespans.[271]

Furthermore, genetic entropy,[272] the inexorable mutation-driven breakdown of the human genome, which increases each generation and is the primary factor responsible for sickness, ageing and death, must have kicked into high gear following the flood.

---

[270] Also called "genetic bottleneck."

[271] Carl Wieland, Living for 900 years http://creation.com/living-for-900-years

[272] Dr. J.C. Sanford, Genetic Entropy and the Mystery of the Genome, FMS Publications 2007

The meat eaten in the centuries following the flood would of course have been raised on a natural diet and free of industrial pollutants, artificial toxins, hormones, etc. So, for those who ate meat sparingly, as no doubt most did, it probably didn't have a big impact on their longevity.

However, overindulgence in carnivory, no matter how "clean" the meat, will cause chronic disease and shorten lifespan. So the question arises, if the addition of meat to the post-flood diet introduced a risk factor, having the effect of causing disease if it were abused, why did God give it to them?

It is impossible to know for sure what His purposes were in giving humans, whom He loved, meat. But we can speculate on some possibilities.

Many creationist scientists and others have asserted, with good evidence, that the post-flood world was much changed from what it had been previously. The immense coal, oil, and natural gas deposits found around the world today are the remains of massive amounts of vegetation which was buried during the great flood. This suggests that the amount of vegetation on the pre-flood earth was orders of magnitude greater than what we see today.[273] It is probable that no deserts existed.

Thus the post-flood earth must have contained far fewer opportunities for the gathering of wild plant foods. And its new and varied environments were probably not nearly as crop-friendly as previously. The newly established seasons would not allow for year-round access to the fruit of the field, and seasonal famines would result.

But many wild and domestic animals can convert grass and other plant matter which are indigestible by humans into edible meat. So it may be that God gave meat to humans at this time as an act of His grace. It helped to ensure that people would be sustained in a wider variety of environments, even places where

---

[273] Gerhard Schönknecht, Too much coal for a young earth? http://creation.com/too-much-coal-for-a-young-earth

little or no plant food consumable by humans could be grown or gathered.

If this suggested explanation is correct, then meat is not only a "feasting food," but for many populations it was probably a "survival food," at least during certain periods of the year.

There are other possibilities as to why God gave meat, which we will not take time to examine here. But in any event, we can be sure that the giving of meat was both part of God's plan for man, to accomplish His purposes, and that it was in some way an act of His love and grace. For God is love. We can trust that He does have a good purpose in all He does and for all who love and trust Him (Romans 8:28).

The significant takeaway from this discussion is that in giving dietary meat to humans there is no reason to suppose that God intended for the privilege to be abused to the point of disease.

Daniel's diet

Let's take a moment to consider the case of Daniel and his three friends' diet test. For religious reasons they didn't want to eat the pagan king's defiled food, but avoiding the royal diet had great physical benefits as well.

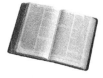

[15] At the end of the ten days [on a whole food plant based diet], Daniel and his three friends looked healthier and better nourished than the young men who had been eating the food assigned by the king. [16] So after that, the attendant fed them only vegetables instead of the food and wine provided for the others.

Daniel 1:15-16

It is apparent that "the youths who ate the king's food" were eating a diet similar to the SAD in regards to the large quantity of meat and paucity of veggies. On their veggie diet, Daniel and his friends fared much better than the others. We know Daniel lived a long life, and it seems likely his healthy diet was at least partially responsible.

A different role

The example above from the book of Daniel is interesting, but it does not represent the normal, common diet found among God's people in the Scriptures. However, we should not conclude from that fact that the Israelites typically ate a diet similar to that which is commonly consumed in the West in modern times.

Processed foods were few: stone-ground whole grain flour, olive oil, wine, honey, perhaps a few others. With the relatively low-tech equipment they had available, there was not a whole lot they could do to ruin the goodness of the whole plant foods God had provided. Olive oil was used sparingly, as it was very expensive. Apart from some wild honey, they had no sugar.

Regarding the Israelites' eating of meat, it is clear that their practice was much different from what we find in rich Western nations – though probably similar to what is still found in the few remote agrarian societies left in the world today. The eating of meat in Bible times played a much different role in the diet than it does in modern society. The Israelites were definitely not on the SAD!

For the common folk, meat consumption was generally a luxury, normally eaten sparingly. Larger quantities were typically only eaten on special occasions of feasting and sacrifice. Meat was not the centerpiece of the everyday diet, responsible for the majority of the calories consumed, as is the norm in many Western countries today.

The nature of meat in Bible times

Additionally, as mentioned earlier, we know that the meat God sanctioned for consumption by people in Bible times was either wild or from domestic animals raised on a natural diet, relatively free of toxins. And it is good to note that God commanded the Israelites to not eat the blood or the fat, two components of meat which are particularly problematic to good health.

It definitely would be a good idea to limit one's meat

consumption to the model of ancient Israel. Eating meat sparingly, avoiding sugar, oils, and other processed foods, and eating a lot of whole plant foods, is also the pattern found in the modern day Blue Zone populations, where people live so long, enjoying good health into old age.

However, considering the nature of the meat generally available to us in the West, which contains many toxins introduced either intentionally or incidentally, it seems the healthiest course would be to limit its consumption as much as possible.

Are all "foods" clean?

Recognizing the nature of the animal food products available in Jesus' day, and the nature of those foods today, helps us correctly interpret and apply the words of the Evangelist when he commented that Jesus declared every kind of food "clean," or acceptable in God's eyes (Mark 7:19).

Of course the issue at hand was ritual defilement, not health. Jesus was saying that the consumption of food was not an issue in determining a person's acceptability in God's sight. But for the sake of this discussion, let's assume that the acceptability of food from a health standpoint was also in view.

So in the context, what sort of "food" was Jesus talking about? Hormone-injected beef? Mercury-contaminated fish? PCB-tainted eggs? Nitrate-infused lunch meat? Sugar-laden ice cream and cupcakes? French fries and doughnuts soaked in damaged, inflammation-causing oil? No. These are foods contaminated with dangerous non-food substances which didn't even exist in foods in Jesus' day. Was He really saying such things were acceptable, that He wanted believers to eat them? Of course not.

The Webster's dictionary defines food this way:

> material consisting essentially of protein, carbohydrate, and fat used in the body of an organism to sustain growth, repair, and vital

processes and to furnish energy[274]

The Sage dictionary on my computer has this:

> Any substance which can be metabolized by an animal to give energy and build tissue… Any solid substance (as opposed to liquid) that is used as a source of nourishment.[275]

Many of the partial foods and other additives we find in processed foods today do not sustain growth, give energy, build tissue or nourish. Not only do they not help our bodies to be healthy, but they actively damage our health. *They are not food.*

Jesus said that all *foods* are suitable for consumption, not all *non-foods*. And when one takes real food and mixes it with some non-food substance which is harmful to the body, the result, in my view, is not really food. And I think it would help us to make healthy food choices if we could mentally reclassify such contaminated foods as "non-food."

Personal convictions

Please don't misunderstand what I am saying here. **If someone wants to consume such things, they of course are not necessarily sinning by doing so.** That is not for me or anyone else to judge. It all depends on how God is working in the individual's life, what He is leading them to do.

> Remember, it is sin to know what you ought to do and then not do it.
> James 4:17

It is not sin for the person who has other convictions. If a person understands the health challenges these foods present, yet believes before the Lord that they have the freedom to eat them, then of course they are free to eat.

My point here is that one cannot find Biblical commands or

---

[274] *Merriam-Webster,* Merriam-Webster online dictionary
http://www.merriam-webster.com/dictionary/food
[275] Sequence Publishing, The Sage English Dictionary and Thesaurus
http://www.sequencepublishing.com/thesage.html

principles which in any way sanction our consumption of foods which contain substances known to be toxic and promote disease. Neither is there Biblical support for the notion that God doesn't care one way or another whether we make healthy lifestyle choices.

I approach this subject much the same way I approach the issue of tobacco use. I know that many believers smoke or chew with a clear conscience. For them it is not sin. But I would still look for opportunities to share with them the health hazards of tobacco use, and encourage them to quit, with much the same spiritual and scientific reasoning I use when it comes to encouraging people live healthier lifestyles in other areas.

That analogy may seem to some to be a bit of a stretch, but **the science regarding the health-damaging effects of the SAD is just as strong as the science regarding the health-damaging effects of tobacco use.** This is hard for most of us to accept, as our culture hasn't yet caught up with the science. Perhaps it will one day, just as it finally caught up with the science on the dangers of tobacco use.

At any rate, I do take Romans 14:4 and other similar Scriptures seriously, that it is wrong to judge another believer when they are acting in faith according to their convictions.

"All things are lawful for me"

When faced with the diet information in this book, and an exhortation to be prudent about our food choices, perhaps some will defend their eating habits by quoting what Paul wrote in 1 Corinthians 6:12: "All things are lawful for me," in other words, "I am allowed to do anything I want." Let's look briefly at the whole verse:

> You say, "I am allowed to do anything"—but not everything is good for you. And even though "I am allowed to do anything," I must not become a slave to anything.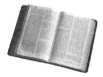

The wording here of the NLT makes explicit the correct interpretation of this verse. Some other versions seem to leave the door open for someone to think the verse actually gives license to do what one pleases, as if God doesn't care about our behavior, that it doesn't impact our spirituality. After all, we're "free in Christ," right?

The Translator's Handbook sheds a bit of light on this passage which helps us come to the correct interpretation of Paul's words:

> Commentators agree that the clause All things are lawful to me was a slogan used in Corinth at that time.... Probably the people who misused this saying thought that because the body did not matter, they could do anything they liked with it.[276]

I have given evidence earlier that our bodies do indeed matter to God (and we will see more on that presently). And the above quoted verse shows clearly that He expects us to take care not to become enslaved by our physical desires for pleasure which hinder His purposes for us.

So let us seriously ask the Lord what He would have us to do regarding this. Could it be that some of our food choices are made because of food addictions, that we are enslaved by what we want to eat? Or are we making decisions in an attitude of a reasoned, wise, humble submission to a lifestyle which is consistent with Biblical revelation, truly healthy, and will afford us the maximum opportunity to worship and serve our Creator and Savior?

"Food was made for the stomach"

Some may also quote the first part of the next verse in an effort to argue that it doesn't matter what foods we eat:

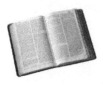

> You say, "Food was made for the stomach, and the stomach for food." (This is true, though someday God will do away with both of them.) But you can't say that our bodies were made for sexual immorality. They were made for the Lord, and the Lord cares about our bodies.
>
> 1 Corinthians 6:13

[276] Paul Ellingworth and Howard A. Hatton, 1993, A Translator's Handbook on Paul's First Letter to the Corinthians, United Bible Societies, New York

As Paul says, the saying quoted by the Corinthians is true. But he goes on to explain that it doesn't apply to the issue of sexual immorality, indicating that they should stop quoting it to justify immoral behavior.

But I would contend that the saying also cannot be applied to gluttony, to the consumption of foods in an unhealthy manner, such as in overindulging in foods which cause harm to the body when consumed in excess. It also wouldn't apply to the consumption of toxic non-foods, as defined in the discussion above.

As Paul says, our food and our bodies are, in light of eternity, temporary, physical objects. But he is in no way suggesting that this fact negates the importance of being good stewards of them. After all, our bodies "were made for the Lord." In fact, what he writes next shows this to be completely contrary to his intent.

The last phrase of the verse is very difficult to interpret, because a literal reading of it makes no sense in English. The NLT says, "the Lord cares for our bodies." That sounds great. However, a literal translation of this phrase, following as much as possible the Greek form, would be "the Lord for the body." What in the world does that mean? It is impossible to know for sure, but it is variously interpreted to mean

- the Lord cares for our bodies,
- the Lord belongs to the body,
- the Lord provides for the body,
- the Lord is for the body to bless and save it
- the Lord is for the body to inhabit and glorify it, and
- the Lord fills the body with Himself.

Though these interpretations differ from each other, together they indicate something very significant to our present discussion. They appear to be unanimous in asserting that the Lord is quite interested in and concerned about our bodies, and in light of that it seems all the more clear that we should be good stewards of them.

Food made acceptable

Paul wrote something interesting to his disciple Timothy, which some may take to indicate that it must be okay to eat any food you want, as long as you pray and are thankful for it.

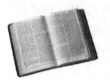

³They [the false teachers] will say it is wrong to be married and wrong to eat certain foods. But God created those foods to be eaten with thanks by faithful people who know the truth. ⁴Since everything God created is good, we should not reject any of it but receive it with thanks. ⁵For we know it is made acceptable by the word of God and prayer.   1 Timothy 4:3-5

Paul here warns Timothy against false teachers who would make legalistic pronouncements about the spiritual value of celibacy and avoiding certain taboo foods. This teaching must be opposed since it is antithetical to the Gospel of grace.

But what does it mean that the food "is made acceptable (sanctified) by the word of God and prayer"? Some commentators suggest that this refers to meat which had been offered to idols and then purchased by the Christian in the market. God's Word says you can eat it with a clear conscience since an idol isn't anything (1 Corinthians 8:4-8), Jesus said it's acceptable (Mark 7:19), and you thank God for it in prayer. Others suggest that whether the food was offered to idols or not, it should be consecrated to God, set apart for holy use, that is, for the nourishing of God's children.

The sort of food prohibition urged by the false teachers is not relevant to the subject of this book. The issue then was not what is healthful. The issue was what is proper to eat from a religious point of view, irregardless of nutritive value. Every food God created is indeed good, and it surely should be received with thanks.

However, the verse does imply that God created meat, and that meat is good to eat and should be received and eaten with thanksgiving. This does raise a valid question about the healthfulness of meat. How can one maintain that there is anything wrong with eating meat in the light of what this Scripture says?

The answer is plain from the issues discussed earlier in this chapter as well as elsewhere in the book. First of all, in the context Paul was addressing, meat comprised a relatively small part of the overall daily menu. Furthermore, it was eaten as part of a diet which was otherwise nearly completely whole food plant based. So the meat would have little negative impact on health, if any.

Secondly we can point out that the verse *does not say* "everything *we call* food is good" or "anything someone sells you that he tells you is food is good," that is, healthful to eat.

For example, our food supply has been contaminated by industrial pollutants such as heavy metals, PCBs and dioxins. As discussed elsewhere in this book, these substances, when ingested, can cause cancer and other diseases.

The meat and milk of all sorts of animals acts as a magnet for these toxins, concentrating them and storing them (see the sidebar in **Chapter 5: PCB concentrations in various food groups**, and note that plant foods contain very little of these toxins). This was not a problem when the Bible was written, but certainly is now.

And toxins are added to foods intentionally as well, as with nitrates and nitrites in processed meats, certain artificial sweeteners, preservatives such as BHA, and other chemical additives in sodas and most other processed foods. So should we consider these foods to be the kind the Bible is talking about when it speaks of the foods God created as being "good"? Did God really create sausage or Coke?

Even apart from toxic chemicals added to foods, whole plant foods are always being intentionally changed into something resembling food, but which is unhealthy to eat, and could even be described as toxic. These partial foods are then combined to make a compound non-food something-or-other. We want to believe it is food, because it tastes better than the original whole foods from which its ingredients were derived. But is it food?

For example, God made the whole foods wheat, beets, and corn. If you eat these foods as whole foods, you can and indeed should receive them with thanksgiving. They will provide important nutrients which your body will use to grow and thrive.

> *Thus doughnuts and similar partial food products cannot be considered to be true food in a Biblical sense.*

But one cannot say that in the same sense God made refined white flour (from wheat), sugar (extracted from beets), and corn oil, three main ingredients which may be used to make doughnuts. People have taken God's good, whole foods, and extracted certain components of those foods, and then combined them together to make a manmade product we call "food." But this product bears little nutritional resemblance to anything God ever made. And in fact it degrades the health of those who eat it.

Thus doughnuts and similar partial food products cannot be considered to be true food in a Biblical sense. And so it follows that it is not valid to use 1 Timothy 4 to support the notion that one can convert such things into acceptable food by praying over them.

Perhaps some would still be reluctant to accept this conclusion. Allow me to share a more stark example which should help get my point across.

Apricot seeds are nutritious food. But they contain cyanide. When eaten as part of the whole seed, the cyanide is not toxic, and in fact it promotes health (see **Chapter 15: Other Topics Related To Health: Vitamin B17**).

But if I were to extract the cyanide from the seed and concentrate it into a pill, would that be "good food"? Of course not. It would be deadly poison. And no one considers deadly poisons to be food.

Just as concentrated cyanide, though a natural substance created by God as part of His good creation, isn't food, so a case can be made that sugar, oil, and white flour, extracted from their respective original whole foods, are not food.

All of these substances damage health when they are consumed in significant quantities. The only difference is that cyanide kills very quickly, while with the others it may take years before the effects of disease are felt.

So when the Bible talks about food, let's be careful to remember what sort of food it is talking about.

Other Scriptures deal with the subject of the believer's liberty in Christ in the area of diet, such as Romans 14. The same arguments laid out above apply there as well: The issue has to do with meat offered to idols, not health. And it has to do with organic meat from animals fed a natural diet, eaten in moderation, not indulgence in the SAD.

What is the true food of the future?

We have discussed issues relating to diet in the past and present. What about the future? The Bible has something to say about that, too.

Isaiah wrote about the changed attitude and diet of carnivorous animals during the Millennial Kingdom age:

> [6]In that day the wolf and the lamb will live together; the leopard will lie down with the baby goat. The calf and the yearling will be safe with the lion, and a little child will lead them all. [7]The cow will graze near the bear. The cub and the calf will lie down 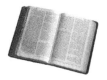 together. The lion will eat hay like a cow. [8]The baby will play safely near the hole of a cobra. Yes, a little child will put its hand in a nest of deadly snakes without harm. [9]Nothing will hurt or destroy in all my holy mountain, for as the waters fill the sea, so the earth will be filled with people who know the Lord.   Isaiah 9:6-9

So what does this Scripture clearly imply about the human diet at that time? Will animals be slaughtered for food? Could such be done under the stipulation that "Nothing will hurt or destroy"?

Furthermore, if formerly carnivorous animals are not allowed, indeed not even disposed, to kill and eat, it seems quite likely that the same rule, and disposition, will hold for humans, and vegetarianism will be the order of the day.

What about the eternal state in the new heaven and new earth? Are there any clues as to our diet there?

The Apostle John had the amazing privilege of seeing what the eternal state will be like:

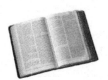

[1]Then the angel showed me a river with the water of life, clear as crystal, flowing from the throne of God and of the Lamb. [2]It flowed down the center of the main street. On each side of the river grew a tree of life, bearing twelve crops of fruit, with a fresh crop each month. The leaves were used for medicine to heal the nations.

[3]No longer will there be a curse upon anything. For the throne of God and of the Lamb will be there, and his servants will worship him.   Revelation 22:1-3

Interesting. Leaves are spoken of as "medicine to heal the nations." Reminds me of the amazing medical miracles which are performed in our day as people switch to a whole food plant based diet, often composed largely of leaves such as kale, collards, and spinach, and find their bodies able to take this super fuel and heal from cardiovascular disease, diabetes, high blood pressure, high cholesterol, PMS, arthritis, and even cancer.

It is evident that in the eternal state, as during the Millennial Kingdom, plant foods will be the only human food.

Of course, we will be so consumed with worshipping our very present and glorious Lord that eating will likely not be an issue we are much concerned with. And in fact some would interpret this verse figuratively, saying it indicates that there will be only good health and abundant blessing from the Lord for all who are in Heaven. Perhaps there will be no actual eating at all.

Some may respond that they had better eat as much yummy

unhealthy food as they can now, because they won't get any later. That's fine. It would just be good to remember that such an approach will also get you there faster, so has a double benefit!

At any rate, my alternative suggestion would be to waste no time, but to begin practicing now our Kingdom and possibly eternal state eating habits.

Hedonism

> *But the fruit of the Spirit is...self-control.*
> *Galatians 5:22-23*

Another way to look at this subject, which we have touched on before, is to recognize the lust for pleasure evident among many believers for what it is: *hedonistic.* **Hedonism is a devotion to pleasure, and it has been a problem in the church ever since it surfaced among the Corinthian believers** (if not before). Hedonism betrays a lack of Spirit-directed and energized self-control.

This hedonistic tendency among Christians manifests itself in many ways. From an obsession with sports; to a preference for sensual, shallow, often self-focused "worship" music over praiseworthy songs with edifying Scriptural lyrics; to indulgence in pornography;[277] this is a serious problem crippling the church.

Of course many pleasures we enjoy are not sinful. After all, Paul told Timothy that God provides what we need so we can enjoy life:

> Teach those who are rich in this world not to be proud and not to trust in their money, which is so unreliable. Their trust should be in God, who richly gives us all we need for our enjoyment. 1 Timothy 6:17

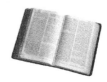

"Those who are rich in this world" describes most of us who live in the West. We can afford so many unhealthy and sinful pleasures that we have indulged our way into a chronic disease

---

[277] Surveys show that 30-40% of protestant clergy struggle with pornography addiction; how much more their flocks!

epidemic. Yes, God provides richly for us everything we need to enjoy the things He wants us to enjoy. But when a drive for pleasure enslaves us, keeping us from doing what we know God wants us to do, that pleasure become sinful.

We must ask ourselves, are we willing to forego a few temporal pleasures for the sake of long-term, even eternal benefit? And of course, when it comes to issues of healthy lifestyle, ultimately it really isn't simply a loss of pleasure, but rather a trading of old, familiar, unhealthy pleasures for new, healthy ones.

Think about the likely prognosis for someone on the SAD: heart disease, cancer, diabetes, obesity, arthritis, dementia, etc. Yet we have seen that a whole food plant based diet holds promise of a dramatic reduction in the likelihood these chronic diseases will strike.

So in reality a person who adopts this way of eating is trading some familiar pleasures for the new pleasures of a healthy diet, plus the much more significant pleasures of enjoying good health into old age, increased time with family and friends, seeing one's grandchildren and even great-grandchildren grow up, an opportunity to have more years to worship and serve God while on earth, etc. **A devotion to this sort of pleasure, arising out of our primary devotion to God and obedience to Him, is a kind of "hedonism" which we can all embrace with clear conscience and God's approval.**

May our Lord help us to be devoted to Him alone, seeking to please and serve Him, even if it means suffering the loss of some of our favorite familiar temporal pleasures.

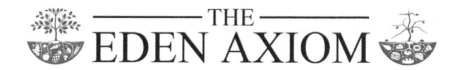

THE EDEN AXIOM

Chapter 14:

Additional Issues To Consider

How many cigarettes?

Regarding reducing intake of sugar, fat, meat & dairy, and processed foods, one doctor had a good analogy. He said his patients ask how much of these unhealthy things are they allowed to eat. He says his answer is the same as when a smoker asks him how many cigarettes they can smoke and still be healthy. The answer is zero.

Of course, partially adopting this diet is better than not changing at all. But one should understand that some chronic disease risk is associated with even a small intake of unhealthy foods and additives, as suggested by several studies. And different people will respond differently to unhealthy foods. Some can live till old age relatively disease free in spite of consuming large amounts of junk foods. But the scientific studies clearly show that more of us would live longer, feel better, and have lower healthcare costs if we adopted the healthy lifestyle I am suggesting.

Maybe not so radical, actually

I realize that deciding to adopt all of these guidelines to the fullest requires a *radical redoing* of one's lifestyle. And most people aren't willing to convert to such a lifestyle, even when they know the facts.

But then, considering the likely alternatives, *is it really that radical?* Let's talk about *radical* for a moment, the *radical experiences* in store for so many of us who aren't willing to give sufficient weight to Bible principles and the scientific facts when it comes to making our lifestyle choices.

- Taking a cholesterol lowering drug that has more potential to harm you than to help you, and could result in permanent muscular damage and pain, diabetes, memory loss, and put you in a wheelchair, *that's radical*.

- Having a balloon catheter inserted into an artery in your groin during an angioplasty procedure to improve blood flow in a plaque-obstructed coronary artery, *that's radical*.

- Lying on an operating table while a surgeon splits your chest open to get access to your ailing heart, and your leg open to get access to a vein for use in a bypass, *that's radical*.

- Giving yourself insulin injections daily, *that's radical*.

- For men, losing your ability to urinate normally, getting a biopsy needle stuck into your prostate, and possibly losing your prostate and sexual function to cancer, *that's radical*.

- For women, having painful and embarrassing mammograms, getting painful needle biopsies, and possibly losing your breasts and/or life to cancer, *that's radical.*

- Having painful gallstones and having your gallbladder removed, *that's radical.*[278]

- Submitting to radiation and chemotherapy treatments and suffering the resulting pain and sickness, *that's radical*.

- Suffering helplessly as your joints swell up and your fingers twist grotesquely with arthritis pain, *that's radical.*

- Losing your mind to dementia and Alzheimer's and living

---

[278] Most gallstones are made up of crystalized cholesterol, along with other materials. It is thought that this is from dietary sources of cholesterol (meat and dairy). In one study non-vegetarians were found to be nine times more likely to suffer from gallstones than vegetarians. Greger, Cholesterol Gallstones http://nutritionfacts.org/video/cholesterol-gallstones/; S.B. Pradhan, Prevalence of different types of gallstone in the patients with cholelithiasis at Kathmandu Medical College, Nepal http://www.ncbi.nlm.nih.gov/pubmed/20071875

out your final years not knowing even your closest loved ones, *that's radical.*

Changing **now** to a whole food plant based diet which has great proven potential to help you avoid these experiences, greater than any drugs or medical procedures, well, **maybe that's not so radical after all**!

Motivation

What will help to motivate you to make wise health choices, and stick with it? Here are a couple of ideas:

1. Consider seriously the issue of the stewardship of your body. In light of what you know to be true regarding the impact of diet and other lifestyle factors on health, ask **God what He would have you to do**.

2. Continue to grow in your understanding of these things. Go to the links referenced in this book and read the articles and watch the videos.

These are the main motivating factors for me. **I want to obey what I believe God is telling me to do. And learning about these things and continuing to learn more makes it relatively easy for me to pursue a healthy lifestyle**.

Heading in the right direction

I realize that many don't respond to this information the same as I do. During a discussion about these things with a doctor, he told me that even if he were convinced that eating the way I suggest would add 10 or 20 years to his life, he would still have to think long and hard about it, and he doesn't know what decision he would make, because he loves eating meat so much.

Frankly, in light of what I believe God wants for His children regarding body stewardship, I have a hard time understanding that sort of thinking.

But, as mentioned in an earlier chapter, it doesn't have to be all or nothing. Even small changes, like eating one extra serving of dark green leafy veggies every day, can make a difference in your health. It is often said that it takes three weeks to form a new habit. Our tastes can change, too, if we will just be persistent for a bit of time.

It may be that some day you will find yourself not even wanting to eat the foods and beverages you used to love, but have come to know are toxic.

The palatability angle

Keep in mind that, though making this radical diet move means you will leave behind many cherished tastes, that doesn't mean your new diet has to be boring or bland. There are innumerable delicious recipes out there for whole food plant based dishes. Help is available. Many vegan cookbooks may be purchased, and countless free recipes are available online. (But choose them carefully. Many are not "whole food" based.) Dr. McDougall's website has hundreds of great recipes.[279] And he and his wife have published four excellent cookbooks. Dr. Esselstyn's Prevent and Reverse Heart Disease Cookbook is highly recommended. Dr. Colin Campbell also has published a couple of plant based cookbooks. Lindsey S. Nixon, "the happy herbivore," has a great book for plant based holiday cooking called Happy Herbivore Holidays & Gatherings. You can easily order these online, or check your local bookstore.

It is worth noting, however, that our culture's focus on what might be called the carnal pleasure of eating could rightly be termed hedonistic, as we discussed in the last chapter. **In the hedonistic cuisine of the SAD the effects on health are of little import.** Or claims of healthfulness are made which are bogus, only asserted to make the junk food seem more attractive.

There is nothing wrong with preparing delicious food for your family to eat, food which they like to eat. But we need to increase the importance of the wholesomeness factor, even if that means sacrificing familiar tastes to some extent. And as you persevere in eating truly healthy foods, which previously you

---

[279] McDougall and Mary McDougall, Recipes
https://www.drmcdougall.com/health/education/recipes/

would not have chosen, you will become accustomed to the new tastes and learn to really enjoy them.

We have heard the phrase "the sauce of hunger," which can make even a plain meal extra tasty. I enjoy the food I eat because it tastes good to me, but in addition to that it is all covered with "the sauce of wholesomeness." Knowing it is promoting good health in my body makes it taste even better.

The economic angle

Some fear that it must be more expensive to eat whole food plant based. But think about it. How much does produce cost per pound? Usually between $1 and $3; some staples such as potatoes, rice and beans, which can make up the bulk of a healthy diet, cost less than $1 per pound.

> *The most effective things you can do to achieve and maintain good health don't have to cost anything.*

Compare that to the price of meat and dairy. How much did you pay per pound for that last fish filet you bought? Or that hamburger? Or block of cheese?

And what did you get for your money? Animal protein, fat, cholesterol, hormones, toxins, along with a few vitamins.

Compare that to what you get when you buy beans, beets, broccoli, bananas or berries. 100% nutrition, with little or no toxic baggage – especially if you buy organic. Thus you can expect fewer sick days in the future, and lower healthcare costs.[280] Considering these facts, which is really a better choice from an economic perspective?

Furthermore, some of the least expensive foods are also the

---

[280] *Corporate Wellness Insights, "The Blue Zones": Linking Behavior, Good Health, and Lower Costs* http://blog.wellnesscorporatesolutions.com/2010/02/blue-zones-linking-behavior-good-health.html

most healthy. For example, potatoes, sweet potatoes, brown rice, and beans. You could literally live almost exclusively on these foods, as they provide nearly complete nutrition. And your food bills would plummet.

Some who decide to go meat free may start shopping for meat substitutes, such as vegan bacon, no-meat hotdogs, soy-protein fake chicken, etc. These products can indeed be expensive. And while they are no doubt healthier to consume than their animal sourced counterparts, they are not whole food, so not ideal. You may wish to consume some of these in a transition period to plant based, but I don't recommend they be part of your diet in the long term, because, as mentioned previously, these types of "fake meats" do pose health concerns.

> *The nutrition aisle, if you want to be healthy, you want to just stay off that aisle.*
> *– Janice Stanger, Ph.D.*

When you shop you should avoid the "health food" or "nutrition" aisle. Avoid it because that is where some of the most expensive food is. But more importantly, avoid it because, while food which is sold as especially healthy may be marginally less unhealthy than other processed foods, *it is often still highly processed food!*

If you want to eat healthy, and eat inexpensively, here are the sections of the supermarket, *the true health food aisles*, which you will normally visit:

- Produce aisle – fresh veggies and fruits
- Whole grains and beans aisle – brown rice, quinoa, whole oats, other whole grains, dried beans, lentils, etc.
- Flour aisle – whole grain flour, corn meal, masa harina corn flour, etc.
- Frozen fruits (including berries) and veggies aisle
- Spice aisle

- Canned beans aisle

There may be a few healthy choices elsewhere in the supermarket, but if you follow the dietary recommendations presented in this book you will spend almost all of your shopping time in the above areas of your supermarket.

Another answer to the economic objection is that most of us really do have the money we need to do what we want to do, to buy the things we want to buy. Think about the money you spend going out to eat, going to movies, getting your nails done, paying for that late model car and your fast internet, cable T.V., Netflix, and fancy smart phone service. If you just stop dropping $5 a day on that Starbucks Caramel Brulée Latte, you could easily afford some real good healthy food! **If good health is a priority for you, and if you really want to be a good steward of the body God created for you, you can be sure you will be able to afford to eat well.**

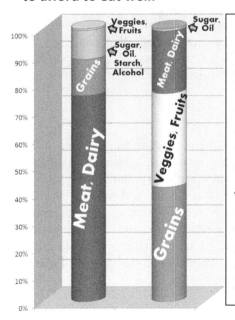

This chart compares the percentage of U.S. government subsidies for industries producing various types of foods (left) with a proportional representation of the number of daily servings recommended by the U.S. government for those same foods. These subsidies enable certain industries to hawk their products extra cheap. What sort of diet is the government really trying to promote?

Sadly, government policy can affect food prices and encourage unhealthy eating. In the U.S., meat and dairy products, as well as sugar and oils, are artificially inexpensive due to large subsidies from the federal government – i.e. from those of us who pay taxes. **If our leaders really wanted to promote good health by encouraging Americans to eat a better diet, and thus reduce healthcare costs nationwide, they would withdraw those subsidies, and if anything subsidize the production of fruits and veggies.** (However, I believe no subsidies would be best of all, since I find no place in our Constitution for government subsidies of any industry. "But they are needed to 'promote the general welfare' of the nation." I guess that's working out real well for us. But I digress...).

The environmental angle

Aside from the personal health benefits, anyone who cares about environmental damage to our planet should consider a whole food plant based diet. This is from the Food and Agricultural Organization of the United Nations (FAO):

> A new report from FAO says livestock production is one of the major causes of the world's most pressing environmental problems, including global warming, land degradation, air and water pollution, and loss of biodiversity. Using a methodology that considers the entire commodity chain, it estimates that livestock are responsible for 18 percent of greenhouse gas emissions, a bigger share than that of transport.[281]

This also from the FAO:

> The livestock business is among the most damaging sectors to the earth's increasingly scarce water resources, contributing among other things to water pollution, eutropication (pollution to bodies of water receiving excessive runoff of fertilizers and sewage) and the degeneration of coral reefs. The major polluting agents are animal wastes, antibiotics and hormones, chemicals from tanneries, fertilizers and the pesticides used to spray feed crops. Widespread overgrazing disturbs water cycles, reducing replenishment of above and below ground water resources.[282]

Raising food animals contributes to more environmental

---

[281] *Food and Agriculture Organization of the U.N.,* Livestock impacts on the environment http://www.fao.org/ag/magazine/0612sp1.htm
[282] *FAO Newsroom,* Livestock a major threat to environment http://www.fao.org/newsroom/en/News/2006/1000448/index.html

contaminants being released into our world than raising plant food. But not only that, raising food animals requires much more land per amount of food produced, as well as eight times more fossil fuels, and contributes much more to land erosion.[283] In many countries livestock production causes a significant amount of deforestation, out of proportion to the amount of food produced, when compared to raising food crops. Grazing and foraging domestic animals are a major contributor to desertification in many countries (which is what the final sentence in the above quote indicates).

Your diet affects the environment

Researchers at Carnegie Mellon University studied the effects of the Standard American Diet and a vegetarian diet on the environment. They found that the environ-mental impact of meat production is so great that if one person on the SAD eats plant based (no animal products) only one day per week, the positive effect on the environment after one year is similar to driving a 25mpg car 1,160 fewer miles. A person eating plant based every day of the year will positively impact the environment similar to driving that car 8,100 fewer miles.

— C.L. Weber et al, Food-Miles and the Relative Climate Impacts of Food Choices in the United States

---

The world's high consumption of seafood poses other significant problems. A large proportion of large fish have disappeared

---

[283] *Cornell Chronicle*, U.S. could feed 800 million people with grain that livestock eat, Cornell ecologist advises animal scientists
http://www.news.cornell.edu/stories/1997/08/us-could-feed-800-million-people-grain-livestock-eat

from the oceans over the past generation, and some say the populations of many species will collapse in the near future.[284] It is simply not sustainable for many people to follow the advice of "experts" who say we should consume more fish. And as discussed previously, fish farming is no solution, whether for the environment or human health.

Animal suffering is of course a major concern of many. And well it should be. In Proverbs we read,

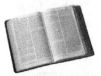

> The godly care for their animals, but the wicked are always cruel.   Proverbs 12:10

Thus it is Biblically legitimate to be concerned about the cruel methods employed in factory farms and slaughterhouses. Were people to witness the immense suffering which these animals often endure, that alone would probably convince many to stop eating meat, if for no other reason than to avoid being a party to the cruelty.[285]

And as to the sheer scope of the suffering, consider that it is estimated that 1,000,000 (yes, one million) animals are slaughtered *every hour* in order to keep Americans on the SAD. If that is how many are killed every hour, how many are living daily in deplorable misery? SAD indeed.

---

[284] Marla Cone, *Los Angeles Times*, Overfishing threatens catastrophe, study finds http://articles.latimes.com/2006/nov/02/local/la-me-oceans-webnov03

[285] The documentary Earthlings has a philosophical premise which Christians cannot embrace, yet if viewed with discernment it will shed vivid light on the stark and horrific realities of the meat production industry, and in the process change how you look at the nice, neat cellophane-wrapped packages in the meat aisle and in your kitchen. https://www.youtube.com/watch?v=ce4DJh-L7Ys

Christian environmentalism

Many Christians are openly skeptical of the reality of any environmental crisis. It's viewed as a liberal issue, or New Age propaganda, or just plain unimportant since this earth will be destroyed after the millennium. What we fail to realize is that Christians have a sacred responsibility to the earth and the creatures within it...

A true Christian environmental ethic...is based on the reality of God as Creator and man as his image-bearer and steward...

Nature has value in and of itself because God created it. Nature's value is intrinsic; it will not change because the fact of its creation will not change...

But a responsibility goes along with bearing the image of God. In its proper sense, man's rule and dominion over the earth is that of a steward or a caretaker, not a reckless exploiter...

Technology puts the creation to man's use, but unnecessary waste and pollution degrades it and spoils the creation's ability to give glory to its Creator. I think it is helpful to realize that we are to exercise dominion over nature, not as though we are entitled to exploit it, but as something borrowed or held in trust. — *Raymond G. Bohlin, Ph.D. in cell biology*
Vice President of Vision Outreach
Probe Ministries

Pregnancy, childbirth and nursing

Pregnant moms can start eating exclusively whole plant foods without worries.[286] This lifestyle is as healthy for babies in the womb and those nursing as it is for anyone!

In fact, a whole food plant based diet has been shown to prevent morning sickness. Some researchers describe this miserable nausea as the body's attempt to eliminate foods which are harmful to mother and baby. Quite frequently these foods are animal products.

Most likely this effect is partially due to the significant reduction in toxic chemical intake when animal products are not consumed.[287] These toxins, which the baby is exposed to whether the mother eats meat or just smells it grilling, frying, broiling, smoking or barbecuing, can cause low birth weight, small fetal head size, and can impair cognitive development later in life.[288] **Pregnant and nursing plant based mothers can take satisfaction in knowing they are eliminating at least 90% of the toxins they would otherwise be passing on to their babies were they still on their old diet!**

Apparently some of the complications and trauma experienced in childbirth are due to poor diets. Some women have found that being on an ultra healthy whole plant diet during pregnancy has enabled them to deliver their babies easily, with relatively

---

[286] Of course, as with all who don't eat animal products, it is important for pregnant and nursing mothers on a whole food plant based diet to take a B12 supplement. One study discussed by Dr. Greger indicated that pregnant vegans may be at risk of iodine deficiency. It is not known, however, whether many of those in the study were on a whole food plant based diet, or just the typical junk food vegan diet. Eating sea vegetables (far and away the best source; 1 tsp. provides your daily needs), cranberries, beans, potatoes and strawberries would prevent any potential deficiency. Pregnant Vegans At Risk for Iodine Deficiency http://nutritionfacts.org/video/pregnant-vegans-at-risk-for-iodine-deficiency-2/

[287] McDougall, *McDougall Newsletter,* The McDougall Diet for Pregnancy https://www.drmcdougall.com/misc/2011nl/jan/pregnancy.pdf

[288] Greger, Meat Fumes: Dietary Secondhand Smoke http://nutritionfacts.org/video/meat-fumes-dietary-secondhand-smoke/

little pain.

And it is important to recognize that your eating habits while pregnant and nursing will usually be transferred to your baby in her preferred food tastes. If you eat a lot of health-damaging junk food, your baby will crave that later when she is on solid foods. If you eat a lot of whole plant foods, your baby will take to that food more readily.

Do your baby a favor. Eat a healthy diet, if for no other reason than your love for her, and your desire for her to live a long, healthy life enjoying the foods which will enable her to thrive.

Healthy habits for your children

If you have children, you now have a wonderful opportunity to help them get started on a life of good health.

Most parents are intentional and strategic in certain areas of childrearing, such as having a regular bedtime, and insisting their children obey and respect them. All too often, however, I have not seen this intentionality when it comes to training children in healthy lifestyle habits.

For example, I have many times seen people serving their toddlers large dessert portions. A child may be just learning to eat solids, yet the parents think it is important that they get their share of whatever sugary treat is available. **In fact what they are doing is building the foundation for a lifelong sugar addition**, setting their children on a course which will likely lead to diabetes, heart disease, obesity, etc.

I know that parents commit this grave error because they love their children and want them to enjoy life, and they don't understand the harm they are doing. They don't realize what is at stake, or understand what a truly healthy lifestyle is all about. But that knowledge deficit must be corrected! Doesn't the principle of love demand this?

If your kids have been accustomed to eating a lot of sweets, white flour, oil and meat, if they have a habit of spending hours every day sitting in front of T.V. and computer games, the transition to the new lifestyle of wise body stewardship may be difficult.

Be careful how you introduce the changes you want to see in your family's diet and other areas of lifestyle. Try to do it in such a way that your children don't develop negative attitudes toward the family's new direction. Go slowly. In some cases resistance might not be avoidable. Don't give up. Pray for guidance, and press ahead, for their sake.

If your children are older and able to understand, it is important to teach them the reasons for the changes you want to make. You want them to support the move and be on board as much as possible. Show them the results of the alternative. Share with them the information in this book in terms they can understand. Talk about relatives and other people they know who are suffering from, or who have succumbed to, chronic diseases. Help them understand why that happened, and the importance of making healthy lifestyle choices.

If your children are good readers, you might have them read this book themselves, or some specific sections of it. Ask them to read it and then explain it to you. Talk it over as a family. Use the Scriptural portions of this book as springboards for family devotions. Ask them what they think the family should do about what you all have learned together. Pray together, asking God for guidance and courage to make whatever changes He is leading you to make.

If as a family you do decide to make some changes, involve the children as much as possible. Look up new whole plant food recipes together. Make shopping lists together and take the kids shopping. Show them how to choose good quality fruits and veggies, and how to read labels intelligently and with discernment. Cook your wonderful new meals together with them, and after eating take a vote on whether or not to keep the recipe.

Carefully leading your children to see the importance of making changes, giving them power to help decide on the direction the family should take, and involving them in implementation, will probably go a long way toward helping them to willingly, even eagerly get on board and be ready for decisive action.

Provide yummy but healthful snacks. (A food dehydrator is a great help in this.) Take a 30 minute walk with your children each day and use the time to memorize Scripture together or talk about other important things. Give them guidance on what interesting and useful things they can do with the hours of time they used to spend glued to a display screen. Model for them and in other ways teach the rewards of investing their time and energies in service to others. Show them that they can enjoy this new lifestyle as you help them understand the significant benefits.

Please, choose now to be intentional regarding training your children in this area. As you model a healthy lifestyle, and talk with them about why you as a family do things the way you do, they will catch it and make it a lifelong habit, which they will in turn pass on to their children.

Sharing with others

If you really catch on to the spirit of the message of this book, if you have understood the significance of the correlation between God's original creation of humans and the perfect lifestyle He established for them in Eden, and the confirmation of this significance which is clearly evident in the results of numerous scientific studies, and if you take seriously the Biblical body stewardship implications for the Christian, you will not only seriously consider embracing the lifestyle, but you will want to share it with others. After all, when you learn something this valuable, even lifesaving, you want those you love to learn it also, and receive the same benefit.

Here are some tips to keep in mind as you interact with family and friends over this important subject.

- Keep it positive. Be cheerful. Let your excitement about your lifestyle show.

- Don't be negative, complaining about the great foods you miss so much but are no longer allowing yourself to indulge in.

- Notice the positive results regarding your health, such as weight loss, improved sleep, or better blood lab numbers, and share these victories with others.

- Don't have a critical attitude toward others' lifestyle choices.

- Be sensitive to others' desire to discuss diet and other aspects of health, or to their desire to **not** do so.

- Keep learning about **why** a whole food plant based diet is the best diet to be on, so that you are ready to share with others in a convincing and interesting way.

- Don't get into useless debates with people whose minds are made up that the diet they are on is fine, even if you know for a fact that it is toxic. Their minds are made up. End of conversation – for now. Pray for them, that they would become more open minded and interested in discussing it in the future.

- Meditate on the spiritual truths undergirding the importance of this lifestyle. Memorize some key Scriptures. You may wish to start with some of the ones discussed in this book. Use them as you share about God-focused wise body stewardship with those who are interested. Who knows? The Lord may use these things to open doors for ministry to others.

- God wants to use you to help others know Him better. And He wants this even more than He wants you to help them change to a healthy lifestyle. So whatever you do, maintain a good testimony with others so that your door of ministry remains open, so that your light shines out into a lost world, that they may see your good works and learn to glorify God in Heaven.

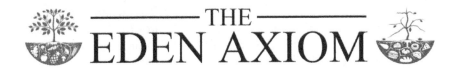

Chapter 15:

Other Topics Related To Health

As we have seen, for good health and long life, diet is king, and exercise, sleep, stress and good relationships with God and others are also very important factors. But there are many more subjects relating to good health which I have learned and which I think are important to understand. I cover some of these in this chapter.

Drugs and medical tests

Keep in mind that I am not a doctor qualified to give medical advice. In the following discussion, as in most of this book, I am merely attempting to share what I have learned, information which has been published by noted medical doctors and researchers. My opinions about what the best medical decision to make might be are based on general trends and probabilities, not on anyone's individual case. It is my hope that you the reader will find this information helpful as you make important medical decisions.

➤ **"Safe" drugs:** Avoid taking any drugs whenever possible. If you think you might need to take a drug, find out what side effects accompany the drug's use, and whether a natural alternative is available. Even the relatively benign NSAIDS (Tylenol, aspirin, Advil, Aleve, Ibuprofen, etc.) can be deadly.

This is from The American Journal of Medicine:

> Conservative calculations estimate that approximately 107,000 patients are hospitalized annually for nonsteroidal anti-inflammatory drug (NSAID)-related gastrointestinal (GI)

complications and at least 16,500 NSAID-related deaths occur each year among arthritis patients alone. The figures of all NSAID users would be overwhelming, yet the scope of this problem is generally under-appreciated.[289]

NSAIDs may temporarily reduce inflammation in order to give your body a chance to heal. But the drugs themselves don't cure anything. And as the quote above indicates, they may do harm as they mask the symptoms of some chronic problem. Yet often doctors will not prescribe an alternative.

An NSAID is anti-inflammatory by definition. So given their dangers, wouldn't the logical course of treatment begin with reducing or eliminating inflammation-causing lifestyle factors? The possibilities are many, such as animal products, oils, sugar, and refined grains; food and environmental toxin sensitivities; and stress. Chiropractic and acupuncture can often help people with chronic pain. A wise doctor will be knowledgeable about all these possibilities and more.

Pain is a symptom, but sometimes a doctor won't make an effort to figure out the reason for the pain. Typically they are allotted a mere 7-10 minutes with each patient, and may have no control over that constraint. So there isn't time to provide the healthcare that really is needed.

We have briefly discussed the dangers of NSAIDS. But these are some of the more benign drugs routinely prescribed by doctors. I think the point is made without going into detail about the myriad much more dangerous drugs commonly used by many, perhaps most, Americans.

➤ **Drugs vs. lifestyle:** Often a disease can be effectively treated by lifestyle modification, yet instead drugs and/or some procedure, such as surgery, is prescribed. But quite often the drug or surgery will not cure the disease, it will simply temporarily relieve the symptoms.

---

[289] G. Singh, *American Journal of Medicine,* Recent considerations in nonsteroidal anti-inflammatory drug gastropathy
http://www.ncbi.nlm.nih.gov/pubmed/9715832

For example, neither statin drugs, heart bypass surgery, nor an angioplasty or stent procedure will ever cure cardiovascular disease. These are merely attempts to put off the inevitable, death by heart failure or stroke. **Lifestyle modification, including changing the diet to include only whole plant foods, and regular moderate exercise, can in fact stop the disease in its tracks.** Furthermore, such a "treatment" is virtually free.

Sadly, all too often with alternative, "natural" medicine practitioners, such as naturopaths, the story is much the same as with conventional doctors. The difference is that instead of pharmaceutical drugs or surgery the solution is often some supplements or other alternative therapy.

Yet, like the M.D., the natural medicine practitioner may not even ask the patient about their diet, whether they exercise, about stress in their life, or how they are sleeping. And often they won't counsel them regarding how they should eat, nor teach them the healing power of a whole food plant based diet.

And naturally so. After all, like doctors, often they are ignorant of how certain foods can adversely affect health, and of the power of whole plant foods to heal.

Also, they may profit by selling supplements to patients, and if the patient becomes healthy through diet and exercise alone, the practitioner loses potential income. Never underestimate the power of a financial incentive.

I have no doubt that many and perhaps most natural medicine practitioners do have good motives, truly wanting to help patients, and not trying to make extra money by selling them unneeded supplements and procedures. But it is a good idea to keep this tendency in mind.

➤ **Drugs and the FDA:** The FDA is supposed to keep Americans safe from dangerous pharmaceutical drugs. There is a process for approving new drugs which drug companies must submit to. However, this process is influenced by politics and money. Much of the FDA's financial support comes from the drug companies. Also, many FDA officials are former drug company officials, and vice versa, so it is impossible for them to be objective. **The foxes are guarding the henhouse, and the hens are in trouble.**

Nowhere has this been more evident than when the FDA has been asked to approve anticancer therapies which originate from outside of the established cancer industry. Dr. Burzynski is a notable example.[290] A gripping documentary was made about Dr. Burzynski's virtual persecution by the FDA.[291] For his novel cancer cure protocol, which was curing many with no dangerous side effects, he was hounded incessantly by the same agency which approves of radiation and chemotherapy treatments which are highly carcinogenic, often ineffective, and often result in severe pain, irreversible damage to the body, and new cancers developing. Obviously politics and big money were involved to provide the motivation for this.

Many drugs have been approved by the FDA thanks to pressure from Big Pharma, only to be taken off the market after patients have been harmed and even killed as a consequence of their use. Vioxx is one notable example of this.[292] Again, the Foxes are guarding the henhouse, and tens of thousands of people who simply wanted pain relief ended up dead. More on the FDA later.

➢ **Imaging tests:** X-rays (dental, chest, etc.), CT and PET scans, mammograms, etc. expose the patient to potentially harmful x-ray radiation, and these cause many deadly cancers each year.

Sadly, the number of CT scans performed each year continues to increase dramatically.

> The use of CT scans, MRIs and other imaging tests has skyrocketed over the last 15 years, leading some experts to raise alarms over the

---

[290] Burzynski Clinic website: http://www.burzynskiclinic.com/
[291] Documentary about the FDA persecution of Dr. Burzynski, Cancer Is Serious Business https://www.youtube.com/watch?v=rBUGVkmmwbk
[292] Drugwatch, Vioxx Recall Information
http://www.drugwatch.com/vioxx/recall/

potential risks of patients' increased exposure to radiation.[293]

Have you ever had a CT scan? Did you know that a CT scan subjects your body to 6-12 times as much x-ray radiation as a standard chest x-ray? Did you know that a CT scan can cause cancer?[294,295]

Of course I am not suggesting these tests should never be done. The risk is small compared with the increased risk of cancer from many other carcinogens, such as those found in grilled and processed meat, which pose a significant threat when regularly consumed. And the risk of not having the scan could be higher than the risk of having it, depending on the situation. The point is to make sure you know what these risks are so you can make an informed decision.

➢ **X-rays and children:** Children are especially vulnerable to damage from x-rays (including CT scans) for the following reasons:

- Children are considerably more sensitive to radiation than adults, as demonstrated in epidemiologic studies of exposed populations.

- Children have a longer life expectancy than adults, resulting in a larger window of opportunity for expressing radiation damage.

- Children may receive a higher radiation dose than necessary if CT settings are not adjusted for their smaller body size.[296]

CT scans are known to increase the probability of serious disease

---

[293] Alice Park, *TIME*, Too Many Scans? Use of CT Scans Triples, Study Finds http://healthland.time.com/2012/06/13/too-many-scans-use-of-ct-scans-triples-study-finds/
[294] *Radiologyinfo.org*, Radiation Dose in X-Ray and CT Exams http://www.radiologyinfo.org/en/safety/?pg=sfty_xray
[295] U.S. Food and Drug Administration, What are the Radiation Risks from CT? http://www.fda.gov/Radiation-EmittingProducts/RadiationEmitting ProductsandProcedures/MedicalImaging/MedicalX-Rays/ucm115329.htm
[296] *National Cancer Institute*, Radiation Risks and Pediatric Computed Tomography (CT): A Guide for Health Care Providers http://www.cancer.gov/cancertopics/causes/radiation/radiation-risks-pediatric-CT

in children:

> Indeed, in a study recently published in The Lancet, scientists found that otherwise healthy children who had multiple CT scans — after falls, accidents or to diagnose infection — were three times more likely to develop brain tumors and four times more likely to be diagnosed with leukemia later on, compared with children who were exposed to less radiation.[297]

So be especially careful that you know the risks and expected benefits associated with any x-ray imaging of your child before you allow such tests be performed.

➢ **Unnecessary imaging tests:** When your doctor recommends you have a screening test it is important that you learn the potential risks of the test as well as the likelihood that it will be of any benefit to you. When the chance of benefit is objectively evaluated, it appears that some commonly recommended screening tests are not necessary, or the percentage of those having the screening who actually derive benefit is so small it does not justify the risks.

Breast mammography is a prime example of this. **Studies have found that women who have regular mammogram screenings die of breast cancer just as frequently as those who don't get screened**, or the difference is statistically insignificant.[298,299,300]

Moreover, many women receive a false positive result, leading to unnecessary anguish and worry. And some of those have useless and traumatic needless biopsies done. So consider

---

[297] Alice Park, *TIME*, Too Many Scans? Use of CT Scans Triples, Study Finds http://healthland.time.com/2012/06/13/too-many-scans-use-of-ct-scans-triples-study-finds/

[298] McDougall, Mammograms and Breast Exams Fail Women Again https://www.drmcdougall.com/misc/pdf/pdf050800nl.pdf

[299] *National Cancer Institute,* Breast Cancer Screening Modalities— Mammography http://www.cancer.gov/cancertopics/pdq/screening/breast/healthprofessional/page5#Section_101

[300] Joann G. Elmore et al, *Journal of the National Cancer Institute,* Efficacy of Breast Cancer Screening in the Community According to Risk Level http://jnci.oxfordjournals.org/content/97/14/1035.full.pdf+html?sid=2f2a6e89-d8a8-4c75-a153-8268aef21da9

carefully whether you want to subject yourself to the pain, expense, and radiation exposure for what some evidence suggests is little chance of benefit.

But even though there is little evidence mammography is helpful, and very unlikely that early detection of a tumor will result in extension of life,[301] the medical community continues to push the message that early detection by such means is the key to fighting breast cancer. I have no doubt that most doctors feel this is the best course to take to truly help women. But in fact the result doesn't seem to be fewer cancer deaths, but rather more cancer patients, and thus more money for the cancer industry. **And what's the real key to fighting breast cancer, which they ignore? Prevention.** Which means adopting a healthy lifestyle, primarily in regards to diet.

Studies have found that women who have regular mammogram screenings die of breast cancer just as frequently as those who don't.

If you do want to get breast imagery done, consider thermography instead of mammography. It does not employ x-rays and is completely harmless.

➢ **Other diagnostic tests:** A PSA test, colonoscopy, biopsy, or imaging test is actually very unlikely to uncover disease early enough to save a life. What many don't realize is that typically the tumor has been growing for several years and may have already spread to other parts of the body by the time it is large enough for a test is able to detect it.

At the same time these tests have the potential to cause much harm – and in fact evidence indicates they do cause harm more often than they help. And this has been known for a long time.

---

[301] McDougall, Early Detection for Cancer Is a Risky Business
https://www.drmcdougall.com/misc/2014nl/aug/early.htm

Note for example this excerpt from an article in the Stanford University News from 2004:

> The most commonly used screening tool for detecting prostate cancer – the PSA test – is virtually worthless for predicting men's risk of contracting the disease, medical school researchers have determined.[302]

Okay, so perhaps the PSA test is worthless, but how can it cause harm? It's just a blood test, after all. It can lead to harm because the results may prompt further testing which is invasive, painful, and which can have serious negative side effects, while at the same time being unlikely to find any cancer which should be treated. See the Mercola and McDougall articles cited below for more on this.[303]

The chances of receiving benefit from some common screening tests are much smaller than you might guess. In fact, studies indicate that the odds of a person's life being extended as a result of a PSA test, mammogram, or colonoscopy are, regardless of the test, much less than 1 in 1000. Yet the odds of harm from undergoing such tests are higher than this. For example, the chances of suffering serious complications from a colonoscopy are estimated to be 5 in 1000.

And of course you can choose to dramatically lower your risk of any of these tests finding disease, and thus make it even more important and safe to avoid submitting to such tests, by adopting a truly healthy lifestyle.

I won't tell you to not get a test recommended by your doctor. But please learn the facts about any screening test your doctor might recommend, evaluate carefully the information, and make an informed and prayerful decision about the best course of

---

[302] Mitzi Baker, *Stanford News,* Common test for prostate cancer comes under fire http://news.stanford.edu/news/2004/september22/med-prostate-922.html

[303] Mercola, Men Who Have this Popular PSA Prostate Cancer Screening Have a Staggering 4-Fold Increase in Serious Blood Infections http://articles.mercola.com/sites/articles/archive/2011/11/07/conventional-prostate-cancer-treatments.aspx

action. Please read the below cited article by Dr. McDougall before submitting to any such tests.[304] The decision is yours, not your doc's.

➢ **Drug studies:** Most research on the effectiveness of drugs is funded by the drug manufacturers themselves. Some require the researchers they hire to sign statements promising to not publicize the study results unless given permission by the drug company. **The drug company has complete control of the results, and can publish or withhold publication at their pleasure**. And they can spin the results to sound more positive than the true facts would warrant. Thus their results cannot often be trusted to be reliable. In fact, surveys have been done comparing drug research studies funded by drug companies with those funded by an independent source. They found that **when a drug company funds a study it is significantly more likely to come up with results which "prove" the drug is safe and effective**.[305,306]

Doctors' knowledge is limited

Why is it that so few doctors make a significant effort to educate their patients regarding the powerful effects the right diet can have on achieving good health? There are several reasons. The first is ignorance. Doctors can't know everything. But why don't they know some of the basics of nutrition that seem so clear to some of us laymen?

➢ **Doctors don't study nutrition:** Good nutrition is foundational to good health. Most of us would assume that medical schools would have as their primary goal to equip future

---

[304] McDougall, *McDougall Newsletter,* Early Detection Testing? Chance of Harm Is 100%; Chance of Benefit Is < 1 in a 1000
https://www.drmcdougall.com/misc/2010nl/feb/early.htm
[305] Greger, Food Industry Funding Effect http://nutritionfacts.org/video/food-industry-funding-effect/
[306] Justin E. Bekelman et al, *Journal of the American Medical Association,* Scope and Impact of Financial Conflicts of Interest in Biomedical Research: A Systematic Review https://iims.uthscsa.edu/sites/iims/files/EthicalIssues-10.pdf

doctors to help their patients achieve good health and stay healthy by a wide variety of means, including through the means of nutrition counseling. Certainly they would if they took seriously the wisdom in Thomas Edison's rather optimistic prediction:

> The doctor of the future will give no medicine, but will instruct his patient in the care of the human frame, in diet and in the cause and prevention of disease.

Very few medical schools in the U.S. offer, much less require, courses in nutrition.

(Perhaps the medical establishment just doesn't think the "future" has yet arrived...)

Yet very few medical schools in the U.S. offer, much less require, courses in nutrition, so few doctors have more than a very few hours of course instruction in this important area, and many have none. My sister's doctor friend, for example, said she had only three hours of nutrition training over the course of eight years of medical school (a three hour *elective* on breastfeeding). Something is wrong with this picture!

Next time you see your doctor, ask them if they studied nutrition at medical school, and if so, how many hours of nutrition courses they took. Unless they specifically pursued an education in nutrition because of a personal interest in the subject, they probably didn't study it much.

It is clear that **most medical schools and most doctors don't believe that good nutrition is foundational to good health**. Or if they would subscribe to that principle, they would not really know what good nutrition is.

➢ **Doctors and drug reps:** Often doctors' medical opinions are formed not only by their official medical training, but also by their ongoing training while they practice, usually spearheaded by drug company representatives seeking to "enlighten" them about the latest therapies. **But of course these reps represent** the financial interests of their respective companies, not the health and wellbeing of patients.[307] So they tell doctors only part of the story. (For example, they might say, "Our fenofibrate drugs are effective at lowering cholesterol," while leaving out the detail that these drugs have not been proven to prevent heart disease or otherwise improve health or lengthen life.)

I would urge you to be cautious about taking a drug just because your doc passes on to you some free samples provided by a drug company rep. Each of us should do our own research and make an informed decision. **There may be a natural alternative out there which is just as effective.** Or more effective, in fact, as in the case of a low-inflammation, whole food plant based diet which will stop and can even reverse heart disease, reverse prostate enlargement and prevent prostate cancer, reverse the progression of type 2 diabetes and arthritis, normalize blood pressure, etc. They have no drugs which can accomplish these things safely and effectively.

➢ **Accurate information about plant-based nutrition is available:** It is not as though it is hard to find authoritative sources or scientific studies demonstrating the powerful effect of whole food plant based nutrition on health. The National Institutes of Health's website PubMed is a source of medical information used by many doctors. Below is the abstract of an article published first in QJM (a leading general medical journal) in 1999, and republished by PubMed. It is a good summary of the medical benefits of avoiding animal products and embracing a whole food plant based diet, and demonstrates that this information is available to doctors. They just generally don't have the motivation or time to seek out this sort of information. (I couldn't resist adding a few notes, in *[bracketed bold italics]*.)

---

[307] Documentary: Cancer: The Forbidden Cures (minute 16:30)
https://www.youtube.com/watch?v=km2cqQNFtEs

Vegetarian diet: panacea for modern lifestyle diseases?[308]

Segasothy M, Phillips PA

Abstract

We review the beneficial and adverse effects of vegetarian diets in various medical conditions. Soybean-protein diet, legumes, nuts and soluble fibre significantly decrease total cholesterol, low-density lipoprotein cholesterol and triglycerides *[as I have found personally]*. Diets rich in fibre and complex carbohydrate, and restricted in fat, improve control of blood glucose concentration, lower insulin requirement and aid in weight control in diabetic patients *[and in fact can make type 2 diabetics completely asymptomatic, if not cured, as proven by Dr. Neal Barnard[309]]*. An inverse association has been reported between nut, fruit, vegetable and fibre consumption, and the risk of coronary heart disease. Patients eating a vegetarian diet, with comprehensive lifestyle changes, have had reduced frequency, duration and severity of angina as well as regression of coronary atherosclerosis and improved coronary perfusion *[as proven by, among others, Dr. Esselstyn's cardiac patients who have adopted a whole food plant based diet[310]]*. An inverse association between fruit and vegetable consumption and stroke has been suggested. Consumption of fruits and vegetables, especially spinach and collard green, was associated with a lower risk of age-related ocular macular degeneration *[since these vegetables provide carotenoid vitamins essential for eye health; plant foods also help prevent damage to and improve the health of the millions of tiny capillaries servicing the eyes; animal products tend to cause inflammation and plaque, hindering the function of these capillaries]*. There is an inverse association between dietary fibre intake and incidence of colon and breast cancer as well as prevalence of colonic diverticula and gallstones *[all plant foods have fiber, no animal products do]*. A decreased breast cancer risk has been associated with high intake of soy bean products. The beneficial effects could be due to the diet

---

[308] M. Segasothy and P.A. Phillips, Quarterly Journal of Medicine, Vegetarian diet: panacea for modern lifestyle diseases?
http://www.ncbi.nlm.nih.gov/pubmed/10627874
[309] Barnard, Dr. Neal Barnard's Program for Reversing Diabetes
http://www.nealbarnard.org/books/diabetes/
[310] Esselstyn, A way to reverse CAD?
http://dresselstyn.com/JFP_06307_Article1.pdf

(monounsaturated and polyunsaturated fatty acids, minerals, fibre, complex carbohydrate, antioxidant vitamins, flavanoids, folic acid and phytoestrogens) as well as the associated healthy lifestyle in vegetarians. There are few adverse effects, mainly increased intestinal gas production *[once your body adjusts to the increased fiber, the problem of gas usually subsides]* and a small risk of vitamin B12 deficiency *[easily dealt with by taking a supplement]*.

➢ **The root of all sorts of evil:** The problem of doctors remaining ignorant of effective plant-based nutrition is, as usual, money (or rather the love of it). Drug companies, as well as the meat, dairy, egg, soda, sugar, edible oil, alcohol and fast food industries (to name a few), have lots of money to invest in promoting the supposed health benefits of, and in downplaying the health risks of, their products. They know that the more money they invest, the more they will make. **So they court medical students from the beginning to help them have a favorable impression of their products.** They provide only the information which casts their products in a favorable light, and medical students and doctors have no time to check out their claims or go searching for a balanced opinion. The dairy industry even courts nursing students, with the goal of recruiting champions of the supposed benefits of lifelong milk and dairy consumption, while not mentioning that most African Americans, and many individuals of other ethnic groups as well, have digestive systems which are unable to properly digest dairy well.[311]

Many doctors are unaware of natural, drug-free cures which laymen use regularly and with consistent success.

➢ **Medical personnel unaware of natural cures:** Often the reason doctors are so quick to prescribe drugs and surgery instead of more benign, natural solutions to medical challenges is that they are simply unaware that alternatives exist. Or they lack confidence in alternative

---

[311] Brenda Davis, Exploding Nutrition Myths
http://www.youtube.com/watch?v=TK36LFVZA7E

therapies because those therapies have not been rigorously tested, and they are not approved of by the American Medical Association nor covered by insurance. It is their medical training which has molded this way of thinking.

This is very sad, because the near automatic prescribing of drugs, procedures and surgeries, without considering legitimate alternatives, does much harm to patients.

➢ **Doctors unaware of d-mannose:** D-mannose is a good example of an effective alternative therapy unknown to most doctors. It is a harmless natural form of sugar found in cranberries and other fruits. It is available in powdered form, and can be dissolved in water and taken to combat urinary tract infections (UTIs) caused by E. coli. The d-mannose passes quickly into the blood, and from there to the kidneys and the urinary tract. It works by making it difficult for E. coli bacteria to stick to the lining of the bladder and urethra. Thus the bacteria are flushed out on urination.[312]

For a person prone to such infections, ½ tsp. of d-mannose per day can reduce the number of infections dramatically, and thus the need for antibiotics. Should an infection occur, ½ to 1 tsp. 3-5 times per day for a couple of days will usually deal with it effectively. This works for any E. coli UTI (80-90% of UTIs are E. coli), and there is no known way for the germs to become resistant and thus render the treatment ineffective.

Yet my doctor, a general practitioner, was unaware of d-mannose, and when I had a severe E. coli bladder infection he had to prescribe an injectable antibiotic. **So instead of taking a few teaspoons of a harmless (and yummy) sugar, I had to stick myself 20 times with a needle over the course of 10 days.**

---

[312] Research Supports D-Mannose for UTIs
https://www.google.com/url?sa=t&rct=j&q=&esrc=s&source=web&cd=18&cad=rja&uact=8&ved=0CE0QFjAHOAo&url=http%3A%2F%2Fwww.d-manoza.com%2Fword%2FResearch%2520Supports%2520D-Mannose.doc&ei=GWo0VbOADNLSoASlrYHgAg&usg=AFQjCNERqkrvlzBuZvbGfUQvqzcjFaSiow&sig2=9gyzZTXcCiLbdRjZJvXiDg

Soon after this a pharmacist told me about d-mannose, and I used it during the next 10 months of urinary catheter use. Typically there is a high risk of UTIs and thus the need for antibiotics whenever a person is using intermittent catheters. But during that time I didn't have to take any antibiotics, though I had many infections. Each one was dealt with easily, quickly, and harmlessly by d-mannose.

Later, I mentioned d-mannose to another family doctor. Though he is very knowledgeable, and an excellent doctor, he also was unaware of it.

I found that all of the urologists I dealt with were aware of d-mannose. But they did not seem to have much confidence in it, and they did not discuss its use till I brought the subject up. **None of their assistants, nurses, or physician's assistants I mentioned it to knew what it was**. Perhaps there is a good reason for all this. But I believe it primarily has to do with the training they received, and the influences on them from colleagues and drug companies.

The standard procedure called for the use of antibiotics, and so that is what was urged on me, in spite of the fact that a better, safer alternative existed. Even if a doctor knows about the effectiveness of treatment with d-mannose, liabilities will play a role in his decision-making, as often there is more fear of lawsuits when standard antibiotic protocol is not followed.

➤ **Doctor unaware of curcumin:** Another natural substance, mentioned earlier, which has powerful anti-inflammatory properties, and has been used to treat serious ailments, is curcumin, found in turmeric. Yet a very knowledgeable medical doctor I mentioned curcumin to had no idea what I was talking about.

Just for laughs...

If healthcare professionals aren't always as well informed as we would like, what about other hospital staff? The following is an actual conversation between myself and the cafeteria lady who brought me my breakfast the morning after I had surgery. I had preregistered for my hospital stay the previous week. One of the bits of info the preregistration nurse asked was regarding food preferences. I explained carefully the foods I can't eat (due to sensitivities). She dutifully typed the info into the computer. But apparently someone missed the memo. Fast forward 8 days...

Cafeteria lady: Good morning. Here's your breakfast.

Me: Thank you. What is it?

French toast.

I can't eat wheat. So I can't eat it.

Oh. (Removes plate cover.) Oh, it's not French toast, it's pancakes. (Starts to leave.)

Well, I can't eat that either, because I can't eat wheat, including wheat flour.

It's not wheat. It's made with white flour.

But white flour and wheat flour are both made with wheat. I can't eat it.

Oh. So you can't eat the raisin bran either? (She's starting to catch on. I become hopeful this conversation will end well.)

Continued next page...

> *...Continued from previous page.*
>
> *No. It's made with wheat bran.*
>
> *So what can I bring you?*
>
> *How about some oatmeal. Raw. Dry. And I can't have that milk on the tray, either. So if you have some grape juice, I'll pour that over it. It's delicious that way.*
>
> *Okay. Do you want some toast with it?*

➤ **Trusting your doctor:** I am not trying to convince the reader to not trust his or her doctors. I use conventional doctors, and they have helped me with medical issues which others could not have cured.

My point is that we must recognize the limitations in any medical discipline. The human body is so complex, and possible ailments are so numerous, that one doctor, or even one whole philosophy of healthcare, such as conventional medicine, can't hope to be able to cover all the possibilities.

So trust your doctor to be sincere about wanting to help you achieve good health. But recognize that there are limits to their knowledge and expertise. No one can know everything. Don't let your doctor pressure you into a therapy that you are not comfortable with. **Get other opinions and seek other solutions.** With the vast resources of the Internet, and your network of friends, you will probably be able to find what you need.

At the end of the day you may realize that the best course of action is to follow your doctor's original advice. But you will do so with more understanding and confidence that you are doing the right thing, and that you didn't miss out on a better therapy.

Doctors' motives for prescribing drugs instead of diet

➢ **Unaware of truth about drugs:** One reason doctors may be ignorant of the true effectiveness of drugs is that, I am told, they typically don't read complete reports on research studies. Who has time for that? **Their knowledge of the expected outcomes of drug therapies often comes from brief abstracts of published studies done by drug companies**, which tend to magnify the efficacy of the drugs and downplay the potential harm the drugs can do. Thus the doctor remains uninformed of the full truth of the potential danger. The real facts may be buried in the full study report, but most doctors rarely read that far.

Sometimes the real facts regarding a drug trial are inconvenient for the drug company, and so are left out of the study report. Thus doctors have no access to this information at all. Naturopath doctor David Getoff tells of a chemotherapy drug study which is a good example of this problem.[313]

A drug company was testing a new chemotherapy drug. The drug company researchers, looking for a favorable outcome, **did not consider in the results the cancer patient subjects who died as a result of taking the chemotherapy drug**. Only those patients who survived to the end of the study period were considered when the results were calculated. Thus the drug was found to have extended patients' lives by four to six weeks. If the 6 or 7 patients whom the drug killed had been considered, the drug would have been found to shorten patients lives by several months, not lengthen them.

But of course this method of arriving at a favorable outcome was quite ethical. After all, the study design clearly stated that all patients who did not remain in the study till its

---

[313] David Getoff, N.D., Nutrition and Health (minute 4:34:20.) https://www.youtube.com/watch?v=TQhlmx7JZ0E. There is much of value in this seminar. However, Dr. Getoff promotes a diet high in animal fat, which the studies cited in this book show clearly to be problematic in many ways.

conclusion would not be factored into the final results.

➢ **Drug company indoctrination, wooing, and pressure:** We discussed this to some extent earlier. This is an interesting quote from the Journal of the National Cancer Institute:

> In 2004, pharmaceutical companies spent an average of $10,000 per practicing American physician on free meals, free continuing medical education (CME) training [read: "indoctrination/ propaganda" - KER], free trips to conferences, and payments for various services, according to data compiled by IMS Health, a company monitoring the industry's finances. Those drug representatives also gave the average doctor an extra $21,000 in free drug samples.[314]

Those figures were doubled from 6 years previously. It is a safe bet that the situation has continued to worsen in the past 10 years.

Doctors don't have time to really research all the pros and cons of some drug therapy, or the latest studies on alternatives to conventional approaches. It's easier to let a drug rep take you to lunch and fill you in on what you should know.

But many pharmaceutical drugs could rightly be called poisons, which are administered in the hope that their therapeutic effects will outweigh the harm they are likely to do to the body. So when a doctor doesn't do adequate research, remains ignorant of the true harm pharmaceuticals can do, and gives in to the urgings of drug reps, he or she violates this provision of the Hippocratic oath:

> I will neither give a deadly drug to anybody who asked for it, nor will I make a suggestion to this effect. Similarly I will not give to a (pregnant) woman an abortive remedy.[315]

➢ **Financial motive:** According to the above cited article from the Journal of the National Cancer Institute, doctors are often

---

[314] John Dudly Miller, *Journal of the National Cancer Institute,* Study Affirms Pharma's Influence on Physicians
http://jnci.oxfordjournals.org/content/early/2007/07/24/jnci.djm097.full.pdf
[315] *GreekMedicine.net,* The Hippocratic Oath
http://www.greekmedicine.net/whos_who/The_Hippocratic_Oath.html

under financial pressure to prescribe certain drugs.

> *Doctors tend to live consistent with their training and convictions, and all too often their conviction is that health is achieved through drugs and procedures; diet receives little serious consideration.*

➤ **Career motive:** Some doctors are required by the clinic or hospital they work for to prescribe a certain amount of certain drugs. For example, **some clinics require their doctors to have a certain percentage of their patients on statin drugs**. One doctor in a video interview I saw testified that she quit working for a clinic for this reason. She wasn't willing to put the required (I believe the figure was) 80% of her patients on statins if that many didn't really need them.

Some patients have testified that their doctors pressured them to take statin drugs, and said they would fire them as patients if they didn't comply. Could this be because the doctors fear for their jobs?

➤ **Personal motive:** One doctor I know, who still takes the conventional approach for the most part, made an interesting comment. He suggested to me something I have come to suspect as I have studied these things: Doctors are unwilling to accept the data regarding diet and health because they personally aren't willing to live lives consistent with the science. **Even if they believe the data, they are still unwilling to change their lifestyle, and they won't inform their patients about the healing powers of a balanced whole food plant based diet because they don't want to be hypocrites.**

Sadly, in so acting, doctors again violate the Hippocratic oath to which they supposedly (or should) subscribe, which states:

I will apply dietetic measures for the benefit of the sick according to my ability and judgement; I will keep them from harm and injustice.[316]

I saw a lot of doctors, nurses and other health care workers in 2013 and 2014, while I was working through my serious health issues, and I was shocked at how many of them were overweight or obese. **But it shouldn't be so shocking. They are simply living out what they believe: health is achieved through drugs and procedures. Diet has little to do with it.** And so they eat what they want and end up fat and unhealthy, and unable to really provide effective preventive healthcare for their patients, because they are not living healthy lifestyles themselves. Very sad.

Drs. Esselstyn, McDougall, Greger, Campbell, Klaper, and Barnard are among the few exceptions. All of them practice what they preach. May their tribe increase.

➤ **Expectation of noncompliance:** One of the biggest obstacles to doctors recommending their patients make more than trivial improvements to their diets is the perception that patients will not consider giving up meat and other toxic food no matter what their doctor says. So why bother talking with them about it? Some have tried, but no one is interested, they say.

One reason for this is that doctors don't take adequate time explaining the importance of making the change, giving information such as that which is contained in this book. They give up after spending perhaps five minutes explaining it to a skeptical patient who has no interest in giving up his chips and burgers. He needs some serious convincing, and the doctor isn't prepared to do that. He doesn't know how, and even if he did, he doesn't have the time.

Another reason patients won't listen to doctors' lifestyle advice is that the doctor himself is not willing to be a role model, a mentor for the patient, who walks the talk. The patient who considers changing his diet has no one to walk with him in the transition, no one who really understands the struggles he will

---

[316] *Ibid.*

face, the opposition from family and friends, the cravings, no one who can really encourage him in practical ways.

Researchers' expectation of noncompliance

Those who research matters of health can also have low expectations regarding the general public's willingness to change their diet for the sake of avoiding chronic disease. Dr. Greger reports that when the National Academy of Science's Institute of Medicine researched trans fat (TFA), they concluded that no intake level was safe. The researchers wrote:

"The present study supports that TFA intake, irrespective of source [i.e. meat, dairy, hydrogenated vegetable oil such as margarine, cookies, etc.], increases CVD (cardiovascular disease) risk... Because trans fatty acids are unavoidable in ordinary, non vegan diets, consuming 0% of energy [i.e. eating no trans fats] would require significant changes in patterns of dietary intake..."

So, that being the case, why did the researchers not recommend a plant based diet? One of the authors of the report, the director of Harvard's cardiovascular epidemiology department explained:

"We can't tell people to stop eating all meat and all dairy products. Well, we could tell people to become vegetarians. If we were truly basing this only on science, we would, but it is a bit extreme."

So their recommendations are apparently based on science plus, and muted by, the perception that the public can't handle the truth.

Again, some doctors are exceptions. Both Dr. Esselstyn and Dr. McDougall have achieved a very high degree of long term compliance to their respective whole food plant based diets, even though the diets are very strict. They hold seminars in which they spend hours or even days going through the science which supports this lifestyle, and even showing patients how to cook tasty food without toxic ingredients. They are role models and mentors to their patients.

Running such seminars is of course expensive, and the financial cost to participants is high. But, again, chronic disease is also expensive. Spending hundreds or thousands of dollars now to learn how to save tens or hundreds of thousands of dollars in the future, not to mention avoid untold suffering and early death, is not an unwise use of money. Really, it is a bargain.

And if you can get the knowledge and motivation you need from their (and others') books, or even from their free articles and video lectures available on the Internet, as I have, it really doesn't have to cost you much, or anything for that matter, apart from some time invested!

Misleading authorities and "experts"

Sadly, many in various fields of the health industry, including government agencies, routinely propagate false notions about diet. In this section we will take a look at a few examples of these, so you can see how conflicts of interest can so easily creep in and lead to distortions of the truths about healthy lifestyles which these groups claim to be propagating.

> **Registered dieticians:** Not surprisingly, a commonly declared mantra of the food industry is "**There are no good or bad foods.**"

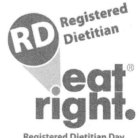

Registered Dietitian Day

"We are concerned there will be a good-food/bad-food approach," said Jim McCarthy, president of the Snack Food [read: "Junk Food" - KER] Association, explaining why he opposes a mandatory rating system [initiated by the FDA]. **"There is no such thing as good or bad food, just bad diets."** [Emphasis added.][317]

This from a man who heads an organization which has as its mandate to get Americans to eat as much junk food as possible.

I guess one would expect such a statement from the junk food industry. Yet diet experts, whom we would expect to be objective, as well as familiar with the latest science on the subject, say virtually the same thing. For example, registered dietitian and American Dietetic Association spokesperson Ruth Frechman said, "There are no bad foods..."[318]

The above referenced article contains a similar statement from the article author, also a registered dietitian:

The truth is **all food** can fit into a healthy diet, even for those with diabetes. [Emphasis added.]

This is an incredibly irresponsible statement. It reassures diabetics and others that they really can keep indulging in their poor eating habits, the ones which caused their diabetes and obesity in the first place.

Presumably these dieticians would caution that one should "limit" junk food, or only eat it "in moderation." But to a food addict, such language is permission from a health authority to not really change eating habits much at all.

As we have seen, most diabetics who adopt a strict whole plant food diet see a marked improvement in their condition, and many are virtually cured of their disease, and need no further insulin or other diabetes meds. But this only happens, or happens most often, if they carefully avoid *all* junk food.

Why don't these registered dietitians mention this important fact for the benefit of their diabetic readers? Instead they

---

[317] *CBS Money Watch,* Candy Makers Fight FDA to Avoid Nutrition Labeling http://www.cbsnews.com/news/candy-makers-fight-fda-to-avoid-nutrition-labeling/

[318] Jill K. Fulk, R.D., L.D., *Ohio Health,* Nutrition: It's a Matter of Fact http://www.medcentral.org/Main/NutritionItsaMatterofFact.aspx

encourage them to go ahead and enjoy their favorite diabetes-promoting foods. *"Moderation is the key."* Whatever that means.

If "bad foods" may be defined as those which erode good health, can the statement **"There are no bad foods"** possibly be true? Well, I suppose so, if the caveat is added, **"unless you eat them."**

➢ **American Dietetic Association:** Not just individual dietitians, but their authoritative 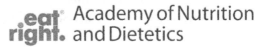 licensing body is also guilty of pumping out misinformation. Also known as the Academy of Nutrition and Dietetics, "the world's largest organization of food and nutrition professionals," states this in their journal:

> It is the position of the American Dietetic Association that all foods can fit into a healthful eating style…. The value of a food should be determined within the context of the total diet because classifying foods as "good" or "bad" may foster unhealthy eating behaviors.[319]

Do you hear the patronizing attitude dripping from those words? We weak-willed and pleasure-driven consumers can't handle the truth about our favorite unhealthy foods, and in fact the truth causes us to make even poorer food choices. So it's best to take the position of denying that any foods are "bad" for us to consume.

Also, and even more amazingly, they declare that should they label certain foods as "good" for us to consume, that, too, might "foster unhealthy eating behaviors"!

Thus this august body of diet and health professionals officially approves of the consumption of toxic foods, at least in moderation. But why? After all,

> **The Academy is committed to improving the nation's health** and advancing the profession of dietetics through research, education

---

[319] Jeanne Freeland-Graves, Ph.D., R.D., Susan Nitzke, Ph.D., R.D., *Journal of the Academy of Dieticians,* <u>Position of The American Dietetic Association</u> http://www.andjrnl.org/article/S0002-8223%2802%2990030-1/abstract

and advocacy. [Emphasis added.][320]

This is what we would expect. But their position on the consumption of foods which are detrimental to health even when consumed in small quantities is not consistent with this stated commitment. Is it just their patronizing attitude which is behind this positon? Apparently the idea that classifying foods as "good" or "bad" will lead people to eat unhealthily is just a convenient excuse. As usual, the real answer is found when you "follow the money."

> The food industry enjoys influential positions in surprising places. The American Dietetic Association (ADA), which, in its own words, is devoted to "improving the nation's health," promotes a series of Nutrition Fact Sheets. **Industry sources pay $20,000 per fact sheet to the ADA and take part in writing the documents**; the ADA then promotes them through its journal and on its website. [Emphasis added.][321]

Just which food industry sources have written these fact sheets? The Berry Board, perhaps? Or maybe the Kale Koalition? No. "The world's largest organization of food and nutrition professionals" needs help in the writing of their Nutrition Fact Sheets from the likes of Wendy's, The Hershey's (chocolate) Center for Health and Nutrition, the Distilled Spirits Counsel, and the Wrigley's (gum) Science Institute, to name a few. Perhaps classifying certain foods as unhealthful and "bad" would antagonize certain corporate partners.

For an in-depth exploration of the ADA's corporate ties and conflict of interest issues, you may wish to read And Now A Word From Our Sponsors.[322]

---

[320] *Academy of Nutrition and Dietetics,* About the Academy of Nutrition and Dietetics http://www.eatright.org/Media/content.aspx?id=6442467510#.VKxkyHtICWQ
[321] Kelly D. Brownell, Kenneth E. Warner, *Yale University, University of Michigan,* The Perils of Ignoring History: Big Tobacco Played Dirty and Millions Died. How Similar Is Big Food? http://www.yaleruddcenter.org/resources/upload/docs/what/industry/Foodtobacco.pdf
[322] *EatDrinkPolitics.com,* And Now A Word From Our Sponsors http://www.eatdrinkpolitics.com/wp-content/uploads/AND_Corporate_Sponsorship_Report.pdf

➢ **American Academy of Family Physicians:** Surely this body would be concerned with our health and prove to be a reliable source of information on diet. However,

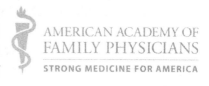

AMERICAN ACADEMY OF
FAMILY PHYSICIANS
STRONG MEDICINE FOR AMERICA

> On October 6, 2009, the American Academy of Family Physicians (AAFP) proudly announced a new corporate relationship with the Coca-Cola company for supporting patient education about healthy eating on the AAFP's public Web site, FamilyDoctor.org.[323]

We have seen above that most doctors are woefully ignorant of basic principles of nutrition. So apparently this group of physicians need help in this area from the likes of Coca-Cola. Unsurprisingly this group also has similar "corporate relationships" with Pepsi and McDonalds. But of course I'm sure that doesn't at all influence any materials they may produce related to "patient education about healthy eating."

➢ **WebMD:** This website is relied upon by many to give helpful information on health, and indeed

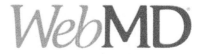

in this book I refer to several helpful articles published there. Yet they approvingly describe a certain diet which promotes the above-mentioned fallacy.

> On this diet, **there are no bad foods, only bad portion sizes**. In other words, you can eat whatever you want -- carbs, meat, fast food, frozen foods, sweets -- as long as you stay within your calorie limits and eat at the right intervals. [Emphasis added.][324]

Of course this diet is focused on weight loss, but the assumption made by the reader will be that they can eat the junk foods they love and still expect to maintain good health. Very sad.

---

[323] Greger, *Nutritionfacts.org,* Academy of Nutrition and Dietetics Conflicts of Interest http://nutritionfacts.org/video/academy-of-nutrition-and-dietetics-conflicts-of-interest/

[324] *WebMD,* The 3 Hour Diet http://www.webmd.com/diet/3-hour-diet

➢ **"Smart Choices" label:** You might see this fancy looking green label on some packaged foods, and get the idea that they are healthy choices. Guidelines have been established for foods with this label, including the maximum amount of sugar, salt, and fat, and the minimum amount of fiber and certain vitamins and minerals.

But consider that these "healthy" guidelines were developed by ten major food producers, including Kellogg's and Pepsi Cola. What might their interest be? Good health or selling product?

So are the guidelines any good? Well, they are if you're one of those food producers and you want to deceive people into buying your products with confidence. For the rest of us, not so much. "Nutritious" "smart choice" foods like Froot Loops, Cocoa Crispies, mayonnaise, and many frozen dinners qualify for this label.

> According to Michael Jacobson, director of the Center for Science in the Public Interest, "you could start out with some sawdust, add calcium or Vitamin A, and meet the criteria."[325]

The lesson here is that we can't trust attractive, authoritative-looking endorsements like this. Read the ingredients label, and put it back on the shelf. Or better, don't venture into any area of the supermarket where the Smart Choices label might be emblazoned on a product.

➢ **The Food and Drug Administration:** One would think that the FDA would be an authority we could trust in matters related to 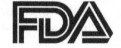 health. And often it is. But financial conflict of interest playing a role in what drugs and food get approved by the FDA, as well as the enormous power drug companies such as Merck have over

---

[325] Dean Andersen, *Spark People*, <u>Froot Loops Qualify for the new "Smart Choices" Label (?!)</u> www.sparkpeople.com/blog/blog.asp?post= froot_loops_qualify_for_the_new_smart_choices_label

FDA decisions, is well documented.[326,327,328]

Quite frequently those making decisions regarding the approval of new drugs have a financial stake in the drug's sales. The FDA has guidelines ostensibly intended to prevent such conflict of interest influencing decisions, on which the life and health of multitudes depend.[329] But waivers are routinely granted to advisory panel members who have a conflict of interest, and thus the decisions regarding which drugs and foods are approved are not infrequently influenced by the financial interests of the food and drug industries.[330]

In addition, many have also seen evidence of conflict of interest and corruption when, as frequently happens, officials and administrators of the FDA, USDA, and other government agencies routinely go to work for food, drug, and biotech companies, and vice versa.[331,332]

---

[326] *Alliance for Natural Health* 2012, FDA's Huge Conflicts of Interest with Big Pharma http://www.anh-usa.org/fda-huge-conflicts-of-interest-with-big-pharma/

[327] Mercola 2009, FDA Admits to Massive Conflict of Interest http://articles.mercola.com/sites/articles/archive/2009/10/13/fda-admits-to-massive-conflict-of-interest.aspx

[328] *Drugwatch,* Vioxx Recall Information http://www.drugwatch.com/vioxx/recall/

[329] For example, Big Pharma giant Merck pressured the FDA into approving Vioxx, a pain medication, in spite of evidence it was not safe. Before it was yanked from the market in 2004, it is estimated that 38,000 people died of heart disease as a result of taking this medication. *Ibid.*

[330] *About FDA,* Percentage of advisory committee members and temporary voting members granted conflict of interest waivers during the quarter http://www.accessdata.fda.gov/FDATrack/track?program=cber&id=CBER-All-commitee-member-waivers

[331] *FDA.gov,* Meet Michael R. Taylor, J.D., Deputy Commissioner for Foods and Veterinary Medicine http://www.fda.gov/AboutFDA/CentersOffices/OfficeofFoods/ucm196721.htm

[332] *Washington Times,* Monsanto petition tells Obama: 'Cease FDA ties to Monsanto' http://www.washingtonpost.com/blogs/blogpost/post/monsanto-petition-tells-obama-cease-fda-ties-to-monsanto/2012/01/30/gIQAA9dZcQ_blog.html

➢ **United States Department of Agriculture:** Many look to the USDA for nutritional guidance. This is the agency of the U.S. government which puts out dietary guidelines such as the "Food Pyramid" and the more recent "My Plate." In a nutshell, their purpose is to promote American agriculture.[333]

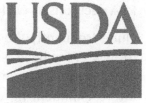

They claim to also be about providing leadership in nutrition, but their nutritional guidelines betray a lack of concern for scientific nutritional evidence in favor of a concern to keep people buying and consuming meat and dairy.

The Food Pyramid, for example, presented the relative amounts of various food groups which should be eaten daily. Included was meat and dairy, as if these were important foods to consume, which contain essential nutrients not available elsewhere. And of course the health hazards associated with consuming these foods was ignored.

The USDA recommendations sometimes lack specifics, and use confusing terminology, similar to what we saw in **Chapter 11** regarding the American Heart Association diet. For example, the "**My Plate**" logo and campaign. This graphic is an improvement over the Food Pyramid, but is still problematic for at least a couple of reasons.

First of all, they imply that one should consume dairy in each meal, as if it is necessary for proper nutrition. We have seen that this is in fact not the case, and in fact that it is hazardous to health (see **Chapter 6: Dairy**

---

[333] *USDA website,* <u>USDA Mission Statement</u>
http://www.usda.gov/wps/portal/usda/!ut/p/c4/04_SB8K8xLLM9MSSzPy8xB
z9CP0os_gAC9-wMJ8QY0MDpxBDA09nXw9DFxcXQ-
cAA_2CbEdFAEUOjoE!/?parentnav=ABOUT_USDA&navid=MISSION_ST
ATEMENT&navtype=RT

for details).

But here again the USDA is bowing to pressure from Big Dairy, instead of acting in the public interest and making truly healthful guidelines consistent with what the science says.

And **secondly**, notice the labels on the four plate sections. Three are specific types of foods. When we see "Fruits," "Vegetables," and "Grains," we have a good idea what it is talking about. But what about "Protein"? What is that? We know "Fruits" are not "Vegetables," and "Grains" are not "Fruits." So what is the implication of having a separate section labeled with the macronutrient "Protein"? One would naturally conclude that the foods in the other food groups don't contain protein, or at least don't contain it in significant, sufficient amounts.

But of course this is not true. One can eat only veggies, fruits and whole grains and get all the protein one needs, even without legumes (i.e. beans, split peas, chick peas, lentils) in the diet.

Even though the protein section is misleading, here the My Plate improves on the Food Pyramid in that meat is not specifically mentioned. Thus the plate is adaptable to either a omnivorous or vegetarian diet.

Interestingly, the year *before* the USDA published the My Plate graphic, the Physicians Committee for Responsible Medicine published their own nutrition plate, the Power Plate, which sports the four whole plant food groups. See the graphic in **Chapter 11: Other diets worth considering**. This plate is the same as My Plate except that the deceptive and dangerous "dairy" circle is left out, and the "protein" section of the plate instead says "legumes." Notice there is protein on every quarter! This is a plate you would do well to fill with food in accordance with its pictures and eat to your heart's content.[334] In fact, your heart will be very content with the *real food* it is receiving. It will

---

[334] *Physicians Committee for Responsible Medicine*, The New Four Food Groups http://www.pcrm.org/pdfs/health/4foodgroups.pdf

thank you for the rest of your long, healthy life.

➢ **American Heart Association:** Mention was made in **Chapter 11** of the clear conflict of interest which the AHA struggles with in making diet recommendations. I will just add a little to that discussion here.

The AHA website lists several dozen corporate sponsors.[335] Most prominent on the list are numerous drug companies, including the giants Bayer, Bristol-Meyers Squibb, Pfizer, and Eli Lilly. Processed food producers such as General Mills are also there. The AHA does not accept sponsorships from candy, alcohol or tobacco companies.

Millions of doctors and regular Americans depend on the AHA for sound health advice. Yet they accept financial contributions from industries which stand to profit if the "right" advice is given. They also allow their "Certified...heart healthy food" label to appear on certain products known to cause heart disease. Read AHA literature with these things in mind.

➢ **The Arthritis Foundation:** The AF claims to be "The largest and most trusted nonprofit organization dedicated to addressing the needs and challenges of people living with arthritis." Their website states: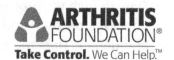

> Our goal is to chart a winning course, guiding families in developing personalized plans for living a full life – and making each day another stride towards a cure (for arthritis).

Under "Treatment" they say,

> There is no cure for RA (rheumatoid arthritis), but there are a number of medications available to help ease symptoms, reduce inflammation, and slow the progression of the disease.[336]

---

[335] *American Heart Association,* Sponsor Thank You
http://www.heart.org/HEARTORG/General/Sponsor-Thank-You_UCM_469280_Article.jsp
[336] *Arthritis Foundation,* Rheumatoid Arthritis: Treatment
http://www.arthritis.org/arthritis-facts/disease-center/rheumatoid-arthritis.php

Note that the first thing they emphasize in the treatment of RA is drugs. Yet no drugs can cure arthritis, and those which promise relief are expensive and have numerous dangerous side effects.

But what the AF doesn't tell the many arthritis sufferers who rely on them for helpful information about their disease is that there *is* ample clinical evidence for a really effective treatment, and for some even a cure, one which is virtually free of charge and unwanted side effects. Moreover, not just a few, but multitudes have found relief from arthritis symptoms using this protocol, many finding themselves cured for all practical purposes. And of course that remedy is simply eliminating animal products and eating whole food plant based.[337]

The Arthritis Foundation in the past has said, *"There is NO special diet for arthritis. No specific food has anything to do with causing it. And no special diet will cure it."* They no longer say this as an official position, apparently, but they do approvingly quote a registered dietician on their website who says, *"...no diet can cure arthritis."* Moreover, they continue the confusion by emphasizing treatment with pharmaceutical drugs instead of food.

However, the AF website does give good advice on reducing inflammation and therefore arthritis symptoms by increasing dietary plant foods, and avoiding certain things such as cheese, meat and omega-6 oils. But I found no recommendations for eliminating these foods entirely for maximum relief.

Furthermore, they recommend increasing consumption of olive oil, which they say is anti-inflammatory. But olive oil is known to cause weight gain, which exacerbates arthritis symptoms.

The AF also recommends fish consumption in spite of its role in promoting inflammation. They claim that fish oil (EPA and DHA) reduces inflammation, and studies have indeed shown it to be

---

[337] McDougall, Diet: Only Hope for Arthritis
https://www.drmcdougall.com/health/education/health-science/featured-articles/articles/diet-only-hope-for-arthritis/

helpful. But borage seed oil (GLA) was found to be just as helpful,[338] and a meta-analysis found that eating fish had no statistically meaningful effect on RA.[339] And toxins in fish, as well as the saturated fat, increase inflammation, of course.[340,341]

The AF website makes brief mention of "a small study" which found that vegetarian and vegan diets can provide relief for some. Otherwise the strongest words one reads promoting the elimination of all animal products for arthritis relief is in comments by readers who have found it to be very helpful!

Strange that the AF all but ignores the best treatment and cure available. Could it be that if people found out how they can get better on their own, they might not need the AF's help or expensive fundraisers any more? Or perhaps they would no longer have as much need for the AF's corporate sponsors, including Johnson & Johnson and other pharmaceutical, supplement, and medical device companies.

So we wonder, is the AF really "addressing the needs and challenges of people living with arthritis"? Should they really be "the most trusted organization" to do this?

➢ **Organizational survival:** Remember that any large organization, such as the ones profiled here, is first of all dedicated to its own survival. Its fundraising often depends on there being large numbers of people whom they can claim as the ones they are dedicated to helping. If a real cure will mean the organization loses constituents, and its reason to exist, they

---

[338] G.W. Reed, et al, *Evidence Based Complementary Alternative Medicine* 2014, Treatment of rheumatoid arthritis with marine and botanical oils: an 18-month, randomized, and double-blind trial http://www.ncbi.nlm.nih.gov/pubmed/24803948

[339] D. D. Guiseppe, et al, *Arthritis Research and Therapy* 2014, Fish consumption and risk of rheumatoid arthritis: a dose-response meta-analysis http://www.ncbi.nlm.nih.gov/pubmed/25267142

[340] Greger, Is Distilled Fish Oil Toxin-Free? http://nutritionfacts.org/video/is-distilled-fish-oil-toxin-free/

[341] Greger, Lipotoxicity: How Saturated Fat Raises Blood Sugar http://nutritionfacts.org/video/lipotoxicity-how-saturated-fat-raises-blood-sugar/

will not want that cure to be found or become known.

Good people work for these outfits, people who really do want to help others, who believe in their cause and methods. But often they don't realize the enormous pressures exerted by conflicts of interest on their organization's policies.

Bottom line: *Know the facts about good nutrition, be careful whom you trust, and don't let anyone, no matter how authoritative they seem to be, deceive you into believing advice which is contrary to the facts, and contrary to sound principles of good nutrition.*

> *It is difficult to get a man to understand something when his job depends on him not understanding it.*
> — *Upton Sinclair*

Cholesterol

There is so much information and misinformation out there about cholesterol. I am by no means an expert, but I hope the following points will clarify for you some of the basics which will help you understand this important substance. Much of this material is controversial. Please remember that these are not my opinions; I am merely reporting what certain authorities in the field have found through solid scientific research.

➤ **Cholesterol is essential – both LDL and HDL:** This fatty compound is essential for human life, and is present in every cell. 25% of the cholesterol in your body is in your brain, which suggests that this substance is quite important for brain health. The cholesterol your body needs is produced primarily in the liver, but also in the brain and in other cells. **All the cholesterol you need you can produce yourself.** You don't need dietary cholesterol to thrive.

➤ **"Good" and "bad" cholesterol:** Much is made of the

difference between LDL and HDL.[342] The one is supposed to be bad for you, because it is more strongly associated with heart disease. The other is good for you as it has a role of eliminating unneeded LDL. Some substances such as fats and oils, especially trans fat, tend to increase your LDL level, others tend to increase your HDL, and having a high LDL/HDL ratio is said to increase your risk of heart disease. Thus the conventional wisdom is that you should make dietary and drug therapy choices based on what will both lower your blood level of LDL and raise your blood level of HDL.

There is some truth to some of these notions, but the situation is not as simple as it is often made out to be. For example, the assumption of many doctors and researchers is that higher HDL concentration in the blood is good, because of its role in disposing of LDL. However, the blood level of HDL has been shown to be irrelevant to its ability to perform this function.[343,344] **Thus, even though a whole food plant based diet will typically result in lower blood levels of both LDL and HDL, this is not a cause for concern.**

Furthermore, a pharmaceutical drug was tested which was very efficient at raising blood levels of HDL, yet the trial was stopped early because **the drug was killing patients**, in spite of the fact that their HDL was rising considerably.[345]

---

[342] It should be noted that technically speaking, LDL and HDL do not refer to two different types of cholesterol. They refer to different types of lipoproteins, or fatty proteins, which attach themselves to cholesterol in order to transport it to wherever it needs to go in our bodies.

[343] Esselstyn, *Experimental and Clinical Cardiology*, The Nutritional Reversal of Cardiovascular Disease, Fact or Fiction? Three Case Reports http://www.dresselstyn.com/Esselstyn_Three-case-reports_Exp-Clin-Cardiol-July-2014.pdf

[344] Amit V. Khera et al, *New England Journal of Medicine*, Cholesterol Efflux Capacity, High-Density Lipoprotein Function, and Atherosclerosis http://www.ncbi.nlm.nih.gov/pmc/articles/PMC3030449/

[345] Matthew Herper, *Forbes*, Failure of Roche HDL Booster is Bad News for Merck and Eli Lilly http://www.forbes.com/sites/matthewherper/2012/05/07/failure-of-roche-hdl-booster-is-bad-news-for-merck-and-eli-lilly/

There is also evidence that the SAD produces an environment in the body which causes damage to the HDL molecule, rendering it incapable of doing its job, and making it a pro-inflammatory agent which promotes injury.[346] Thus **many people with high HDL blood levels still suffer from cardiovascular disease.**

I don't believe it should be necessary to understand all the details about LDL and HDL in order to have optimal cholesterol levels and avoid heart disease. There have been in the past and there are to this day many societies where heart disease is very rare, where they live long, healthy lives free of heart disease. Yet no one in these places has even heard about cholesterol. Why is it that we must be so worried about this substance?

If you are on the SAD, there may be reason for you to worry about cholesterol. But it is clear that for most people who eat a whole food plant based diet, and make a good effort to live by the other healthy principles I have discussed in this book, they can forget about their cholesterol. Their bodies will take that great fuel they are feeding it and regulate their various cholesterols to their optimal levels, levels just right for them, without them even having to think about it. I can't say this is necessarily true for everyone. But normally, for most of us, I believe there is ample evidence that this is the case.

➢ **"Fluffy" and "dense" LDL:** Some also consider the difference between "large/fluffy" LDL and "small/dense" LDL to be of great importance. Again, for a person on a whole food plant based diet, it doesn't matter, because their diet will contain no cholesterol at all. Even for meat eaters, the difference is only marginal, that is, studies have found that food sourced "fluffy" LDL appears to be only a little less dangerous than food sourced "dense" LDL.[347] The point is, both promote poor health, and both can be avoided by not eating foods containing cholesterol,

---

[346] Navab, et al, *Nature Reviews,* Cardiology HDL and cardiovascular disease: atherogenic and atheroprotective mechanisms
http://www.ncbi.nlm.nih.gov/pubmed/21304474
[347] Greger, Does Cholesterol Size Matter? http://nutritionfacts.org/video/does-cholesterol-size-matter/

i.e. animal products.

➤ **Especially bad dietary cholesterol:** There is a type of cholesterol which is especially dangerous, according to Dr. Duane Graveline. This is *oxycholesterol*, cholesterol which has been oxidized. Cholesterol is oxidized by being exposed to oxygen. And that happens whenever cholesterol-containing substances, such as meat and dairy products, are exposed to the air.

Oxidized cholesterol has been shown to cause significant vascular disease, as it does serious damage to endothelial cells, promoting the formation of plaque. This is why in early cholesterol experiments, when rabbits were fed rabbit feed loaded with extra cholesterol, they were so quick to develop arterial disease. The cholesterol in their feed, having been exposed to the air, had become oxycholesterol.

The most significant exposure of dietary cholesterol to the air is in milk and egg powder. Powdered eggs were found to contain 60 times as much oxycholesterol as fresh eggs. And it is important to note that probably most processed food products which contain eggs and/or dairy contain dried, powdered forms of these foods, since they are so much cheaper than fresh.[348] Is there any end to the reasons to avoid processed foods?

➤ **Plants and cholesterol:** No plants or plant products contain cholesterol. However, when plant products such as oils are processed and/or cooked in certain ways, this may produce a product such as trans fat which when consumed stimulates a jump in blood cholesterol levels, and more importantly, a jump in inflammation and damage to endothelial cells. Hence the importance of a *whole food* plant based diet, which by definition avoids extracted fats and oils, whether from plant or animal sources.

➤ **Dietary cholesterol:** Many experts say that when you eat cholesterol, i.e. animal products, your body compensates and

---

[348] Dr. Duane Graveline, M.D., M.P.H., Cholesterol: The Good and the Bad
http://www.spacedoc.com/cholesterol_good_bad.html

scales back production, so that your blood levels of cholesterol remain fairly stable. That may be true for some people, but for many it is not true, as their total cholesterol level drops when they switch to eating only plants, that is, when they eat no cholesterol.

For example, eating an omnivorous diet I was getting an overdose of cholesterol, and my liver apparently didn't notice and adjust, since my total cholesterol level was up at about 300. A whole food plant based diet brought that figure down to 182 within 18 months.

And this is by no means an unusual result. Dr. McDougall tested the cholesterol levels of over 1600 patients in a study to see the effect of diet on several health parameters. After just seven days of eating as much as they wanted of only whole plant foods, the patients' cholesterol levels had dropped by an average of 22 points. (They also lost an average of 3.1 lbs., and the blood pressure readings of participants with hypertension went down by an average of 18/11 mmHg. Nearly 90% were able to get off their blood pressure and diabetic meds.)[349]

People whose cholesterol is in a more "normal" range on an omnivorous diet, when they switch to a whole food plant based diet commonly see their cholesterol drop to below 150, which is the magic number which many doctors look for since it is often associated with an extremely low chance of cardiovascular disease.

➤ **Cholesterol and saturated fat:** One can find some studies which conclude there is no relationship between dietary saturated fat intake, cholesterol levels, and vascular disease risk. Proponents of low carb diets such as Atkins latch onto such evidence to justify their approach to achieving weight loss and good health.

However, it appears that their argument is based on the results

---

[349] McDougall, The McDougall Program Cohort: The Largest Study of the Benefits from a Medical Dietary Intervention
https://www.drmcdougall.com/misc/2014nl/oct/141000.htm

of cross-sectional observational studies. Dr. Greger explains how this is an invalid conclusion, since cross-sectional studies do not have the power to detect such a relationship. Rather,

> ...the appropriate [study] design demonstrating or refuting the role of diet in coronary heart disease is a dietary change experiment. And those dietary change experiments have been done, they implicate saturated fat, and hence the lower saturated fat guidelines from basically every major medical authority.[350]

Please see the referenced Greger video for an explanation of the difference between these types of studies.

Dietary saturated fat from animal sources has been shown repeatedly to raise blood cholesterol and inflammation and promote vascular disease.[351,352] See more on saturated fat in **Chapter 7: Animal fats**.

➢ **Cholesterol and heart disease:** Though there appears to be a correlation between high cholesterol and cardiovascular disease, some in the field are convinced that it isn't the cholesterol in and of itself that causes the disease. Here is what they say: A person eats meat and dairy, which contain animal protein and saturated fat. These substances cause inflammation in the body. This inflammation stimulates the liver to produce more cholesterol, because the cholesterol is needed to deal with the inflammation.

> Cholesterol level reflects chronic inflammation in your body; the more inflammation you have, the higher your total cholesterol tends to be. Your body makes cholesterol to "patch up damages" from this ongoing inflammation.[353]

The result of the inflammation in the blood vessels is damage to

---

[350] Greger, The Saturated Fat Studies: Set Up to Fail
http://nutritionfacts.org/video/the-saturated-fat-studies-set-up-to-fail/
[351] Ibid.
[352] Greger, The Saturated Fat Studies: Buttering Up the Public
http://nutritionfacts.org/video/the-saturated-fat-studies-buttering-up-the-public/
[353] Mercola, Making Sense Out Of Your Cholesterol Numbers
http://articles.mercola.com/sites/articles/archive/2010/08/10/making-sense-of-your-cholesterol-numbers.aspx

the endothelium and the formation of plaque. This process involves cholesterol, and thus this substance is assumed to be the cause of the problem.

If the inflammation theory is correct, it may be more accurate to say that inflammation, not high cholesterol, causes plaque and cardiovascular disease. Or possibly it is a combination of the two factors. In any case, a focus on blood cholesterol numbers, rather than on inflammation, seems to have led doctors to the wrong solution: the reduction of cholesterol levels via the use of drugs, especially dangerous statin drugs. The right solution, of course, is to emphasize the severe restriction of inflammation producing foods like meat, dairy, sugar, oils, and refined flour.

A person with arterial plaque may remain asymptomatic as long as the plaque stays put, and doesn't build up to the point of seriously restricting blood flow. But further damage to the endothelium due to a poor, inflammation-producing diet, may cause the plaque to break loose and block the artery, causing angina, heart attack, stroke, etc. **Thus it seems the most critical factor in avoiding heart disease is maintaining a healthy endothelium, not achieving low blood cholesterol.**

➢ **Palliative care:** Many doctors are doing their best to help their patients. But others in the industry continue to promote the cholesterol-centric approach to treating cardiovascular disease risk, primarily because there are billions of dollars to be made selling cholesterol-lowering, blood thinning, and other cardiovascular disease-related drugs,[354] as well as in performing stent and angioplasty procedures and heart surgeries.

They support their promotion of these drugs and procedures with scientific studies which show they work. But do they? Really? Well, yes, I suppose they work better than doing nothing. But do they cure, or do they just help a person live longer in a diseased state? And do they give the patient the

---

[354] Rachel Cooper, *The Telegraph,* Statins: The Drug Firms' Goldmine http://www.telegraph.co.uk/health/healthnews/8267876/Statins-the-drug-firms-goldmine.html

impression that all that can be done is being done, and so he doesn't look further, to discover that a much more effective treatment is available?

Cardiologists know how to do palliative care, relieving some of the pain and stress of heart disease while they wait for the inevitable. But they don't know how to cure. Their patients still suffer and die of heart disease. **The most charitable explanation of this that I can think of is that the cardiologist doesn't know that the primary cause of the problem is toxic food, and that the only cure is healing food, along with other lifestyle changes, not drugs and medical procedures.**

➤ **The end of an industry?:** If Americans en masse adopted a heart-healthy whole food plant based diet, the cardiology departments of every hospital and medical school would collapse for lack of patients.

But, sadly, that's not likely to happen any time soon, because it seems that most people would rather pop pills and submit to invasive procedures than change their lifestyle, and the people to whom they entrust their medical care continue to keep them in the dark. If they knew all the facts, however, such as that the drugs and surgeries can't stop the disease, while a radical change in diet can, I suspect that many would opt for the diet strategy.

➤ **Statin drugs – Miracle cure?:** Statin drugs such as Lipitor and Crestor are often hailed as the miracle cure for high cholesterol, and therefore heart disease. They certainly are effective at lowering cholesterol. But do the lower cholesterol numbers themselves help prevent heart disease?

As we have seen, there is reason to doubt this. In fact, some researchers now suggest that statin drugs work at preventing cardiovascular disease (to whatever small measure they do) not primarily because they lower cholesterol in the blood, but rather because of their anti-inflammatory effects – though perhaps the latter is the cause of the former. But if it is indeed a lowering of inflammation which is helpful, and considering the well-known dangers of statin drugs, wouldn't it be more prudent to recommend a more safe anti-inflammatory treatment protocol – like a change in diet, perhaps?

> **Effectiveness of statin drugs:** In evaluating the effectiveness of a drug or other therapy, researchers and doctors consider the number of patients which must be treated by the therapy before there can be an expectation that one patient will benefit. This is known as the Number Needed to Treat (NNT). If a given drug helped every patient who took it for a given condition, the NNT would be 1. If it helped 25% of patients, the NNT would be 4. So you can see that the higher the NNT, the less effective the treatment, and the more important the consideration of unwanted side effects becomes.

Anywhere from 30 to 100 people must be treated with a statin drug before one will derive benefit. Yet all of them are at risk of painful and debilitating side effects.

Studies have shown that the NNT for statin drugs is anywhere from 30 (for heart disease patients) to 100 (for healthy people). And these figures assume the patients are taking statin drugs for several years, i.e. it's only after several years on the drugs that one person in 30 to 100 is expected to benefit.[355]

You read that right. If you are a healthy person, without heart problems, but a statin drug is prescribed for you, you have only about one chance in 100 of that drug providing any benefit to you at all. i.e. sparing you of a cardiac event such as a heart attack.

Now, if a treatment is cheap or free, and totally benign and without side effects, then it might be wise to submit to it in

---

[355] Andrew Thompson, Ph.D. and Norman J Temple, Ph.D., *Journal of the Royal Society of Medicine,* The case for statins: has it really been made? http://www.ncbi.nlm.nih.gov/pmc/articles/PMC1079612/

order to reduce the risk of a serious health problem by even a small amount. But statin drugs are not benign, and they are not cheap. So a cost benefit analysis should be done before taking statin therapy. You must decide if the known cost to your wallet, and the likely cost to your health, is worth the tiny chance of benefit.

In fact, all who take statins are at risk for side effects. These include muscle pain and weakness, CoQ10 deficiency, liver damage, and other problems.

While drug companies and doctors commonly assert that only a very few suffer side effects from taking statins, many critics have found evidence that the number of those reporting side effects in the published studies is much lower than the number in the real world. Not only that, but

> A recent study, with electron microscopy and biochemical approaches, examined the muscle tissues of patients on statins. They found muscle cell damage in over 70% of people on statins, *even when they had no complaints of pain.*[356]

So statin therapy is unlikely to help you, and quite possibly will harm you.

Just how ridiculously low the effectiveness of statin drug therapy is can be easily seen when one compares it with the effect of diet changes. For example, a certain statin drug therapy was estimated to be 3.1% effective in preventing symptoms of heart disease over a 6 year period. However, Dr. Esselstyn has reported that his heart attack proof diet has proven to be over 20 times more effective than that! Over 99% of his heart patients who followed his diet faithfully (each of whom had serious heart disease) avoided further cardiac events over an average study period of 3.7 years (one person had a stroke), while 62% of those which did not stay on the diet had

---

[356] McDougall, Who Should Take Statins?
https://www.drmcdougall.com/misc/2007nl/may/statins.htm

such events.[357,358] Which therapy would you choose? Yet doctors rarely give patients a choice.

➢ **Statin drugs – How they work:** Statin drugs work by hindering the body's ability to produce cholesterol, primarily in the liver and brain. But it is not only cholesterol production that is hindered.

Wherever cholesterol is produced, whether in the liver, brain, or elsewhere, the process involves a long chain of compounds, each one forming the foundation for the next. Cholesterol is just one of the several final products of this chain. **Statin drugs interfere with this chain early on, so that the rest of the chain is affected, including the synthesis of other important compounds besides cholesterol.**

> From CoQ10, to dolichols, to normal phosphorylation and to selenoprotein synthesis, all are affected by the broad reach of statins. Side effects on muscle, nerve and memory functions are not some extremely rare, almost unique, problem. They are all but inevitable with the use of mevalonate inhibitors.[359]

The diagram below should help make this connection clear.

In the above quote Dr. Graveline mentioned Coenzyme Q10, or CoQ10, an antioxidant which is critical for cellular energy. Much has been written in the past few years about the dangers of CoQ10 deficiency. Statin drugs cause this dangerous condition.

Dr. Graveline was NASA flight controller for the Mercury and Gemini program in the 1960s, and later served as a scientist astronaut.[360] He suffered temporary memory loss as a result of statin drug use (Lipitor), and has since done extensive research into the side effects of statin drugs. He had this to say regarding statin drugs' interference in CoQ10 production:

---

[357] Greger, The Actual Benefit of Diet vs. Drugs
http://nutritionfacts.org/video/the-actual-benefit-of-diet-vs-drugs/
[358] Esselstyn, A way to reverse CAD? http://www.jfponline.com/fileadmin/qhi/jfp/pdfs/6307/JFP_06307_Article1.pdf
[359] Dr. Duane Graveline, M.D., M.P.H., Lipitor® Side Effects
http://www.spacedoc.com/lipitor_side_effects.htm
[360] Spacedoc.com, Duane Graveline M.D. M.P.H. Biography
http://www.spacedoc.com/Graveline_bio.htm

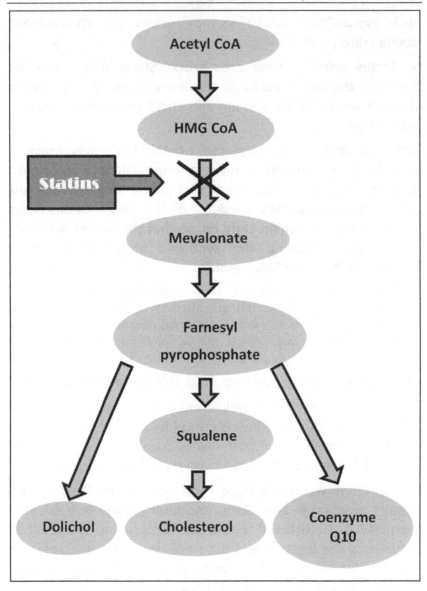

The implications of this were well known to the pharmaceutical industry from the very beginning of statin development. CoQ10 is arguably our most important essential nutrient. Its role in energy production is to make possible the transfer of electrons from one protein complex to another (within the inner membrane of the mitochondria) to its ultimate recipient, ATP (adenosine triphosphate.)[361]

ATP is the body's "energy currency," critical for all metabolic functions. If something hinders its production in sufficient quantities, energy production is bankrupt, and numerous serious complications can result. Please read Dr. Graveline's full article if you would like to better understand the danger this situation presents to the statin drug user.

As you can see from the chart, synthesis of the compound **dolichol** is also suppressed by statin drugs. Dr. Graveline wrote about this problem as well:

> The dolichols are another area of collateral damage from statin use. This class of compounds is involved in an intricate process of cellular activity involving message transport.
>
> Proteins manufactured there in response to DNA directives are packaged into transport vesicles that are shuttled across the cytoplasm to their various destinations. Without dolichols there would be intracellular chaos as various proteins could not be directed to their proper target and would, in effect, be dead-lettered. The post office analogy, though childishly simple, comes very close to describing dolichol's function as we understand it today.[362]

We know how inconvenient it is when the U.S. Post Office doesn't work well. How much more serious it is when our body's own intracellular "post office" malfunctions!

➢ **Statin drugs – The fructose problem:** Fifty percent of table sugar is fructose. Over 55% of high fructose corn syrup is fructose. Most sugar sweeteners found in food contain fructose.

This fructose, when consumed in concentrated form, i.e. from a source other than whole plant foods, is treated much like a toxin in the body. The liver is the organ which metabolizes most of the fructose. But statin drugs hinder the liver's ability to perform this function. If your liver is not able to metabolize the fructose

---

[361] Dr. Duane Graveline, M.D., M.P.H., Statins and CoQ10 Deficiency
http://www.spacedoc.com/statins_CoQ10.htm
[362] Graveline, A Critical Review of Statins
http://www.spacedoc.com/statins_a_critical_review.htm

Taking a statin drug increases a person's risk of Alzheimer's by over two and a half times.

you eat, it will continue to be like a toxin in your body. But your body has a back-up plan, thanks to our wise Creator.

When statin drugs render the liver unable to metabolize fructose, the skeletal muscles assume the responsibility. This deals with the problem of unprocessed fructose in the body, but it also wears out the muscle cells. In effect, the muscle cells sacrifice themselves to prevent a greater danger – the continued presence of high levels of fructose in the blood. That is why muscle weakness and pain is sometimes a side effect of statin use, and 70% of statin users were found to have muscle damage. In effect, **statin drugs accelerate the body's aging process.**[363] Some experience so much muscle weakness that they end up in a wheelchair as a result.[364]

➤ **The importance of cholesterol in the body:** The liver produces cholesterol for a reason. Your body needs it. It is critical for vitamin D synthesis, sex hormone synthesis, dealing with inflammation, and many other things.

God designed the liver, and created it to produce cholesterol (among other functions). **Before we take a drug that hinders God's intended function, we better be very sure we know what we're doing!**

Cholesterol is also important for proper brain function. In fact, 25% of the cholesterol in your body is in your brain. But cholesterol produced in the liver cannot cross the blood brain

---

[363] Stephanie Seneff, Ph.D., How Statins Really Work Explains Why They Don't Really Work
http://people.csail.mit.edu/seneff/why_statins_dont_really_work.html
[364] Jo Waters, *The Daily Mail,* The other side of statins: They've saved countless lives - but now doctors fear for some, the side effects could be devastating http://www.dailymail.co.uk/health/article-1262130/Statins-Doctors-fear-effects-devastating.html

barrier. So the brain is also an important manufacturer of this life-giving substance.

The problem is that some statin drugs not only work to hinder cholesterol synthesis in the liver, they also work in the brain. Not only cholesterol, but also dolichols and CoQ-10 production is affected. This helps explain why statin users are at increased risk of memory loss and other debilitating brain problems.

Senior MIT research scientist Stephanie Seneff, Ph.D., wrote about the likely connection between statin use and Alzheimer's revealed in a population based medical study:

> More alarmingly, people who used to take statins had a hazard ratio of 2.54 (over two and a half times the risk to [sic] Alzheimer's) compared to people who never took statins.[365]

In her article she explains the suspected mechanism of this effect. And she adds that it appears that once the statin drug has gotten the process of Alzheimer's going, stopping statin use does not stop the progression of the disease. The deterioration of the patient's cognitive function continues till death.

So really, should we be messing with the chemistry God built into our bodies, destroying the delicate balance of how important compounds are produced, by throwing a statin wrench into the works, for the purpose of limiting the amount of cholesterol in the blood, with the goal of preventing a disease which some evidence indicates cholesterol doesn't cause in the first place? And all that when simply changing the diet would accomplish the desired reduction in inflammation, cholesterol levels and vascular disease without the bad side effects!

Of course many doctors and others will disagree with this characterization. **The data is available for you to peruse. You decide what is right for your health.**

➢ **Statin drugs – Other side effects:** So far we have discussed a few of the side effects of statin use, the most common of which

---

[365] Stephanie Seneff, *Spacedoc.com,* A Recipe for Alzheimer's Disease
http://www.spacedoc.com/recipe_alzheimers_disease

is muscle pain and weakness.

Many more have been documented. These include increased risk of myotoxicity[366] (damage to energy-producing mitochondria), increased liver enzymes (a sign of damage to the liver), cataracts, mood disorders, dementias, hemorrhagic stroke, peripheral neuropathy (numbness, weakness, burning pain, and loss of reflexes in the limbs) and new-onset diabetes.[367]

Diabetes alone is bad enough, but it in turn increases the chances the patient will develop heart disease. So the drug which is prescribed to prevent heart disease can in certain people actually encourage it to develop!

Did your doctor tell you about all these possible side effects before you agreed to take statin drugs? Probably not. Mine certainly didn't.

Some doctors aren't aware of all of the possible side effects, nor the true likelihood their patient will suffer any one of them. But even if they are familiar with the side effects, often they are convinced that heart disease is more worrisome than the side effects of statins. So they don't fully inform the patient, lest the latter decide out of fear to not take the drug.

➤ **A couple of questions for your doctor:** If your doctor tells you that you need to begin taking a statin drug, or if he already has you on one, you might consider asking him these questions:

- Why is it that millions of Americans need statin drugs, while billions of people in the past lived long lives free of cardiovascular disease, without ever taking a statin pill?

- And why is it that in many cultures today, heart disease is rare, yet no statins are used?

---

[366] A. N. Baer, R. L. Wortmann, *Current Opinion in Rheumatology,* Myotoxicity associated with lipid-lowering drugs
http://www.ncbi.nlm.nih.gov/pubmed/17143099
[367] C. N. Bang, P. M. Okin, *Current Cardiology Reports,* Statin treatment, new-onset diabetes, and other adverse effects: a systematic review
http://www.ncbi.nlm.nih.gov/pubmed/24464306

Is heart disease a statin-deficiency disease? No, it is a whole plant food deficiency disease. When whole plant foods do not comprise the total diet, they are replaced to some degree or another by foods which not only lack the protective properties of whole plant foods, but also contain substances which actively promote vascular disease.

While the NNT of statin drugs is anywhere from 30 to 100, the NNT of the one truly effective therapy for cardiovascular disease is 1.

Every person who adopts a whole food plant based diet will benefit and lower their chance of suffering from heart disease, as well as all other vascular diseases – stroke, Alzheimer's, macular degeneration, backache, etc. **Every. Single. One. Period.** That's not to say every single one will be completely cured. But every one will benefit to some extent, many dramatically. The clinical evidence is clear.

"Ask your doctor of whole plant foods might be right for you."

But alas, there is no way to make gobs of money selling produce, while billions of dollars are made by selling expensive drugs and medical procedures and surgeries. And they advertise their products and services constantly, while the real cure remains relatively obscure, and is entirely unknown to most people. When was the last time you saw an ad for kale or potatoes?

➢ **Fenofibrate fail:** I would like to share with you my experience with cholesterol lowering drugs as an example of what can so often happen when doctor and patient are not sufficiently informed.

Several years ago a doctor put me on Lipitor because my cholesterol level was over 300. I knew very little about this drug, but the doctor told me it could damage the liver. So after starting Lipitor I had my liver checked as per normal procedure. No damage detected. So far so good.

However, just a few weeks later a friend told me his experience with the same drug. After being on it for a while his urine turned brown. "I was peeing out my liver," he said. That's when I determined to never pop another statin pill. I knew there had to be a better way to manage high cholesterol and heart disease risk.

I made a somewhat halfhearted attempt to increase my exercise level and reduce cholesterol intake, all without noticeable impact on my cholesterol numbers.

Some years later another doctor saw my cholesterol numbers and wanted me to take a statin. I declined. So he suggested a drug called fenofibrate to lower my cholesterol. He said it is more benign than statins, and works like a sponge to mop up cholesterol in the blood. It was effective at lowering my cholesterol (to 227). And I spent a lot of money buying this drug over the years.

Then, in 2013, I learned that **fenofibrate drugs actually do cause some bad side effects.**[368] Furthermore, there doesn't appear to be any solid evidence that, **in spite of their ability to lower cholesterol, they can prevent vascular disease or decrease overall mortality.**

So why did I spend several hundred dollars over several years, risking my health taking this drug? Because a well-meaning doctor, believing he was helping me, recommended it. But that recommendation was based on what I now believe to be an unsupported theory that lowering cholesterol artificially with a drug will lead to better health. Meanwhile for years I missed out on the only truly effective high cholesterol and vascular health therapy: eating the diet God originally designed for humans.

➢ **Optimal cholesterol level:** The medical establishment tells doctors and the public what the optimal cholesterol levels are, ostensibly for the purpose of preventing heart disease and saving lives. However, there is a huge potential for conflict of

---

[368] *Drugs.com*, Fenofibrate http://www.drugs.com/fenofibrate.html

interest in setting these standards. Pharmaceutical companies stand to make or lose billions of dollars depending on what decisions are made. For example, if the threshold for a "healthy" total cholesterol level is lowered, statin drug prescriptions will rise sharply. And these same drug companies contribute large amounts of money to the American Heart Association and other medical authorities who set the standards. Can the standards decided upon really be objective? Hardly.

Complicating the issue is the fact that **the healthiest cholesterol level is different for each person.**[369] Many people with relatively low cholesterol suffer from heart disease, and many with relatively high cholesterol never have heart problems.

So how can it be right to set a "one size fits all" standard? If one person could live a long, healthy life with a total cholesterol of 250, why is it that the medical establishment would want to urge on him a statin drug which will potentially cause him harm?

Your cholesterol level reflects what your body is doing, following the chemical mechanisms God built into it, to deal with the influences on it from food, toxins, stress, etc. Improve those inputs toward good health, and your cholesterol levels will normalize, not to some global standard set by an interest-conflicted medical establishment, but to a level optimal for you as an individual.

Eating a whole food plant based diet allows your body to establish its own natural, normal and healthy cholesterol level.

Nutrients and supplements

We have discussed in this book the importance of obtaining your nutrients in the context of whole foods. Supplementing vitamins, minerals, and other nutrients individually, or even in a multi-nutrient supplement, is usually unnecessary and unhelpful, and sometimes maybe even harmful (and almost always expensive). One can get all the nutrients one needs in a whole

---

[369] Greger, The Saturated Fat Studies: Set Up to Fail
http://nutritionfacts.org/video/the-saturated-fat-studies-set-up-to-fail/

food plant based diet, with the exception of only one or two. And this is not just one layman's opinion. Rather it is the consensus of many experts in the field of medicine and nutrition.[370]

➤ **Importance of vitamin D:** Vitamin D is critical to good health. Dr. Mercola notes:

> At least 2,000 genes, or nearly 10% of your genes, have been identified that are directly influenced by vitamin D, which in turn impact a wide variety of health issues, from preventing the common cold and flu to inhibiting at least 16 different types of cancer. There's even evidence linking vitamin D to the process of brain detoxification of heavy metals such as mercury.[371]

➤ **Vitamin D and pregnancy:** The Institute of Medicine recommends that pregnant women get 600 mg of vitamin D per day.[372] Yet in one study of vitamin D levels in women at the time of giving birth, half of them were found to be deficient, even though they were consuming the recommended amount. Furthermore, 65% of their newborn babies were deficient, and thus in danger of rickets and other diseases.[373]

This is also concerning because low vitamin D levels in pregnant women are associated with a high incidence of preeclampsia, [374] formerly called toxemia, a possibly fatal complication of pregnancy characterized by high blood pressure and other factors.

---

[370] McDougall, Just To Be on the Safe Side: Don't Take Vitamins https://www.drmcdougall.com/misc/2010nl/may/vitamins.htm
[371] Mercola, Important Cod Liver Oil Update http://articles.mercola.com/sites/articles/archive/2008/12/23/important-cod-liver-oil-update.aspx
[372] Amanda Gardner, *WebMD,* Are You Getting Enough Vitamin D and Calcium? http://www.webmd.com/osteoporosis/features/are-you-getting-enough-vitamin-d-calcium
[373] J.M. Lee, et al, *Clinical Pediatrics,* Vitamin D deficiency in a healthy group of mothers and newborn infants http://www.ncbi.nlm.nih.gov/pubmed/17164508
[374] Christopher J. Robinson, M.D., M.S.C.R., et al., *American Journal of Obstetrics and Gynecology,* Maternal Vitamin D and Fetal Growth in Early-Onset Severe Preeclampsia http://www.ncbi.nlm.nih.gov/pmc/articles/PMC3136573/

Another study found that vitamin D deficiency resulted in increased odds of a woman in labor needing to give birth by cesarean section.[375]

Are you pregnant or planning on becoming pregnant? Be sure you know the level of vitamin D in your blood, and if it is low, get more sun, and/or consider taking a D3 supplement.

➢ **Impact of vitamin D levels on chronic disease:** Many more studies indicating a connection between vitamin D deficiency and serious disease could be cited. A chart at GrassrootsHealth.net graphically displays the results of several of these, showing that low D is associated with increased risk of breast cancer, ovarian cancer, colon cancer, non-Hodgkin's lymphoma, type 1 diabetes, multiple sclerosis, heart attack, kidney cancer, endometrial cancer, rickets, falls (women), and fractures.[376] GrassrootsHealth.net has a wealth of information on vitamin D and health, including what the optimal vitamin D levels are, and how much you might need to supplement should you not be able to get adequate sunlight.

> *The best way to keep your vitamin D level where it should be is to get lots of midday sun exposure.*

➢ **Vitamin D from sunlight:** A type of cholesterol in your skin is converted into vitamin D when your skin is exposed to

---

[375] A. Merewood, et al., *The Journal of Clinical Endocrinology and Metabolism,* Association between vitamin D deficiency and primary cesarean section http://www.ncbi.nlm.nih.gov/pubmed/19106272

[376] *GrassrootsHealth,* Disease Incidence Prevention by Serum 25(OH)D Level http://www.grassrootshealth.net/media/download/dip_with_numbers_8-24-12.pdf

sufficiently strong UVB rays.[377] If you are not getting 15-30 minutes of strong sun exposure per day, and not taking a vitamin D3 supplement, your vitamin D levels may well be too low for optimum health.

That estimated time is only for light-skinned people, however. The darker your skin, the more sun exposure you need. Very dark-skinned people who don't get several hours of strong sun exposure per day tend to be deficient in vitamin D.

Some have suggested that the high incidence of diabetes, heart disease, cancer, and certain other chronic diseases among those in northern latitudes is partially attributable to lack of vitamin D. Others point out that those who live in northern latitudes tend to eat less fresh fruits and vegetables and more meat and dairy, and this may be a better explanation for the demographics of chronic disease. It seems likely that a combination of both factors is at least partly responsible.

➢ **How strong must the sunlight be?:** So how strong does the sun exposure have to be in order for vitamin D to be produced in the skin? First of all, the sun has to be shining! If it's cloudy, no vitamin D is made.

Regarding how high the sun must be in the sky, here's a very simple rule of thumb: Adequately strong sun exposure is available when your shadow is shorter than you are when you are standing up on level ground. During the summer in southern latitudes of the U.S., that is between about 10 am and 3 pm. In winter months, and in more northern latitudes, the time window during which you can get adequately strong sun exposure for vitamin D production narrows.

---

[377] Whether it is sunny or cloudy, UVA rays from the sun are always present outside during the daytime. They can even penetrate glass and light clothing, and thus you can get a sunburn unexpectedly. UVA rays do not produce vitamin D in your skin. UVB rays are only present in significant quantities when the sun is shining near midday. UVB rays can also cause burning. It is UVB rays which produce vitamin D. But glass filters out UVB rays and prevents D production.

If you live anywhere north of 37 degrees north latitude, during much of the year it is impossible to get adequate amounts of D from sunlight alone, unless you get a lot of sun in the summer months.[378,379]

Thankfully, vitamin D is stored in the body. So if you get good sun exposure during the summer, your vitamin D level may remain adequately high through the winter. Many experts recommend that people get their D levels checked in late winter in order to determine if they have an insufficiency of this nutrient.

Inadequate sun exposure and thus low D levels in the body is considered by many to explain (at least partially) not only why people in northern latitudes tend to get more chronic diseases[380,381,382], but also why people are more likely to get sick during the winter, and why there are more chronic diseases generally in populations as they become increasingly modern and tend to spend the middle part of the day inside, in classrooms, working in factories and offices, and sitting around in their homes. And the use of sunblock compounds the problem (see below).

Of course, no matter how strong the sun is shining, skin covered by clothing will not produce vitamin D. So if you are out in the full sun, but with long pants or a long dress, and long sleeves,

---

[378] The 37th parallel runs approximately from just south of San Jose, CA, to a bit north of Las Vegas, NV, and along or near the northern borders of AZ, NM, OK, AR, TN, and NC.
[379] *Harvard Health Publications,* Time for more vitamin D
http://www.health.harvard.edu/newsweek/time-for-more-vitamin-d.htm
[380] *Vitamin D Council,* Inflammatory bowel disease
https://www.vitamindcouncil.org/health-conditions/inflammatory-bowel-disease/
[381] *American College of Gastroenterology,* US research confirms latitude variation in incidence of chronic digestive diseases
http://www.eurekalert.org/pub_releases/2011-10/acog-urc102711.php
[382] *Diabetes Life,* Why is Everyone Getting Diabetes and Prediabetes?
http://www.dlife.com/diabetes/type-2/diabetes-causes/colberg/causes_of_diabetes?page=2

you're not getting any D. Short pants and short sleeves, even bare shoulders if possible (and adequately modest), will help you get your D.

➢ **Vitamin D from food sources:** Many suggest that in order to get adequate amounts of vitamin D you should eat fish, cod liver oil, eggs, D fortified dairy, and other animal product sources of this nutrient. It is true that these animal sources can provide vitamin D. However, consider whether the benefit of the small amount of D you will get from such sources is not outweighed by the potential long term harm these foods will do to your body.

A significant amount of vitamin D is available from just a few non-animal product foods, primarily mushrooms and tofu. But you would have to eat several cups of these per day to be adequately supplied. Enjoy.

➢ **D from artificial light:** Certain types of UV tanning beds can provide the exposure one needs to produce adequate vitamin D in the skin. Be sure to use a safe tanning bed; some types are bad for the skin.[383] But of course tanning beds are not a practical solution for most.

Unfortunately, those who run nursing homes are often not well informed about the need for D. And so the old people in their charge, sitting inside day after day, decline in health rapidly as their vitamin D levels decrease. The result is that now it is estimated that 80% or more of nursing home patients are vitamin D deficient.[384]

A previously cited article by Stephanie Seneff implicates vitamin D deficiency in the progression of Alzheimer's, certainly a concern to old folks.[385] And studies have shown that artificial indoor UV lighting can help old folks' vitamin D levels improve

---

[383] Mercola, Vitamin D Resource Page
http://www.mercola.com/article/vitamin-d-resources.htm
[384] *Inspired Nutrition,* Ultraviolet Light
http://www.inspirednutrition.com/ultraviolet-light.html
[385] Stephanie Seneff, *Spacedoc.com,* A Recipe for Alzheimer's Disease
http://www.spacedoc.com/recipe_alzheimers_disease

dramatically.[386] Of course spending some time outside, with some wrinkled skin exposed, would be even better therapy, improving vitamin D levels as well as brightening their day.

> **Vitamin D supplementation:** Adequate sunshine is the healthiest way to get your vitamin D. You would be wise to make an effort to take advantage of sunny spring, summer, and fall days by getting outside around the middle of the day and soaking in some nourishment.

But if you can't get enough sun exposure, it is probably a good idea to supplement with vitamin D3 pills. Some doctors and researchers have noted health problems associated with D supplementation.[387,388] But it seems the weight of evidence indicates that supplementing to raise blood levels of D is safer than living with D deficiency.

Recommendations regarding how much D3 should be taken as a supplement vary widely, from 600 to 10,000 IU daily. Unless one is getting a good amount of sunshine, based on the most reliable recommendations I have heard, it seems best to take a minimum of 2000 IU daily. If your D level is low, it may be necessary to take 5,000-10,000 IU D3 per day.

It is important to understand that each person's body responds differently to supplementation. One person may be able to maintain a healthy level on 2000 IU per day, while another person needs more than double that. The only way to verify is to test the blood.

Of course the recommended dosing is based on what target

---

[386] Ran Zhang and Declan P Naughton, Vitamin D in health and disease: Current perspectives http://www.nutritionj.com/content/9/1/65
[387] A.M. Heikkinen, et al, *European Journal of Endocrinology*, Long-term vitamin D3 supplementation may have adverse effects on serum lipids during postmenopausal hormone replacement therapy http://www.ncbi.nlm.nih.gov/pubmed/9405029
[388] P. Tuohimaa, et al, *International Journal of Cancer,* Both high and low levels of blood vitamin D are associated with a higher prostate cancer risk: a longitudinal, nested case-control study in the Nordic countries http://www.ncbi.nlm.nih.gov/pubmed/14618623

level of D in the blood is considered ideal, and the experts vary widely in their opinions of that as well.

Some take a D3 supplement only during the winter. This is helpful if your summer sun exposure is adequate to keep your D at a healthy level while strong sunlight is available, but not adequate to enable your body to store enough to keep the level up through the winter.

Be sure and take your D3 supplement during your biggest meal of the day. This significantly helps proper absorption over taking it between meals.

➢ **Ideal vitamin D level:** As you can see, it is important to make an effort to get adequate sun exposure. If you do get a lot of sun, you probably have a healthy vitamin D level in your body. If you don't get much sun, you should have your blood tested, because your D level is likely deficient, and as we have seen this puts you at risk of chronic disease – a risk significantly mitigated, however, by a lifestyle based on Biblical principles of good health.

So what is the ideal vitamin D level you want to see when you have your blood tested? As mentioned earlier, the experts disagree regarding this, but after surveying the recommendations of several sources it appears a level of between 40 and 60 ng/ml is best.[389,390]

Many suggest the level can go up to 100 or even 150 ng/ml without danger of toxicity.[391] But on the other hand, Dr. Greger cites a study which indicates 30 ng/ml is the best level for optimum overall mortality reduction.[392] This particular study

---

[389] *GrassrootsHealth,* Recommended Range http://www.grassrootshealth.net/
[390] The statement by the U.S. Institute of Medicine that no beneficial effect is associated with blood levels over 30 ng/ml is contradicted by many studies.
[391] *Vitamin D Council,* Am I getting too much vitamin D? http://www.vitamindcouncil.org/about-vitamin-d/am-i-getting-too-much-vitamin-d/#
[392] Greger, Vitamin D and Mortality May Be a U-shaped Curve http://nutritionfacts.org/video/vitamin-d-and-mortality-may-be-a-u-shaped-curve/

indicated that both lower and higher levels were associated with greater overall mortality risk.

Note that if you do more study on this subject, you may notice that there are two units which are commonly used to measure blood levels of vitamin D: In the U.S. ng/ml (nanograms/milliliter) is most commonly used. But in other countries nmol/L (nanomoles/liter) is more common. If you see a figure in nmol/L, divide by 2.5 to get the ng/ml figure.

➢ **Sun exposure and skin cancer:** For many years Americans have been told that any sun exposure is bad for your skin, and if you don't protect yourself you risk skin cancer. If we think Biblically we must question such an assertion. The Israelites were out in the desert for 40 years, yet nowhere is it written that God warned them against sun exposure. We can only assume they had plenty, yet we see no evidence of an outbreak of skin cancers.

Such observations from the Bible don't prove that the so-called experts in our day are wrong. But they do encourage us to dig deeper to find out if their seemingly unlikely pronouncements are really true.

It is in fact true that overexposure to the sun's rays can cause skin cancer. But still, optimal levels of vitamin D derived from the proper amount of sun exposure has also been shown to actually protect from skin cancer.[393] Furthermore,

> …although increased UVB exposure may result in an increase in non-melanoma skin cancers these are relatively easy to cure and have very low mortality rates compared with the internal cancers vitamin D appears to protect against.[394]

In Norway, being so far north, people receive relatively little sun exposure, and so researchers there are especially concerned

---

[393] *Vitamin D Council,* Vitamin D, UV exposure, and skin cancer in a nutshell http://www.vitamindcouncil.org/blog/vitamin-d-uv-esposure-and-skin-cancer-in-a-nutshell/

[394] *News Medical* 2008, Researchers say health benefits of sunshine outweigh the skin cancer risk and might help you live longer http://www.news-medical.net/news/2008/01/07/34041.aspx

with the issue of vitamin D's impact on health.

> The scientists at the U.S. Department of Energy's Brookhaven National Laboratory and colleagues at Norway's Institute for Cancer Research in Oslo, say the health benefits from some sun exposure are far larger than the skin cancer risk.
>
> Lead researcher Johan Moan says modest sun exposure gives enormous vitamin D benefits and though certain foods contain vitamin D, the body's main source is from the sun.
>
> Moan has estimated that doubling the sun exposure for the general population in Norway would also double the number of annual skin cancer deaths to about 300 but that 3,000 fewer people would die from other cancers and he believes the benefits could also be significant for people in other countries.[395]

So the bottom line is that **it is healthy to get a lot of sun exposure, as long as you don't get a sunburn.** Moen suggests that optimal daily sun exposure is half of the time it takes an individual to burn.

➢ **Sunblock:** Using sunblock keeps your skin from producing vitamin D, and no doubt sunblock contributes to the dangerously low levels of vitamin D prevalent among Americans, and thus contributes toward chronic disease.

These assertions are disputed by the majority of doctors and other authorities on the subject. The recommendation is even given that everyone wear sunblock every day just in case you happen to go out in the sun![396]

Not only does sunblock inhibit vitamin D production in the skin, but it also contains harmful chemicals which soak in and get into your blood. In fact, sunblock has been blamed for *causing* cancer![397]

---

395 *Ibid.*

396 *News Medical,* Skin Cancer Awareness Month and Melanoma Monday: Mount Sinai experts to share vital skin cancer tips http://www.news-medical.net/news/20140426/Skin-Cancer-Awareness-Month-and-Melanoma-Monday-Mount-Sinai-experts-to-share-vital-skin-cancer-tips.aspx

397 Joe Martino, Avoid The Toxic Sunscreen & Try Coconut Oil Instead http://www.collective-evolution.com/2014/04/18/avoid-the-toxic-sunscreen-try-coconut-oil-instead/

If you have been in the sun long enough that you fear you will become burned, **use good quality, cold pressed coconut oil as sunblock.** I have found it to be effective, but of course you still can burn if you are out in the sun too long, even when using coconut oil.

➢ **Sunshine – Other benefits:** Some studies indicate that increased time out in the sun keeps the metabolism humming along well. A slower metabolism means you are at greater risk of weight gain. So more sun may help you stay at a healthy weight.

Time spent out in the warm sunshine can also help improve circulation, quality of sleep, and mood. And Stephanie Seneff, Ph.D., of MIT, makes a convincing case for the relationship between inadequate sun exposure and Alzheimer's risk.[398]

We were created to spend at least part of our day, each day, out in the sunshine. It is no surprise that we find that this is an important feature of a healthy lifestyle.

➢ **Vitamin B12:** B12 is an essential nutrient in the body, but it is not produced by any plants or animals. It is made by bacteria.

In the past, when people weren't so germ-conscious, adequate amounts of B12 were obtained from non-chlorinated drinking water, as well as from some inadequately cleaned vegetables and meat, because bacteria which produce B12 live in water, soil and in meat. Also, animals store B12 in their muscles, providing a source for meat eaters.

But now, with our water supply being sterilized of all bacteria (with chlorine and filtration), and our plant foods being grown in a more sterile manner and thoroughly washed before eating, those who don't eat meat can vary rarely end up with a B12 deficiency.[399]

B12 is often found in vitamin fortified packaged foods, so that is

---

[398] Stephanie Seneff, *Spacedoc.com,* A Recipe for Alzheimer's Disease
http://www.spacedoc.com/recipe_alzheimers_disease
[399] McDougall, Vitamin B12 Deficiency—the Meat-eaters' Last Stand
https://www.drmcdougall.com/misc/2007nl/nov/b12.htm

a possible source. But be careful, since usually the ingredients include partial, refined foods, which it is best to minimize in the diet as much as possible.

It is thus advisable for those on a plant based diet to take a B12 supplement. A 500 or more mg tablet (up to 2500 mg) once weekly is the easiest and cheapest way to do this. Or you can take a B-complex multivitamin containing B12 if you wish, but if you have a well-balanced whole food plant based diet you will get all the other B vitamins you need in the food you eat. Generally you should only take a B-complex (or any other supplement, for that matter) if you have a specific medical reason for doing so.

If you adopt a plant based diet, don't slack on the B12. Take this very seriously. The deficiency may not show up for several months or years, and is even unlikely to be a problem for you. But if you do develop a deficiency, the symptoms are very serious. Whenever you have a blood test, you should request that they check your B12 and D levels to ensure they are in the healthy range.

➢ **Calcium:** In the U.S. we often hear that we need to be sure we are getting enough calcium, lest we suffer from osteoporosis later in life, and an increased likelihood of fractures.

Osteoporosis is indeed an increasing problem in Western cultures. It is characterized by a loss of bone mass. In the U.S. it results in more than 1.5 million fractures per year, including 300,000 broken hips.[400] (And an estimated 30% of people over 65 end up dying within 12 months of suffering from a broken hip!) It is indeed a serious problem.

So one of the first questions often asked by people who are wondering about a whole food plant based diet is, "Where do you get your calcium?" Many believe they need a calcium supplement, a lot of dairy, or some drug to avoid osteoporosis

---

[400] Harvard School of Public Health, *The Nutrition Source,* Calcium and Milk: What's Best for Your Bones and Health?
http://www.hsph.harvard.edu/nutritionsource/calcium-full-story/

and fractures, especially in their senior years. After all, the bones are made up primarily of calcium, right? So to keep them strong you should consume a lot of calcium, right? Wrong, and wrong again.

First of all, only about 10% of your bone mass is calcium. The rest is other minerals and tissue cells. While we do need to consume calcium in our diet, we don't really need nearly as much as we are commonly told.

The principles derived from the Eden Axiom suggest that we should be able to get all the calcium we need from plant foods; neither animal products, nor calcium supplements, nor drugs should be required. And we find that the science of human nutrition indicates this is indeed the case.

One strong line of evidence for this is that women in rural areas of poor countries often have six to ten babies during their lifetimes, nurse each one for about two years, consume no dairy products or calcium supplements, and yet suffer no osteoporosis. How can that be? Their calcium intake may be only 300 mg/day, yet obviously it is sufficient for their needs.

The likely reason their bones are able to stay healthy with so little calcium is that **they eat relatively little animal protein, they get plenty of sunshine, and they are physically active.**

There is evidence that excess animal protein intake causes calcium to be lost by the body.[401] The exact mechanism of calcium loss is disputed by some, but what can't be denied is that 300 mg of calcium per day is sufficient in the context of the right lifestyle.

Why is it that according to the National Institutes of Health an American woman in the same situation (bearing and nursing babies) "needs" 1300 mg/day,[402] over **four times** as much

---

[401] McDougall, Osteoporosis
https://www.drmcdougall.com/health/education/health-science/common-health-problems/osteoporosis/
[402] It is interesting to note that the World Health Organization, which is not heavily influenced by the U.S. dairy industry, recommends only 500 mg/day.

calcium as the rural subsistence farmer? Not only that, but after being frightened by the NIH into guzzling milk and calcium pills her whole life, the American woman may still end up with osteoporosis.

Furthermore, we can see the folly of thinking humans need milk and/or supplements by asking this simple question: Where do cows, who have much more massive bones than humans, get their calcium? How about elephants?

No animal consumes milk after infancy. Yet herbivores eating their natural 100% plant diet never get osteoporosis. **Herbivores all get their calcium from plants alone. And we, too can get all the calcium we need from plants**.

It is only when we humans eat too much meat and other unnatural foods, get little sunshine, and live sedentary lives, that osteoporosis shows up. This argues strongly for the notion that plants are our natural diet, the diet we were created to be on.

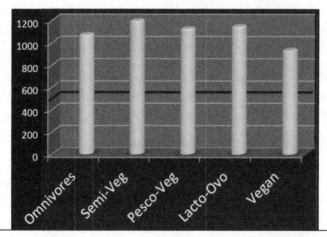

The above chart features data from the Adventist Health Study 2. The black line represents the World Health Organization recommendation of 500 mg of calcium per day. As we can see, even vegans get plenty of calcium.

Though the focus is usually on calcium, that is not the only nutrient needed for healthy bones. Vitamin D is critical, as are several other minerals, including boron (eat your apples, pears, grapes, raisins, flaxseed, almonds, apricots, avocados!), phosphorus (eat your soybeans, lentils, seeds and nuts!), and magnesium (eat your green leafys, beans and seeds!). **And all of these are abundantly supplied in a well balanced whole food plant based diet.**

If you look at the calcium content of foods relative to calories, you will find that many whole plant foods are great sources. For example, whole milk has 1.9 mg of calcium per calorie. Compare that to raw kale, 2.6; raw turnip greens, 5.8; raw beets, 5.5; raw bok choy cabbage, 7.4.[403]

Many argue that calcium from plant sources is not absorbed as readily as that from dairy. This may be true. But then one doesn't need nearly as much when animal products are off the menu. The bottom line is that calcium needs are easily supplied by a whole food plant based diet, with none of the drawbacks of consuming dairy.

The notion that we need to supplement our diet with calcium pills, or we need to consume dairy, is obviously not based on sound science. It is propagated by supplement and food producers and their supporters who wish to convince people that they need their products for good health.

➢ **Protein:** Another common question of those who don't eat animal products is, "Where do you get your protein?" The best answer is similar to the one asked about calcium: "The same place other herbivores get their protein. From plants, of course." **It is easy to get all the protein your body needs from vegetables, whole grains, beans, nuts and seeds.**

Protein is made up of amino acids, special molecules needed by the body to build new tissue and carry out numerous metabolic functions. There are several types of amino acids, and many of them, the essential amino acids, must be obtained from food.

---

[403] Vanessa A. Farrell, Linda Houtkooper, *Arizona Cooperative Extension,* Calcium and Calorie Content of Selected Foods
http://extension.arizona.edu/sites/extension.arizona.edu/files/pubs/az1128.pdf

There is a common misconception that animal protein has all the amino acids, but plant foods are deficient in one or more amino acid,[404] and thus they are considered to be incomplete protein sources. Thus it is said that one should be careful to eat various plant foods in proper combination to obtain complete protein. But this notion is a myth.

Whole plant foods are not incomplete protein, they are not deficient in any essential amino acids. You don't have to worry about matching up certain foods in order to get the right mix of amino acids.[405]

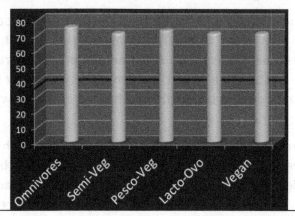

The above chart features data from the Adventist Health Study 2. The black line represents the World Health Organization recommendation that males get 38 g of protein per day (the requirement for women is lower). As we can see, there is very little difference between the amount of protein each group consumes, and even vegans get plenty.

But how much protein do we really need? It would be instructive to know how much protein is in breast milk, since that is the

---

[404] There are nine different essential amino acids, which together are called protein. They are "essential" because they are needed by the human body but the human body does not synthesize them.

[405] McDougall, *McDougall Newsletter* April 2007, <u>When Friends Ask: Where Do You Get Your Protein?</u>
https://www.drmcdougall.com/misc/2007nl/apr/dairy.pdf

perfect God-designed food for growing healthy babies.

It turns out that 5% of the calories in breast milk are from protein. Now, let's compare that with some common plant foods: sweet potatoes: 6%; potatoes: 11%; oats: 16%; beans: 28%.

So, assuming we can utilize the protein in plant foods at least almost as well as a baby can utilize the protein in her food, we should be just fine eating only plants. And in fact such is the case. **It is impossible for a person to suffer from protein deficiency if they are eating a whole food plant based diet and getting enough calories**. There are even successful athletes on this diet, including body builders who are able to develop very large muscles and compete professionally.[406]

If you are on a plant based diet you should take a vitamin B12 supplement. If you get enough sunshine this is the only supplement you really need!

"Protein deficiency" is another term for "starvation." And no one filling their belly several times a day with whole plant foods has ever suffered from that condition!

➢ **Just two nutrient supplements:** If you have a well-balanced whole food plant based diet, and get adequate sunshine, the only nutritional supplement which will most likely be necessary is B12. If you don't get much sun, D3 is probably needed as well. But no other vitamin or mineral supplements are needed. You can get everything you need in the fruits, vegetables, whole grains, beans, nuts, and seeds you eat. I believe this is true for most people. But of course some individuals may have a medical reason that they need other supplements.

---

[406] Abigail Geer, 5 Plant-based Athletes That Blow The Protein Myth Out of the Water http://www.onegreenplanet.org/natural-health/5-plant-based-athletes-that-blow-the-protein-myth-out-of-the-water/

➤ **Other supplements:** There are other supplements which may be called for in some circumstances. But always look for a food source first. Whole foods can often provide the nutrients you want, making the supplements unnecessary. Studies have consistently found that the nutrients in whole foods are more effective for achieving good health than the same nutrients delivered in a pill. However, the concentration desired to address a certain ailment isn't always available in food.

My wife's eye doctor recommended she take a certain nutritional supplement to protect her eyes from macular degeneration. I looked up the supplement to find out what nutrients it contained. Then I looked at the nutrient profile on some of the fresh greens we normally eat. **It turned out she was already getting the nutrients she needed for her eyes.**

A doctor prescribed a selenium supplement for me. But it turns out the same amount of selenium may be obtained by eating eight Brazil nuts. Guess what source of selenium I opted for.

Our doctors never asked us what our diet included so they could determine if we needed the supplement. Perhaps they don't even know how one can be adequately nourished by plants alone.

Keep in mind that while a supplement may be helpful or even necessary to improve or maintain the health of those who eat animal products, in many cases it won't be needed by those eating only plants.

For example, a man may develop BPH (non-cancerous enlargement of the prostate), and its associated symptoms of difficulty urinating and urinary retention. So a prostate support supplement such as saw palmetto and/or a drug like Flomax may be helpful to ease the symptoms.

However, the evidence indicates that usually BPH is caused by a diet rich in animal products (especially chicken and eggs) and white flour. Thus stopping the assault on the prostate and instead eating a whole food plant based diet can correct BPH. That therapeutic diet should include a good dose of flaxseed meal, which has been shown to have a powerful healing effect.[407]

But instead of recommending such a diet to their BPH patients, doctors will usually prescribe the supplement, or worse, a pharmaceutical drug or surgery. That is what their training says they should do. Of course, depending on the exact nature of

> *Meats cooked at high temperatures, and their fumes, contain cancer-causing substances.*

the problem, surgery may eventually be necessary. But diet therapy should certainly be considered first.

The bottom line is, always be cautious when it comes to vitamin, mineral, and other supplements. Please read Dr. McDougall's helpful article, Just To Be on the Safe Side: Don't Take Vitamins.[408]

Cooking

> **Eating foods raw vs. eating foods cooked:** Most food eaten by Americans is cooked. Yet with many if not most plant-sourced foods, raw is much better, providing much more nutrition. **Generally it's best to eat plant foods raw whenever you can.** To accomplish this it's good to get in the habit of eating several servings of fruits (including berries whenever possible), and a big salad (including a variety of dark leafys like spinach and kale, plus broccoli, cauliflower, carrots, tomatoes, avocado, nuts, ground seeds, etc.), every day.

That said, it is also true that while plant foods do lose some nutrients when cooked, some nutrients are actually enhanced in the cooking process. Cooking also softens cell walls, liberating more of the goodness of their contents. Tomatoes are the most

---

[407] Greger, Prostate vs. Plants http://nutritionfacts.org/video/prostate-versus-plants/
[408] McDougall, Just To Be on the Safe Side: Don't Take Vitamins https://www.drmcdougall.com/misc/2010nl/may/vitamins.htm

well known plant food which gains important nutrients when cooked. Of course, some foods must be eaten cooked, such as beans, rice, potatoes, sweet potatoes, etc. So enjoy your cooked veggies, but **remember to try to eat a lot of raw veggies, fruits, nuts, and seeds each day.**

➤ **Cooking at high temperatures:** When you do cook, it is best to use the lowest temperature possible. Studies have shown that **the higher the temperature rises over the boiling point, the more dangerous chemicals are produced**, increasing the consumer's risk of cancer and other diseases. This is especially true of meats cooked at high temps, and eating some cooked meats (fried, broiled, grilled, barbecued and smoked) can cause DNA damage, and thus cancer, due to substances in the meat similar to those found in tobacco smoke.[409]

As discussed previously, breathing the fumes from meat cooked at high temperatures, such as broiling, grilling, frying, smoking and barbecuing, poses a significant health hazard due to the carcinogenic nitrosamines which enter the lungs.

Slow cookers are a good way to cook, as well as boiling or steaming.[410,411] Baking at as low a temperature as possible is also a good option.

A good dehydrator is the ultimate low-temp "baking" machine. If you dehydrate foods at below 120 degrees they maintain their living enzymes, which makes them healthier to eat.

➤ **Microwaving:** There is a lot of controversy regarding microwaving foods, whether it poses any health risks or not. I have not researched this a lot, but my conclusion so far is negative. (A friend of ours has researched it a lot, and he says microwave ovens have only one use: to fill a trash can with.)

---

[409] Greger, Estrogenic Cooked Meat Carcinogens
http://nutritionfacts.org/video/estrogenic-cooked-meat-carcinogens/
[410] Greger, Reducing Cancer Risk in Meat Eaters
http://nutritionfacts.org/video/reducing-cancer-risk-in-meateaters/
[411] Greger, Estrogenic Cooked Meat Carcinogens
http://nutritionfacts.org/video/estrogenic-cooked-meat-carcinogens/

Microwaves can cause toxins from food packaging to contaminate foods. Microwaving foods destroys some of the nutritive value, and can even change food molecularly to make it unhealthy.

> **A study done in Europe showed that microwaving changes the molecular structure of foods,** making them depressive to the immune system, therefore I highly advise against the consumption of foods cooked defrosted or re-heated in a microwave if you are trying to improve your health and immune system.[412]

In addition, microwave ovens emit relatively high levels of electromagnetic radiation (EMF). Whenever a microwave oven is running, unhealthy levels of this radiation are being pumped into the bodies of all within several feet. The radiation emitted from a running microwave oven, at one foot away, can be in the range of 400 milligauss. Some claim that a mere 4 milligauss has been linked to leukemia (but I haven't found the documentation to support this).

Some say these are not significant dangers. But we prefer not to risk it simply to save a few seconds or minutes in food prep time, so we do not use a microwave oven. If you do use a microwave, consider leaving the room when it is running. Children and pregnant mothers should not operate them at all.

As indicated above, there is a lot of controversy about this, so I encourage you to do your own research, looking at both sides.

It is important to keep the microwave issue in perspective. The evidence that eating animal products, sugar, oils, fried foods, chemical additives and other toxins, leads to chronic disease is overwhelming. The evidence of the health dangers of microwave ovens and eating microwaved food is not as clear. To avoid microwave cooking for health reasons while continuing to eat unhealthy foods seems to me to be inconsistent.

---

[412] David Getoff, N.D., If You Have Cancer http://www.naturopath4you.com/ IfYouHaveCancer.htm.

GMO and organic

➢ **Genetically modified organisms:** GMO foods are becoming hard to avoid. It is said that 96% of corn in the U.S., for example, is GMO. There are nine GMO crops grown for sale in the U.S.: soy, corn, cotton (oil), canola (oil), sugar beets, zucchini, yellow squash, Hawaiian papaya, and alfalfa. It is also good to know that most GMO soy is fed to farm animals, while most non-GMO soy is sold for direct human consumption. GMO wheat has never been approved by the FDA.[413]

Some GMO foods may be harmless. But many say that there is good evidence at least some are harmful. And not enough testing has been done to verify safety, while testing which suggests harm is suppressed.

Kevin O'Leary, the multimillionaire proponent of GMO and defender of Monsanto, a chemical company which is making billions of dollars as the leader in the GMO industry, had an interesting discussion with 14 year old Rachel Parent, an anti-GMO activist.[414] Parent was calling for long-term studies on the safety of GMO foods. O'Leary told her, "We're in a long-term study. You're eating GM food whether you like it or not." The cohost of the program added, "We're the lab rats."

Yes, we are the lab rats. And many claim that the disturbing results of the experiment are starting to come in.

> Most GM crops are engineered to tolerate a weed killer called Roundup®, whose active ingredient is glyphosate. These crops, known as Roundup-Ready crops, accumulate high levels of glyphosate that remain in the food. Corn and cotton varieties are also engineered to produce an insecticide called Bt-toxin. The Bt-toxin is produced in every cell of genetically engineered corn and ends up in corn chips, corn tortillas, and other ingredients derived from corn. A recent analysis of research suggests that Bt-toxin, glyphosate, and other components of GMOs, are linked to five

---

[413] However, there are many research fields growing strains of GMO wheat. So the potential is high that non-GMO wheat will be contaminated.
[414] *The Lang and O'Leary Exchange,* 14 year old Rachel Parent Educates Kevin O'Leary on GMO's https://www.youtube.com/watch?v=7H3Spe03oyg

conditions that may either initiate or exacerbate gluten-related disorders:

- Intestinal permeability[415]

- Imbalanced gut bacteria

- Immune activation and allergies

- Impaired digestion

- Damage to the intestinal wall[416]

So it is possible that GMO foods actually cause gluten intolerance, even though the specific crop causing the condition may not contain gluten.

Some studies have shown that when small mammals are fed a GMO diet, by the third generation they become sterile and suffer other abnormalities.[417] Worldwide birthrates are dropping at startling rates, and some claim GMO foods are part of the reason.[418]

Evidently it is not the glyphosate itself which is most dangerous. Tests have shown little harm from it directly. In fact, Monsanto has done tests which show that glyphosate isn't so bad, and

---

[415] Intestinal permeability, also called leaky gut, refers to a condition resulting from a damaged large intestinal wall. This can lead to a host of autoimmune diseases (note "antibody reaction" in the following quote), as well as other problems. "The spaces in between the cells that line the intestines are normally sealed. These tight junctions are called desmosomes. When the intestinal lining becomes irritated, the junctions loosen and allow unwanted larger molecules in the intestines to pass through into the blood. These unwanted substances are seen by the immune system as foreign (because they aren't normally present in blood). This triggers an antibody reaction." Cathy Wong, N.D., *About Health,* Leaky Gut Syndrome/Intestinal Permeability http://altmedicine.about.com/od/healthconditionsdisease/a/TestLeakyGut.htm
[416] Jeffrey M. Smith, Are Genetically Modified Foods a Gut-Wrenching Combination? http://responsibletechnology.org/glutenintroduction
[417] *Institute for Responsible Technology,* Genetically Modified Soy Linked to Sterility, Infant Mortality http://www.responsibletechnology.org/article-gmo-soy-linked-to-sterility
[418] Hethir Rodriguez, C.H., C.M.T., *Natural Fertility Info,* Research Indicates That GMO Could Be a Cause of Infertility http://natural-fertility-info.com/gmo-infertility.html

then concluded that Roundup must be safe. However, Roundup contains many toxic compounds besides glyphosate, and the toxicity of the total concoction is actually quite significant.[419] So avoiding Roundup treated food is indeed a good idea.

Why we know GM foods are safe

Monsanto is the company that told us that PCBs were safe, and they were convicted of actually poisoning people in the town next to the PCB factory, and fined $700,000,000. They told us that Agent Orange was safe. They told us that DDT was safe. And now they are in charge of telling us if their own genetically modified foods are safe, because the FDA doesn't require a single safety study. They leave it to Monsanto.

— Jeffrey Smith
Executive Director, Institute for Responsible Technology

Monsanto should not have to vouchsafe the safety of biotech food. Our interest is in selling as much of it as possible. Assuring its safety is the FDA's job.

— Phil Angell
Director of Corporate Communications, Monsanto

Ultimately, it is the food producer who is responsible for assuring safety.

— FDA, "Statement of Policy:
Foods Derived from New Plant Varieties"

---

[419] Greger, Is Monsanto's Roundup Pesticide Glyphosate Safe? http://nutritionfacts.org/video/is-monsantos-roundup-pesticide-glyphosate-safe/

But again, as with microwaving, it is important to keep the possible dangers of GMO in perspective. There is overwhelming evidence that eating unhealthy types of foods causes disease in most people, while the current evidence indicates that the chance of GMO-induced harm, though very real, is much lower.[420] **Thus it is clearly inconsistent to be meticulous about avoiding GMO foods, while at the same time making animal products and partial foods a prominent part of one's diet.** Even a moderate level of these unhealthy foods in the diet probably represents a greater threat to health for most people than GMOs.

There is much controversy on this subject, with billions of dollars to be made or lost depending on public perceptions, legislation, and the outcomes of scientific studies. **For now it seems the prudent thing to do is to avoid eating GMO when possible.** Since much animal feed is GMO, one of the easiest ways to avoid GMO is to simply avoid eating animal products.

➢ **Organic:** There is controversy regarding whether organic foods are worth the extra cost. To be labeled organic they must be grown without synthetic chemicals, must be grown on land that has not had chemical fertilizers, pesticides, or herbicides used on it for three years, and the crops must not be GMO.

However, some certified organic foods may not actually be GMO free. This is because organic crops may be contaminated by GMO crops grown nearby via seeds blown in the wind or cross-pollination. One would think such contamination would disqualify the crop from being considered organic. But as long as the organic farmer makes a reasonable effort to avoid this contamination (whatever that means), they are still allowed to keep the "Organic" label on their product. So the "Organic" label alone is no absolute guarantee the product is not GMO.[421]

---

[420] Greger, <u>GMO Soy and Breast Cancer</u> http://nutritionfacts.org/video/gmo-soy-and-breast-cancer/

[421] Gary Null, Documentary: <u>Seeds of Death</u> (minute 13:40) https://www.youtube.com/watch?v=eUd9rRSLY4A

Some studies show organic produce to contain higher nutrient levels, but there are no requirements regarding replenishing soils with natural fertilizers, compost or minerals, so organic produce may not always be more nutritious than their non-organic counterparts.

Some say that the most important foods to buy organic are high oil seeds and nuts, since the oils tend to concentrate the pesticides used in non-organic farming. I don't know if this is true, or of any studies proving a link between high oil pesticide laden seeds and nuts and disease.

As with GMO, to be consistent, a person who is careful to only choose organic foods for health reasons will also avoid consuming animal products. In the large amount of research I have done I have seen that the science implicating the consumption of animal products as the cause of chronic disease is stronger than the science supporting the health benefits of eating organic.

So yes, do eat organic whenever possible. But don't fret if certain organic foods are unavailable, or too expensive. The move to whole food plant based will make a tremendous difference in your health, while eating organic is just the icing on the cake. (Poor metaphor, perhaps!)

➢ **Plant nutrition trumps pesticides:** Some may wonder if eating more plants might tend to expose a person to more dangerous chemicals. After all, we all know that tons of pesticides and herbicides are dumped on crops every day.

However, in comparison to the hormones, bacteria, industrial pollutants and other toxins which are commonly present in red meat, poultry, fish and dairy, plant foods are relatively pristine. Eating organisms which are lower on the food chain is a distinct advantage!

Not only that, but **the benefit to your health from plant foods will tend to compensate for any danger from pesticides you may ingest.** The increased nutrition, especially the phytochemicals, provide protection from synthetic chemicals which might otherwise pose a health hazard.

Additionally, preliminary studies appear to show that the phytochemicals also confer protection from other toxins in our environment such as dioxins and DDT.[422]

And another study found that chlorophyll, the green pigment in plants, is able to block the body's absorption of cancer causing aflatoxin, which may be present in peanuts products which have (or have had) mold on them.[423]

Researchers in another study estimated that if half the population of the U.S. increased their fruit and vegetable consumption by one serving each per day, perhaps ten people would get cancer as a result of the extra consumption of pesticides. That's bad. **However, an estimated 20,000 cases of cancer would be prevented by the extra healthy food consumed** (and unhealthy food not consumed, since it would be displaced by the extra servings of plant food). That's good. **Very good.**

How much cancer would be prevented if we increased our consumption of whole plant foods by more than one serving? Up to all the servings of food we eat? And how many other diseases would be prevented?

➤ **Grow your own:** The best source of fresh plant foods is your own garden. That is often the only way you can guarantee you are getting synthetic-chemical-free food grown in rich healthy soil. So if you have a little land you can dedicate to growing vegetables, make use of it! Gardening is a great way to get some exercise and healthy sunshine as well!

Obesity

➤ **A Western phenomenon:** In America roughly one third of the population is overweight and one third is obese. **Recently**

---

[422] Greger, Plants vs. Pesticide http://nutritionfacts.org/video/plants-vs-pesticides/
[423] Greger, Eating Green to Prevent Cancer http://nutritionfacts.org/video/eating-green-to-prevent-cancer/

published figures stated that every state except Hawaii has an obesity rate of 30% or more. Some states, including Louisiana and Mississippi, have rates over 40%.[424]

It is unprecedented in the history of the world that such a high proportion of a nation's population would have a weight problem. But should we be surprised? It is the result of tainted dietary guidelines from corporate-sponsor-controlled government and non-government agencies, slick wall-to-wall advertising of unhealthy foods and beverages, and an overly-gullible public, ready to purchase and devour whatever new processed meat, dairy, sugar and fat concoctions Big Food will pitch to it.

In the past, obesity was limited to only the rich classes, who could afford so-called "rich" diets which included a large proportion of animal products, and fewer "cheap" foods such as grains, leafy greens and potatoes.

But tragically, today the poor suffer from obesity proportionally more than the rich.

- Based on a large national study, body mass index (or BMI, an indicator of excess body fat) was higher every year between 1986 and 2002 among adults in the lowest income group and the lowest education group than among those in the highest income and education groups, respectively (Truong & Sturm, 2005).

- Wages were inversely related to BMI and obesity in a nationally representative sample of more than 6,000 adults – meaning, those with low wages had increased BMI as well as increased chance of being obese (Kim & Leigh, 2010).[425]

---

[424] Rachael Rettner, *Fox News,* U.S. States Are A Lot Fatter Than We Thought http://www.foxnews.com/health/2014/11/20/us-states-are-lot-fatter-than-thought/. Others report somewhat lower rates. It is difficult to get accurate figures. Often they are obtained by telephone surveys, but some have reported that respondents tend to overestimate their height, and thus lower than reality BMIs are calculated.

[425] *Food Research and Action Center,* Relationship Between Poverty and Overweight or Obesity http://frac.org/initiatives/hunger-and-obesity/are-low-income-people-at-greater-risk-for-overweight-or-obesity/

The evidence indicates that the easy availability of cheap, high calorie foods, combined with welfare programs which tend to encourage less work and physical activity, have contributed to this disturbing trend.

➤ **A significant risk factor for chronic disease:** The most important reason to lose weight is that obesity is a significant risk factor for many diseases. Principal among these is type 2 diabetes. Simply losing weight can cure some people of diabetes,[426] and significantly reduce your risk of other obesity-related diseases as well. And a whole food plant based diet lifestyle is a great way to lose those dangerous pounds once and for all!

➤ **Body Mass Index:** Your BMI is the ratio of your weight to your height. A person's BMI number gives important information about their general state of health.

There are risks associated with low BMI:

> A body mass index, or BMI, below 18.5 means a person is underweight and this is associated with health complications such as bone loss, decreased immunity, cardiac problems, and infertility.[427]

But high BMI is much more common in the West and of much greater concern.

> If your BMI is high, you may have an increased risk of developing certain diseases including high blood pressure, heart disease, high cholesterol and blood lipids (LDL), Type 2 Diabetes, sleep apnea, osteoarthritis, female infertility, gastroesophageal reflux (GERD) and urinary stress incontinence.[428]

Two thirds of the people in the U.S., over 205 million people, are thus at risk of the above diseases based on their BMIs alone.

---

[426] McDougall, Diet, Drugs and Diabetes - One Hundred Years of Missed Opportunities https://www.youtube.com/watch?v=iosoXlr3ZVI
[427] Gina Battaglia, Health Risks of Low BMI
http://healthyeating.sfgate.com/health-risks-low-bmi-5687.html
[428] East Carolina Family Practice Center, What is BMI and Why is BMI Important? https://www.ecu.edu/cs-dhs/fammed/customcf/resources/nutrition/what_is_BMI.pdf

To calculate your BMI you can go to this website, which has a BMI calculator. Simply enter your height and weight and click to calculate. http://www.nhlbi.nih.gov/health/educational/lose_wt/BMI/bmicalc.htm

Or you can calculate it manually using one of the following formulas:

BMI = mass in kilograms / (height in meters)^2

BMI = weight in pounds x 703 / (height in inches)^2

So if a man weighs 170 lbs. and is 70 inches tall (5'10"), his BMI would be:

BMI = $(170 \times 703 / (70)^2) = 24.4$

Another way to learn your BMI is to consult a BMI chart. The chart on the next page also tells you what your BMI figure means.

Where does the above calculated BMI fit on the underweight/ ideal weight/overweight/obese continuum? The BMI chart should make that clear. This person with a BMI of 24.4 is right on the edge of being overweight.

➢ **The diet dilemma:** The person described above should try to lose from 10 to 20 pounds to reach his ideal weight for optimal health.

But dieting to lose weight rarely works in the long term. Part of the reason is that many diets include unhealthy foods which encourage unhealthy pounds to stay on. Additionally, the dieter doesn't adequately understand why certain foods should stay off the menu. They don't know which foods they really should avoid, and why. They aren't convinced of the seriousness of choosing the right foods, and are unaware of the damage the junk food they love is really doing to their bodies, the disease it is causing and will cause for them and their families.

Body Mass Index

Zone labels shown across the chart: **UNDERWEIGHT**, **HEALTHY**, **OVERWEIGHT**, **OBESE**, **EXTREMELY OBESE**

WEIGHT lbs →	100	105	110	115	120	125	130	135	140	145	150	155	160	165	170	175	180	185	190	195	200	205	210	215
kgs →	45.5	47.7	50.0	52.3	54.5	56.8	59.1	61.4	63.6	65.9	68.2	70.5	72.7	75.0	77.3	79.5	81.8	84.1	86.4	88.6	90.9	93.2	95.5	97.7
HEIGHT ft (cm)																								
5'0" (152)	19	20	21	22	23	24	25	26	27	28	29	30	31	32	33	34	35	36	37	38	39	40	41	42
5'1" (155)	18	19	20	21	22	23	24	25	26	27	28	29	30	31	32	33	34	35	35	36	37	38	39	40
5'2" (158)	18	19	20	20	21	22	23	24	25	26	27	28	29	30	30	31	32	33	34	35	36	37	38	39
5'3" (160)	17	18	19	20	21	22	23	23	24	25	26	27	28	29	30	31	31	32	33	34	35	36	37	38
5'4" (163)	17	17	18	19	20	21	22	23	23	24	25	26	27	28	29	29	30	31	32	33	34	35	35	36
5'5" (165)	16	17	18	19	20	20	21	22	23	24	25	25	26	27	28	29	30	30	31	32	33	34	35	35
5'6" (168)	16	16	17	18	19	20	20	21	22	23	24	24	25	26	27	28	28	29	30	31	32	33	33	34
5'7" (170)	15	16	17	18	18	19	20	21	22	22	23	24	25	25	26	27	28	29	29	30	31	32	33	33
5'8" (173)	15	15	16	17	18	18	19	20	21	22	22	23	24	25	25	26	27	28	28	29	30	31	31	32
5'9" (175)	14	15	16	17	17	18	19	20	20	21	22	23	23	24	25	25	26	27	28	28	29	30	31	31
5'10" (178)	14	15	15	16	17	17	18	19	20	20	21	22	22	23	24	25	25	26	27	27	28	29	30	30
5'11" (180)	14	14	15	16	16	17	18	18	19	20	21	21	22	23	23	24	25	25	26	27	28	28	29	30
6'0" (183)	13	14	14	15	16	16	17	18	18	19	20	21	21	22	23	23	24	25	25	26	27	27	28	29
6'1" (185)	13	13	14	15	15	16	17	17	18	19	19	20	21	21	22	23	23	24	25	25	26	27	27	28
6'2" (188)	12	13	14	14	15	16	16	17	17	18	19	19	20	21	21	22	23	23	24	25	25	26	27	27
6'3" (191)	12	13	13	14	14	15	16	16	17	18	18	19	19	20	21	21	22	23	23	24	24	25	26	26
6'4" (193)	12	12	13	14	14	15	15	16	17	17	18	18	19	20	20	21	21	22	23	23	24	25	25	26

For many, knowing some of the important facts about these things, and being committed to doing what is right from a stewardship standpoint, makes eating the right foods, and saying no to the wrong ones, a lot less difficult.

Do you find it difficult to refuse to smoke cigarettes? Or to sniff glue? Most of us would say no, it's easy to avoid such things. But why is it so easy? Many people find the use of such substances pleasurable.

But you can easily say no, and at least part of the reason is because you truly believe there are dangerous health consequences. Another part of the reason is that you aren't addicted to them. But perhaps you are addicted to sugar, oil, meat, etc. The same principle holds for all addicts: Understanding the health-damaging effects of your addiction plays a major role in helping you kick the habit. So keep learning!

For the man above with a BMI of 24.4, his goal of losing 10-20 pounds (and improving his health overall) will very likely be reached if he follows the lifestyle principles I am suggesting in this book. See **Chapter 11: Diets**, for more on dieting.

➢ **BMI and various dietary habits:** Researchers compiled BMI figures of people with various dietary habits to determine which type of diet tended to produce the healthiest BMI.[429] Data from people on five types of diets were compared. The findings were as follows:

Regular meat eaters......................28.8

Occasional meat/dairy eaters.......27.3

Pesco-vegetarians..........................26.3

Lacto-ovo vegetarians...................25.7

Vegans..23.6

---

[429] Serena Tonstad, M.D., Ph.D., et al, <u>Type of Vegetarian Diet, Body Weight, and Prevalence of Type 2 Diabetes</u> http://www.ncbi.nlm.nih.gov/pmc/articles/ PMC2671114/ This study also found that the more animal products were consumed, the more likely the person would have type 2 diabetes.

BMIs of 25 to 30 indicate the person is overweight. So according to this survey, only those on a plant based diet, consuming less than one serving of meat or dairy per month, have an average BMI in the ideal weight range (18-24). Even vegetarians are normally overweight. The average person on the SAD is dangerously close to being obese, and thus has a high risk of developing serious chronic disease.

Notice that even the vegans, with an average BMI of 23.6, are close to being in the overweight category. How can this be? This is evidence that many are "junk food vegans." I suspect that for most of these their primary reason for choosing their diet is moral (they don't wish to be a party to animal cruelty), not good health. So they eat a lot of sugar, oils and processed foods.

Regarding BMI it is good to recognize that it gives an approximate estimate of a person's health as it relates to body weight. Certainly a person can be in good physical shape and be at their correct personal weight, with a BMI near the overweight range. But that would be relatively rare, a person with a very stocky build.

Tobacco use

We all know tobacco use is not a healthy lifestyle habit, and this book was written with the assumption that the reader does not smoke or chew. However, perhaps it would be good to discuss it briefly. I hope the reader will find the few things I share on this subject to be interesting and helpful.

There is no record of tobacco use in the Bible. So we can assume that God did not give it to humans for their use in Eden, or even later for that matter. Tobacco use was unknown by Europeans until Columbus discovered natives of Cuba using it. It was introduced to Europe for the first time in the early 1500s.

Some will argue that God created tobacco, so we should use this gift and enjoy it. Of course God created the tobacco plant for a reason. But it was not to help us get deadly diseases. Using it in a way which is harmful to the body is an abuse of God's creation.

Tobacco has many medicinal uses. It has been used as a tooth whitening ingredient in toothpaste, for headache relief (breathing the smell of the fresh leaves), for colds and fevers, applied as a poultice, and for many other ailments.[430]

The health-damaging effects of smoking and chewing tobacco are well known. Cigarette smoking alone causes about 480,000 deaths annually in the U.S., and 3,000,000 worldwide. Smokers can expect any of several types of cancers, stroke, COPD (emphysema), diabetes, etc. Users of chewing tobacco can expect oral cancers, gum disease, tooth loss, etc.

> Tobacco leaves and the smoke generated when they are burned contain over 4 thousand chemicals, the best known of which is nicotine, first isolated from tobacco leaves in 1828 by Posselt and Reimann. It is the nicotine that causes smokers to become addicted to tobacco, and the chemical itself is lethal in small doses…
>
> (Some of the) harmful contents of tobacco smoke (include) the carcinogenic polycyclic aromatic hydrocarbons and N-nitroso compounds; irritant substances such as acrolein; benzene; formaldehyde; ammonia; acetone; acetic acid, and carbon monoxide.[431]

When a person smokes, nicotine is absorbed into the bloodstream from the lungs and quickly makes its way to the brain, and to every other organ as well.

In the brain the nicotine joins to nicotine receptors, which have been hungrily crying out for a fix. Thus the tobacco user is a sort of slave to these nicotine receptors, and each puff is an automatic reaction to the receptors demanding another dose. A smoker may smoke several cigarettes without consciously thinking about what they are doing.

The more one smokes, the more nicotine receptors are stimulated to appear in the brain. Thus the greater the hunger for nicotine becomes. This is addiction.

---

[430] Anne Charlton, Ph.D., *Journal of the Royal Society of Medicine,* Medicinal uses of tobacco in history http://jrs.sagepub.com/content/97/6/292.full
[431] *Ibid.*

For chewing tobacco, the process of addiction, and the health hazards, are much the same – though chewing delivers more nicotine than smoking.

Tobacco use poses a significantly greater risk to health than obesity. Many fear that if they quit smoking they will gain weight. It is true that the average smoker does gain some weight when they quit. However, the positive effect on their health of quitting smoking far outweighs the negative effects of putting on a few extra pounds.

And while the former tobacco user is in the mood to make positive lifestyle changes, they can also move toward a whole plant food diet, and seek ways to reduce stress (stress makes quitting as well as weight loss more difficult). These changes will make any significant amount of weight gain extremely unlikely!

If you smoke, I urge you to make that life-changing decision to quit now. I know it is an extremely difficult addiction to break. But God can give you the strength to do it, if you are willing and determined, and trust in His help. If for no other reason, quit for the sake of those around you whom you love and who love you. Your habit is killing them as well.

Toxins in water

➢ **Fluoride:** Fluoride has no known use in the human body, but rather is toxic. It is classified as a drug by the FDA.[432] Paul Connett, Ph.D., wrote:

> There is not one single process in the human body that needs fluoride to function properly. There is no evidence that fluoride is an essential nutrient. On the other hand there are many biological components and processes that are potentially harmed by fluoride, e.g. fluoride inhibits enzymes, switches on G-proteins, etc....[433]

---

[432] The FDA has asserted this repeatedly. This letter from the FDA to the Honorable Ken Calvert is just one example: http://www.fluoridealert.org/wp-content/uploads/fda-2000a.pdf
[433] Paul Connett, Ph.D., FDA and OTC Fluoride (slide presentation) http://www.fda.gov/downloads/drugs/newsevents/ucm392708.pdf

He adds that

> The level of fluoride in mothers' milk is EXTREMELY LOW
> (0.004 ppm, NRC , 2006, p. 40). A bottle-fed baby in a fluoridated
> community (0.7–1.2 ppm) is getting 175–300 times the fluoride
> dose that a breast fed baby gets.[434]

If fluoride waste from aluminum, steel and other industries were
dumped in rivers the polluters would go to jail. But when it is put
into our water supply so that we drink it, it is supposed to be
good for our teeth. In fact it is not.

Fluoride consumption is known to cause dental fluorosis
(discoloration of the teeth), and to accumulate in the bones,
making them more prone to break. There have been several
studies which implicate fluoride in lowering IQs.[435] Yet the
powers that be insist on "medicating" everyone with fluoride
without their consent, without a doctor's prescription, and
without any controls on dosage!

Here are some measures you may want to take to reduce
fluoride exposure for you and your family:

- Find out if your water supply is fluoridated. Even if the city
  doesn't add fluoride, the water may contain it naturally.

- Try to avoid drinking fluoridated water.

- Consider installing a water filtration system which removes
  fluoride. (See **Water filtration**, below.)

- Do not brush with fluoride toothpaste.

- Do not let your dentist give you or your children fluoride
  treatments.

Remember, most medical professionals really do want to help
you the best way they know how. But they can't know
everything, and can make mistakes. In past centuries physicians
would often drain blood from patients, as it was thought to be

---

[434] *Ibid.*

[435] Joseph G. Hattersley, *The Journal of Orthomolecular Medicine,* The Case
Against Fluoridation http://orthomolecular.org/library/jom/1999/articles/1999-
v14n04-p185.shtml

therapeutic. But now we know that is not true. Many current therapies, such as fluoride treatment for teeth, will one day be considered rather barbaric, too.

At any rate, cutting back, especially cutting out completely, added sugar and animal products from your diet, will prove to be much more beneficial to your teeth than any fluoride water, toothpaste, or syrupy goop in a dentist's office.

➤ **Chlorine in tap water:** Chlorine is another toxic substance which should not be consumed in any form, whether liquid or gas. It is so dangerous that it was used as a chemical weapon by the Germans in WWI:

> According to the fieldpost letter of Major Karl von Zingler, the first chlorine gas attack by German forces took place before 2 January 1915: "In other war theaters it does not go better and it has been said that our Chlorine is very effective. 140 English officers have been killed. This is a horrible weapon ...".[436,437]

When you drink tap water, you are most likely drinking chlorine (and probably fluoride). Chlorinating drinking water helps prevent water-borne diseases, which is good. But in preventing acute infections, it may cause chronic disease.

Ingested chlorine kills good bacteria in your gut. Many claim this encourages candida overgrowth, which can cause significant health problems.[438,439]

---

[436] *Academic Dictionaries and Encyclopedias,* Chemical weapons in World War I http://en.academic.ru/dic.nsf/enwiki/11525563#cite_note-8

[437] Aksulu, N. Melek (May 2006). Die Feldpostbriefe Karl v. Zinglers aus dem Ersten Weltkrieg (PDF). *Nobilitas, Zeitschrift für deutsche Adelsforschung Folge* IX (41): 57: "Rousselare 2 Januar 15 ... Auf anderen Kriegsschauplätzen ist es ja auch nicht besser und die Wirkung von unserem Chlor soll ja sehr gut sein. Es sollen 140 englische Offiziere erledigt worden sein. Es ist doch eine furchtbare Waffe...."
http://perweb.firat.edu.tr/personel/yayinlar/fua_241/241_26862.pdf

[438] *Leakygut.co.uk,* Leaky Gut Syndrome
http://www.leakygut.co.uk/Candidiasis.htm

[439] Dr. John Humiston, M.D., Candida Risk Factors
http://candidamd.com/candida/exposures.html

When you take a hot shower with chlorinated water, you inhale chlorine gas. When chlorine enters the body as a result of breathing, swallowing, or skin contact, it reacts with water to produce acids.[440] The acids are corrosive and damage cells in the body on contact.

> *Chlorinated water is associated each year in America with thousands of cases of cancer.*

Tests comparing the effects of non-chlorinated and chlorinated drinking water on chickens found that the chlorine drinking group developed arterial plaques, while the control group didn't. This same effect in humans has been noted as well.[441]

To make matters worse,

> A…meta-analysis found chlorinated water is associated each year in America with about 4,200 cases of bladder cancer and 6,500 cases of rectal cancer. Chlorine is estimated to account for nine percent of bladder cancer cases and 18 percent of rectal cancers. Those cancers develop because the bladder and rectum store waste products for periods of time. (Keeping the bowels moving regularly lowers such risk.) Chlorinated water is associated, too, with higher total risk of combined cancers.[442] [See the article for footnote references to the research.]

Of course, as with any substance, the toxicity depends on the dose. The low levels of chlorine ingested from tap water or breathed in a shower don't often produce acute harmful effects. However, for some sensitive individuals it can cause serious problems in the short term. And the above referenced studies, and many more, make it clear that for all of us the cumulative

---

[440] New York State Department of Health, The Facts About Chlorine https://www.health.ny.gov/environmental/emergency/chemical_terrorism/chlorine_general.htm

[441] Joseph G. Hattersley, *The Journal of Orthomolecular Medicine* Vol. 15 2000, The Negative Health Effects of Chlorine http://www.orthomolecular.org/library/jom/2000/articles/2000-v15n02-p089.shtml

[442] *Ibid.*

effect of chlorine exposure will be harmful to one degree or another. So I advise avoiding chlorinated water whenever possible.

See the section on **Water filtration** below for some ideas on how to reduce your exposure to chlorine in drinking and shower water.

➢ **Chlorine in swimming pools:** Pools of course typically contain a lot of chlorine. Again, this cuts down on dangerous disease-causing pathogens. But considering that this substance is toxic, and how readily it is absorbed into the body via the skin, lungs and mouth, why would we assume that swimming in it is harmless?

When I was a child, my sister, our cousins and I would spend hours on Saturdays swimming in my grandparents' pool. We had a great time! But I also remember that the longer we swam, the more my chest would hurt whenever I took a deep breath after we were done. At the time I assumed that was due to the L.A. smog. But now I believe it was actually the chlorine. I played hard in the smog in other contexts with no chest pain.

Indoor pools are the worst, of course, since the chlorine gas evaporating off the water is much more concentrated in the air near the pool, and the main way chlorine is absorbed into the body is via the lungs. Indoor swimming pool areas can be virtual gas chambers.

A study done in Europe examined the relationship between the prevalence of public pools and childhood asthma. The study's conclusion was as follows:

> The prevalence of childhood asthma and availability of indoor swimming pools in Europe are linked through associations that are consistent with the hypothesis implicating pool chlorine in the rise of childhood asthma in industrialised countries.[443]

---

[443] M. Nickmilder, A. Bernard, *Journal of Occupational and Environmental Medicine,* Ecological association between childhood asthma and availability of indoor chlorinated swimming pools in Europe
http://oem.bmj.com/content/64/1/37.short

Exposure to chlorinated swimming pools has been linked to development of melanoma.[444] And of course, it would also be linked to the problems associated with drinking chlorinated water, noted in the previous section.

If someone wants to swim in chlorinated pools, that is fine. But it would be good if everyone knew of the dangers so they could make an informed decision.

There are safe alternatives to chlorination of pools, such as hydrogen peroxide. Hot tubs may be disinfected with colloidal silver. But these methods are more expensive in the short term; disinfecting a pool with chlorine may be more expensive in the long term, however, because of the ultimate health care costs which may result.

Swimming is a very healthy activity, probably one of the best ways to get exercise. But the evidence I have seen of the dangers of swimming in chlorinated swimming pools makes me wonder if the only truly healthy swimming can take place in lakes, rivers, and the ocean.

➤ **Pharmaceuticals in tap water:** Medications can go through a person and end up in the sewer. People also dispose of pills in the toilet. So **the drugs get into the water supply and are not filtered out at water treatment plants**, which are primarily concerned with making sure there are no germs or particulates in the water. Thus tap water often contains lots of pharmaceuticals, such as antibiotics, anti-convulsants, mood stabilizers, sex hormones, and NSAIDs (non-steroidal pain killers). They are normally in the water in small quantities, but it is unknown what the cumulative effect of ingesting them over a long period is.

➤ **Water filtration:** Unless your water supply is a good local well, with no chlorine or other toxins added, you should consider investing in some sort of water purification system for your

---

[444] Joseph G. Hattersley, *The Journal of Orthomolecular Medicine* Vol. 15 2000, The Negative Health Effects of Chlorine http://www. orthomolecular.org/library/jom/2000/articles/2000-v15n02-p089.shtml

house.

If you decide to drink distilled water, you will want to invest in a water distillation system, which will be more economical in the long run than buying it by the gallon. You should get one with a carbon filter, which will remove volatile gasses during the condensation process.

There are a number of different non-distillation water filtration options to consider. Again, buying a filtration system will be more economical in the long run than buying drinking water by the gallon.

There are large, whole house water filter systems, as well as "point of use" systems. The latter is a smaller filter system which is attached to any faucet or shower head where you need pure water.

What is needed is a filter which will remove fluoride, chlorine, and pharmaceuticals. Brita-type filters may remove some chlorine, and improve taste, but they do not remove fluoride or pharmaceuticals. You need either a reverse osmosis (RO) filter system, a high quality gravity filter system, or the filter system sold by Pure Effect Filters,[445] which is the one we use when in the States.

Unlike RO systems, the Pure Effect system retains helpful minerals, and it doesn't waste any water when filtering (RO systems waste a significant amount). The Pure Effect system is a bit expensive, but much cheaper per gallon than buying filtered water, and I believe the health benefits are worth it. There may be other, better systems out there; do some research and see what you find.

Of course, you can buy your drinking water by the gallon. The cheapest way to get good drinking water is to buy "bulk" or "refill" reverse osmosis water (such as Culligan) at a supermarket, where it usually goes for anywhere from $.25 to $.40 per gallon.

---

[445] www.pureeffectfilters.com

Shower head filters are available starting at about $40. These can help you avoid the gas chamber effect of showering with chlorinated water.

Be sure to change the filter cartridges on schedule as indicated by the manufacturer.

A few more facts and tips

➢ **Essential oils:** I want to briefly mention essential oils, as they have been gaining in popularity in recent years, and considering the information I share in this book about dietary oils, some may be wondering if and how essential oils fit into a whole food plant based lifestyle. An essential oil is a

> highly volatile substance isolated by a physical process from an odoriferous plant of a single botanical species. The oil bears the name of the plant from which it is derived; for example, rose oil or peppermint oil. Such oils were called essential because they were thought to represent the very essence of odour and flavour.[446]

Essential oils are medicinal, not nutritional. Normally they are used in very small amounts, and either consumed by mouth (mixed in water or taken in a capsule), smeared or massaged into the skin, or diffused into the air so they may be breathed. Some are effective but safe antimicrobials, and so are used in cleaning solutions.

Different essential oils have different properties and are used for a wide variety of purposes, such as flavoring, to give a nice smell to perfumes, cosmetics and soaps, to disinfect, to affect moods, and to heal from various ailments. Some popular essential oils and oil blends are thieves, lavender, peppermint, frankincense and lemon.

A few specific ways essential oils are commonly used:

- Tea may be made with thieves oil, lemon and honey. Many say drinking this tea is helpful in reducing the cold's

---

[446] *Encyclopedia Britannica,* <u>Essential Oil</u>
<u>http://www.britannica.com/EBchecked/topic/193135/essential-oil</u>

severity and duration. (My wife is among them.)

- Diluted thieves oil may be vaporized to help disinfect the air in the house and prevent colds, flu, etc. from passing between family members.

- Lavender oil may help calm allergic reactions when the vapors are inhaled. Many also use it to deal with pain, anxiety, and depression.

- When driving a long distance the driver may smear a little diluted peppermint oil on the chest or neck to help maintain alertness.

Essential oils vary considerably in quality and purity, depending on the brand. While a high quality brand may be able to achieve impressive and consistent results, a cheaper one may not. "You get what you pay for."

I believe essential oils can be helpful, and when used correctly they certainly are a better choice than medications and other toxic chemicals. But like any medicinal product, for optimal health they should not be used in an attempt to correct health issues caused by the continued consumption of a toxic diet. They may help relieve some symptoms, but they are wholly incapable of counteracting the permanent damage a bad diet inflicts, and preventing the chronic diseases which will naturally result. Of prime importance is to get yourself on a truly health promoting diet, as well as making other healthy lifestyle choices. Beyond that you may find that essential oils can help you to further achieve the best health possible.

If you want to learn more about essential oils, I suggest you contact our friend Sharon Koehn through her Young Living Essential Oils website.[447] Sharon and her husband Mark are great folks with a lot of knowledge about essential oils and how to use them effectively.

---

[447] Website of Sharon Koehn, Young Living representative: http://essentialjoys.younglivingconnect.com/

➢ **Eating in restaurants:** The increase in obesity and chronic disease in the developed world has paralleled the decrease in cooking and eating at home and the increase in eating out. This is no coincidence. It is no surprise that studies show that those who eat more home-prepared meals are markedly healthier than those who eat out often, eat a lot of takeout, or eat a lot of packaged food like frozen pizzas, TV dinners, etc.

You have little control of what goes into your meal when you eat out, even if you order side dishes like steamed veggies. At Cracker Barrel I once asked what was in their veggie side dishes. Almost all of them contained bacon or bacon fat, including the spinach and the cooked apples! Remember, restaurants will put in the food whatever will keep people coming back for more, so taste is paramount, *not* your health.

During his 40+ year career, Dr. Michael Klaper, M.D., has repeatedly seen first hand the physical devastation caused by unhealthy diets. He knows full well that restaurants provide some of the worst the SAD has to offer. Here he shares his heart regarding how to handle eating out:

> Restaurant food is ethnic flavored salt, sugar, and fat, served with seared flesh or over cooked vegetables… You're going to have to (eat at restaurants sometimes,) there are social pressures, etc…. (But) don't kid yourself that anything healthy is happening in those kitchens. It's not. And you don't want to eat a whole lot of it… I have gotten my restaurant eating down to as seldom as possible. Less is more when it comes to restaurant meals.

> You know what I do before I go out to eat? I eat! I have a salad or a bowl of soup before I go so I'm not famished when I get there, and I don't polish off half the basket of bread before the waiter gets there. Order as healthfully as possible, order the vegetable soup, the steamed greens, eat it and get the heck out of there as soon as you can.[448]

---

[448] Klaper, *VegSource* 2012, <u>Olive Oil Is Not Healthy</u>
https://www.youtube.com/watch?v=OGGQxJLuVjg

Some restaurants are catching on to the health conscious consumer's desires, and an increasing number are offering vegetarian and vegan options. Cracker Barrel, for example, has, according to their website, a very attractive vegetable plate with corn, broccoli, carrots, cauliflower, and a sweet potato. Doesn't look like any of those are prepared with bacon fat, but I would ask to be sure – and maybe take a peek in the kitchen to really be sure. I would also ask whether they can prepare the sweet potato without added sugar and butter – a real challenge for some restaurants. If they can't, you may want to pass it up.

> *Restaurant food is ethnic flavored salt, sugar, and fat, served with seared flesh or over cooked vegetables.*
> *— Dr. Michael Klaper*

Don't be shy about asking your server if they have a vegan or vegetarian menu. If there is a good-looking, almost all-vegetable dish, except that it has cheese and/or eggs on it, ask your server if they can leave those ingredients off and instead substitute extra avocado or broccoli or whatever.

Be wary of "vegetarian" or "vegan" menu items which may be prepared with lots of oil and/or sugar.

Don't get uptight if in spite of your best efforts to explain your wishes to your server you end up with a meal with lots of oil, or a salad with some cheese. Just eat however much of it you want, and move on. A little off-the-menu food semi-occasionally won't make any significant difference in your health in the long run, while letting yourself get stressed over it will. (Not to mention make those around you uncomfortable, and sorry you ever started this new lifestyle.)

But the bottom line is that it is best from a health standpoint to keep the frequency of your visits to restaurants down to only semi-occasionally or less. Save yourself some money, and save your health. Eat home-cooked meals as much as possible.

➢ **Coconut oil – Skin moisturizer:** Use a natural oil such as coconut oil to moisturize your skin. Coconut oil is a good choice because, some say, it nourishes the skin. **Hand lotions have chemicals which will absorb into your skin and get into your blood.** Read the label. Do you know what those strange chemical terms mean? Do you know what those chemicals do when they enter your blood? Do you really want them in your blood?

➢ **Hard lotion:** Coconut oil tends to be absorbed quickly, and your skin can soon be dry again (if you have skin as dry as mine). Skin moisturizer actually should remain on the skin, to keep the skin's natural moisture in. Lotion bars or "hard lotion" is a good solution. It can be made from 1 part coconut oil, 1 part shea butter, and 1 part beeswax, heated and mixed together and poured into small containers or small muffin cups. (You can add some yummy smelling essential oil if you wish.) It keeps skin moist a long time, and it is totally natural and healthy. Check out this website if you want a recipe with step-by-step instructions: http://wellnessmama.com/4770/lotion-bars/.

➢ **Rebounding:** Jumping on a mini-trampoline, commonly called a rebounder, is a great way to exercise. Try simply jumping, doing jumping jacks, etc. You can do some jogging in place on a rebounder, especially to get your heart moving, but be sure to do at least 20 minutes of jumping as well. This kind of jumping is said to get your lymph moving. A certified lymphologist wrote:

> The body has a built-in need for activation. The lymph system, for example, bathes every cell, carrying nutrients to the cell and waste products away. Yet the lymph is totally dependent on physical exercise to move.

> Without adequate movement, the cells are left stewing in their own waste products and starving for nutrients, a situation that contributes to arthritis, cancer and other degenerative diseases. Vigorous exercise such as rebounding [jumping on a therapeutic mini-trampoline] is reported to increase lymph flow by 15 to 30 times. Also, bones become stronger with exercise.

> Vertical motion workouts such as rebounding are much different and much more beneficial and efficient than horizontal motion

workouts, such as jogging or running.[449]

You can easily adjust your exertions from the equivalent of an easy walk up to a brisk run. And rebounding is much easier on the knees than jogging or running. After decades of hard running my knees started to hurt whenever I ran more than 30 minutes or so, and after running even a short distance I had a hard time walking up stairs. But I can rebound as long as I please, and then briskly climb a flight of stairs, all with no pain.

Rebounders can cost up to $700 for the German made bungee suspension Bellicon. You can also get cheap ones for under $40, such as at Walmart. As usual, you get what you pay for. These cheap ones only work for children; even though they may be rated for up to 250 lbs., the springs, mat, stitching, and other parts will break when used by adults.

The first rebounder I bought was The Urban Rebounder, which costs a little over $100. It is probably the best brand in that price range.

If you can spend more, the ReboundAIR is highly rated, and after much research it is what I bought (the Urban Rebounder is in Guinea, and I'm not currently). The best price I could find for the quarter fold model is about $340 on eBay.[450,451] It is relatively quiet, has a much nicer bounce than the cheaper units I have tried, and is much easer to set up than other folding rebounders. And, very importantly, it is the only rebounder with a lifetime warranty. If anything breaks on it ever, the company will replace

---

[449] See the full article, which describes many more health benefits of rebounding, at http://www.wellbeingjournal.com/rebounding-good-for-the-lymph-system/. This is just one of many such articles that have been written on this subject. I can't promise that all the claims made in the article are scientifically verifiable, but if even half of them are true, rebounding is definitely something anyone interested in good health should look into. (As far as I can tell, the author does not sell rebounders!)

[450] Website for ReboundAir: https://www.reboundair.com/vhosts/rebound-aerobics/products1.htm

[451] Quarter fold ReboundAir rebounder on eBay http://www.ebay.com/itm/281462925564?_trksid=p2060778.m2749.l2649&ss PageName=STRK%3AMEBIDX%3AIT

the part free of charge. This is important, because some parts on any rebounder can break, leading to expensive and time-consuming repairs. And even parts on the expensive Bellicon wear out, including the bungees, but that company only provides a very limited warranty.

Rebounders are much lighter and more portable than other comparable exercise equipment; they can be stored under a bed or in a closet. And they are relatively low-tech, not needing to be plugged in, which is a plus. And they provide a better overall workout than other equipment of comparable cost.

Kids love rebounding, and it is a great exercise for them, especially when they are unable to get outside and run around during cold winter months.

If you think you can't fit a workout into your day, but you always make time to watch the evening news or a morning show, you can easily rebound while you watch. (Often I will watch a sermon or health-related lecture online while I rebound.) And you can rebound with small hand weights, combining your cardio workout with your weight-bearing exercise.

Note that rebounding isn't for everyone. A few people may find it makes their neck or back hurt, or gives them a headache. Higher quality models have a better, more even bounce which will reduce the risk of such problems.

➢ **Vitamin B17:** Many seeds contain a compound often called vitamin B17 (though it is not a vitamin, as it is not a compound which your body requires for proper functioning). B17 contains cyanide and another toxic substance. Proponents of B17 say that these toxins are kept bound up in the molecule until it comes in contact with cancer cells, where chemicals on the surface of the tumor cause the toxins in B17 to be released and kill the cancer.[452] The details of how this works are of course very complex, but that is the gist of what happens, as I understand it.

---

[452] *Worldwithoutcancer.org.uk,* Welcome to Worldwithoutcancer.org.uk
http://worldwithoutcancer.org.uk/

The medical establishment has discounted these claims, and asserted that eating seeds with B17 is in fact dangerous. But if this were so there would be many sick and dead people as a result, since there are multitudes who consume them on a regular basis. And there are many who claim that far from being harmed, they were cured from cancer as a result.

The anti-cancer drug laetrile is essentially concentrated B17. Though it is safe, it is tightly regulated by the FDA and very difficult to obtain. Interesting, when you consider that chemotherapy and radiation treatments are carcinogenic and cause much suffering and death, and yet are the gold standard for cancer therapy.

Some claim that regularly consuming B17 can help the immune system dispatch any little cancers which frequently occur in all or bodies, and thus prevent tumors from developing. Others of course dispute this claim.

My personal belief from all I have read on the subject is that eating these seeds is at worst harmless, and at best it may prevent cancer. And since seeds contain other nutrients, I make it a point to eat B17 containing seeds. The hearts of apricot seeds have the highest concentration of B17, and other stone fruit seeds (peach, nectarine, plum, cherry) and apple seeds contain it as well.

➢ **Children with chronic disease:** We have seen that clinical studies confirm that a whole food plant based diet can keep artery-clogging plaque from forming. But the fact is that **most people on the SAD already have vascular disease before they graduate from high school.**

Dr. Esselstyn was a doctor in the armed forces during the Vietnam war. He and his colleagues did autopsies on many American servicemen killed in action, as well as on many Vietnamese. These autopsies revealed that 80% of the Americans, whose average age was 20, had coronary artery disease,[453] while only a small percentage of the Vietnamese did.

Childhood obesity is becoming a huge problem in the West. Some clueless parents are basically weaning their babies at McDonalds. The term "infant obesity" is increasingly being used of obese infants, who are commonly born to obese mothers, but rarely diagnosed as obese by their physicians.[454] The dietary sins of the fathers are being visited on their children. "My brothers, these things ought not to be so!"

Type 2 diabetes used to be called "adult onset diabetes," because it tended to strike only adults, who had been eating the SAD for many years. But this is no longer an accurate designation, because the SAD is getting so bad, children are eating it starting earlier and earlier, and they are spending more and more time sitting around inside in front of video screens and less and less time running around outside playing. An alarming number are becoming type 2 diabetics while still young.

Cancer rates among children are also rising, especially leukemia. We have seen that consumption of processed meats – hotdogs, sausage, etc. – are a significant cause of leukemia. Other features of the SAD are also carcinogenic. And chemical exposure from household cleaners and household pesticide use is a significant contributor as well.[455]

Please protect your children from these dangers. The sooner a child switches to a whole food plant based diet, and the more you can limit exposure to household toxins, the better.

➢ **Gut bacteria – Good and bad:** There are literally trillions of bacteria, or microflora, in your colon (large intestine). Some of these are pathogenic, promoting disease, while others are

---

[453] Esselstyn, Huffington Post Interview
http://www.dresselstyn.com/huffpost.htm
[454] D.P. McCormick et al, *Journal of Pediatrics,* Infant obesity: are we ready to make this diagnosis? http://www.ncbi.nlm.nih.gov/pubmed/20338575
[455] Christina Jewett, *California Watch,* As adult cancer cases drop, rates go up among children http://californiawatch.org/dailyreport/adult-cancer-cases-drop-rates-go-among-children-16538

beneficial, assisting in the digestion of food and absorption of nutrients. One key to maintaining good health is to maximize the amount of good bacteria, while minimizing the amount of bad.

A diet containing added sugars tends to increase the amount of bad bacteria, plus candida fungus. A high meat diet also shifts the balance the wrong way, as explained by Dr. McDougall:

> The partially digested remnants of our meals, after arrival in our large intestines, become the foods for our microflora. Each species of bacteria survives best on specific kinds of nutrients. In short, "friendly" bacteria prefer to dine on plant-food remnants, and pathogens thrive when the diet is low in plant foods and high in meat and other "junk food." Therefore, what we choose to eat determines the predominance of the bacteria species that will live in our gut. By changing from a diet based on animal and highly processed foods to whole plant foods, you can suppress the growth of harmful bacteria and stimulate those that are beneficial. Major alterations in the microflora take place within one to two weeks of changing a person's diet.[456,457]

A probiotic can be helpful in increasing the amount of good bacteria in the gut.

> Probiotics have been found to inhibit intestinal bacterial enzymes involved in the synthesis of colonic carcinogens. There are many mechanisms by which probiotics enhance intestinal health, including stimulation of immunity, competition for limited nutrients, inhibition of epithelial and mucosal adherence, inhibition of epithelial invasion and production of antimicrobial substances.[458]

Many report health conditions clearing up after starting on a good quality probiotic. Also, if you have to take antibiotics, be sure and take a good probiotic for a while after you finish the

---

[456] R. Peltonen et al, Applied Environmental Microbiology An uncooked vegan diet shifts the profile of human fecal microflora: computerized analysis of direct stool sample gas-liquid chromatography profiles of bacterial cellular fatty acids http://www.ncbi.nlm.nih.gov/pubmed/1482187

[457] McDougall, Beneficial Bowel Bacteria – Our Neglected Friends https://www.drmcdougall.com/misc/pdf/pdf050800nl.pdf

[458] Rial D. Rolfe, The Journal of Nutrition, The Role of Probiotic Cultures in the Control of Gastrointestinal Health http://jn.nutrition.org/content/130/2/396S.short

drug, because the antibiotic will kill not only the pathogenic bacteria, but also the good bacteria in your gut.

Many eat yogurt or drink milk-based kefir to replenish their probiotics after an antibiotic. This may be helpful temporarily, but of course it carries the health-eroding baggage that always comes with dairy. I also understand that the bacteria from yogurt does not establish itself in your gut permanently. This indicates that it is not native to the human gut, and thus not the best solution. So clearly it is better to find a non-dairy alternative.

Good quality probiotics can be expensive. Aside from a period following antibiotic use I doubt they are normally needed, except perhaps by meat eaters and those eating a lot of sugar, oils, and processed foods. A whole food plant based diet tends to support a healthy population of healthy bacteria in the gut.

> **Gut bacteria – Meat based and plant based:** As stated above, when a person changes their diet to whole food plant based, their gut bacteria adjusts. The species of bacteria which like to dine on meat are different than the ones which like to dine on plants. So the former will die out in the gut of a 100% plant eater, and the latter will thrive. Furthermore, **as the gut bacteria of a meat eater chews on the meat he eats it will produce substances which are harmful to blood vessels, leading to heart disease.** Dr. Esselstyn explains how this works:

By adjusting your diet to one of only whole plant foods, you can eliminate vascular disease-causing bacteria from your gut.

Omnivores possess intestinal bacteria which metabolize lecithin and carnitine from these foods into trimethylamine N-oxide (TMAO) that promotes vascular injury. Increased plasma levels of TMAO were associated with 2.5-fold increased risk of a major adverse cardiovascular event even after adjustment for traditional risk factors. However, those who strictly consumed plant foods were not able to manufacture TMAO even when challenged with the main dietary sources (steak and/or labeled carnitine), because they did not possess intestinal bacteria capable of producing TMAO.[459] [See the article for footnote references to the research.]

How cool. **By adjusting your diet you can eliminate vascular disease-causing bacteria from your gut,** and thus it follows that you would experience a reduction in risk of heart disease, stroke, Alzheimer's, and other diseases caused by endothelial damage.

➢ **Genes and disease:** Some will protest against the emphasis of this book, telling stories about some relative who ate lots of bacon and burgers and died happy and healthy at 93 years old. Which of course, they say, proves that it's the genes, stupid.

It is true that the occasional person will punish their bodies with junk food, yet still live till a ripe old age. But some smoke cigarettes till they are 100, too. Do we therefore conclude that smoking is actually harmless, and lung cancer and emphysema (COPD) are genetic? Of course not. Why? Because the scientific evidence based on the health histories of multitudes of smokers and non-smokers shows clearly that smoking often causes these diseases, and others, anecdotal evidence to the contrary notwithstanding.

Genes can influence how likely it is a person will get a given chronic disease. But they are only a minor influence. **In the case of cancer, for example, it is estimated that only 5-10% of cases can be blamed on genes.**[460]

Heart disease is also often blamed on genes. "He has bad genes. His father died of a heart attack at 44, and he's doomed to the same fate." Though genes may play a role, the more powerful contributor to heart disease, as well as to cancer, is the "inherited" food culture, which tends to be passed down from

---

[459] Esselstyn, Nutritional Reversal of Cardiovascular Disease
http://doctorklaper.com/medcap-images/Esselstyn-Nutritional-Reversal-of-Cardiovascular-Disease.pdf
[460] Greger, Hot Dogs and Leukemia http://nutritionfacts.org/video/hot-dogs-leukemia/

parent to child. **Typically I will eat what my parents ate, unless I make a conscious choice to do otherwise.**

This brings us to our responsibility as parents raising the next generation. Not only will the healthy lifestyle choices you make for your family benefit your family's health this year and the next, but those choices are modeling for your children how they should live. If you teach them why you eat the way you do, and the dangers associated with the alternative, **they will likely embrace the lifestyle and live it for the rest of their lives.** In this sense good health can be "genetic."

➢ **Smoothies:** I find smoothies to be a great way to get many servings of fruits, veggies, and seeds each day. Some say drinking smoothies is healthful. The claim is that blending increases the nutrient value of the food, because it liberates more nutrients from the plant cells than would be available to your body if you only chewed the food.

However, according to others, blending up fruits and veggies does not improve their nutritional value, and some claim it actually makes them less nutritious. Dr. Esselstyn and others suggest that it is better to avoid drinking smoothies because blending fruit separates the sugar from the fiber. Then when you drink it that sugar is dumped into your stomach too fast, without adequate mixing with saliva, as would be the case if you chewed it all up yourself. The effect is thus similar to drinking juice or other sugary beverages: insulin spikes, inflammation, vascular damage, etc.

So what do I do? I still eat smoothies. Notice I said eat, not drink. Here's my suggestion. When you make a smoothie, only blend the ingredients a little, just enough to get them chopped up and well mixed. The result should actually end up quite chunky. Then be sure to thoroughly chew each "bite" before swallowing.

A Ninja blender model which has a blade "tree" with several blades sticking out along its length, instead of the common blade "flower" at the bottom of the blender pitcher, is perfect for making chunky smoothies.

> ➢ **Juicing:** If you feel you must drink juice, juicing at home is a better alternative than drinking store bought juices. The juice is much fresher and more nutritious than store bought.

However, any juice is by definition partial food, not whole food, and food is made to be eaten whole as much as possible. When you eat fruit and veggies whole, as you chew and saliva is mixed with the food, the process of digestion begins. This, along with the fiber in the food, causes the food to be digested properly, releasing the sugars more slowly into the blood.

But when you drink juice this process is short circuited. As mentioned above, **the rapid absorption of the sugars is stressful and inflammatory to the body. Additionally, polyphenol phytonutrients bound to the fiber are lost in juicing, thus you miss out on important nutrients you need.**[461]

However, it should be recognized that there are many who say they have been healed from cancer and other serious chronic diseases by drinking carrot and other veggie juices. The claim is that modern produce has fewer nutrients than in past ages due to depleted soils. Thus one needs to eat more to get the same amount of nutrition as before. Juicing vegetables concentrates the nutrients, so you can consume a much higher quantity of nutrients than would be possible if you were to eat the whole food. This nutrient boost is said to enhance your immune system, allowing your body to heal itself, including fighting cancers.

Note: While juicing veggies can apparently be helpful, juicing fruits is not recommended, as it results in a significantly high amount of concentrated sugars entering the stomach and being absorbed too quickly by the digestive process. This is not considered to be healthful. Eat your fruits.

I don't know if there is specific scientific evidence to prove the therapeutic effect of drinking fresh vegetable juices. But there is good scientific data on the beneficial effects to the immune

---

[461] Greger, <u>Juicing Removes More Than Just Fiber</u>
<u>www.nutritionfacts.org/video/juicing-removes-more-than-just-fiber/</u>

system of increasing plant food intake, so it makes sense that upping the nutrients through drinking veggie juice would increase the effects even more.

If you do juice, it is a good idea to add back into the juice some of the separated pulp, even to the point of making it necessary to "chew" the juice a bit before swallowing. Thus you will get the benefits of juicing, the nutritional and fiber benefits of the pulp, and a more health-friendly digestive process.

Though it is evident that for healthy people juicing is not necessary, juicing of vegetables may be warranted in certain cases as a disease therapy. Since vegetables have much less sugar content than fruit, the drinking of veggie juice is less problematic health-wise. And the downside of eating a partial food is counterbalanced by the potential healing properties of the concentrated vegetable nutrients. You may even find your vision improve after drinking carrot and other veggie juices for a while, as I did. See the section on the Hallelujah Diet in **Chapter 11** for more discussion of this subject.

➢ **Chewing food:** Adequate chewing of food is fundamental to good health. In their busy, stress-filled lives, people tend to rush through meals, wolfing down their food like our dog used to wolf down whole weaver birds which I shot with a BB gun. One gulp and she was ready for the next one. That is fine for a carnivore like a dog, but not so good for humans! **We need to learn to relax and take our time to chew thoroughly, virtually liquefying our food before swallowing it.**

Purdue University professor Dr. Richard Mattes explained the importance of thorough chewing:

> Particle size [affects the] bioaccessibility of the energy of the food that is being consumed. The more you chew, the less is lost and more is retained in the body.[462]

If you don't chew thoroughly, you are wasting food. It is like

---

[462] Elizabeth Renter, Chewing Food Increases Energy Availability and Nutritional Potency http://naturalsociety.com/chewing-food-up-increases-energy-availability/

dumping a portion of it in the trash (or the toilet). Food is expensive. Why make it more expensive by wasting some of what you eat?

Chewing thoroughly also means you spend a longer time eating, and your full stomach has a better opportunity to tell your brain in time that you are full. **Thus adequate chewing can help you eat less and lose weight.**

Also, when relatively large chunks of food pass into your intestines, they provide a place for bacteria to grow, which can cause bloating, gas, diarrhea, and other intestinal discomforts.

Here are some good chewing tips I came across:

- Take smaller bites of food to begin with (it's easier to chew smaller morsels)
- Chew slowly and steadily
- Chew until your mouthful of food is liquefied or lost all of its texture
- Finish chewing and swallowing completely before taking another bite of food
- Wait to drink fluids until you've swallowed[463]

I would add this one:

- Finish chewing and swallowing before you talk

Talking while chewing is not only rude (at least in our culture), it will result in you being in a hurry to swallow, and your food will not be adequately masticated (chewed up).

Chew your food thoroughly. This one change may make a difference in your health.

---

[463] Mercola, 7 Important Reasons to Properly Chew Your Food
http://articles.mercola.com/sites/articles/archive/2013/07/31/chewing-foods.aspx

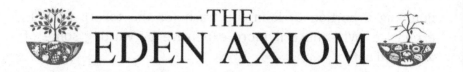

Conclusion: A Radical Lifestyle of Body Stewardship

Chapters 5 through **9** identify five primary lifestyle factors which are necessary in order to attain and maintain good health. At the end of **Chapter 9** I suggested an equation which adds up these factors such that the sum would be the level of health a person would expect to attain as they seek to improve their lives in these areas. Each element was connected by a plus sign.

However, this may give the impression that one could potentially do well in most areas, but very poorly in one or two, and still maintain reasonably good health. This is not true, at least not over the long haul.

For example, if you are only getting four hours of sleep a night, the other areas have no power to compensate for that lack and keep you healthy. If you eat the SAD, but are physically active throughout the day, sleep soundly, manage stress well, and have great relationships with God and people, you will still be unhealthy. You might not feel it today or tomorrow, but eventually it will cause chronic disease.

So the situation can really be more accurately symbolized if we instead multiply the five elements by each other, calculating a "health product" rather than a "health sum." And let's change the order to create an easy to remember acronym:

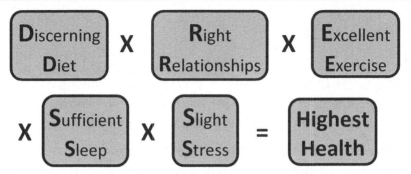

Consider the significance of the multiplication signs. If any one of the five values drops to a very low level, no matter how well you are doing in the other areas, your state of health will be diminished considerably. So please, pay attention to each area. Trust God for the strength, wisdom and drive to successfully address any which are lacking. Each is very important.

Now let's take a look at the acronym in the equation: **DRESS**. The verb **dress** has many meanings. Here are a few from my dictionary:

- *Give a neat appearance to* – These lifestyle principles will improve our appearance.

- *Apply a bandage or medication* – These lifestyle principles protect our bodies and allow them to heal.

- *Cut down rough hewn lumber to standard thickness and width* – These lifestyle principles will allow us to achieve our ideal size.

- *Cultivate, tend, as a garden* – These lifestyle principles are the best way to cultivate health and tend our bodies.

- *Arrange in ranks (as in soldiers preparing for inspection by an officer)* – When we practice these lifestyle principles, intentionally ordering our lives with a desire to be good stewards of the bodies God has created for us, it meets with His approval.

- *Dress or groom with elaborate care* – We take elaborate care to stay healthy; it's worth it!

- **_Put a finish on_** – These lifestyle principles will enable us to finish life well.

Perhaps these thoughts will help you to not forget the five lifestyle factors which are central to optimal health. Simply remember to **_DRESS for success!_** (Corny, I know. But hopefully the corniness will help you remember.)

And remember why we know these five factors are important: They were all present in Eden, the perfect environment God originally created for humans. At that time, before sin had entered mankind and the world, they all worked together to support the perfect health of Adam and Eve. We also see the importance of each of these areas born out by the findings of modern medical science.

Therefore we believe that as we pay attention to these principles from Genesis 1-3, even now in our day and in our context, we can enjoy, in the will of God, the good health we desire and He desires for us.

To be sure, some of the positive lifestyle changes we may realize we should aim for are indeed quite radical in our culture, especially in the area of truly healthy eating. Yet we can press forward undaunted, because this lifestyle is based on solid evidence and settled convictions.

And of course this isn't simply so we can have our "best life now." That would be a shallow, temporal goal. We wish to live this radical lifestyle for the purpose of body stewardship, making the responsible choice to nurture this amazing gift we have been given, the gift of our bodies. And that for the purpose that we might be enabled to worship and serve our Creator all the more until He takes us home to be with Him.

I really am thankful for the interest in this book which so many have shown. It gives me hope that many will take its lessons to heart, even if change in some of these important lifestyle areas is hard.

If you have questions about anything in this book, would like more ideas about switching to plant based eating or shaping other areas of your lifestyle, or have found errors in what I have written, please let me know. I am still learning and growing in these areas, of course, so I welcome any input which may be of help to me as well.

The Eden Axiom is the self-evident truth that God's original lifestyle design for humans really is the wisest one to aim for as we seek to serve and honor Him. The weight of evidence from scientific research strongly confirms that this is true, especially in our modern times.

The world, and those in the church who don't understand these things, say this is a radical lifestyle, and they doubt the need to be so "extreme." But we have seen the evidence that such a lifestyle accords with being wise stewards of the bodies God has entrusted to us.

If you agree, and the Lord is leading you and your family to make positive lifestyle changes, I pray He will give you the strength of conviction to carry them out, for the sake of your good health and, more importantly, His glory. May we all be faithful stewards of what He has given us!

> Dear friend, I hope all is well with you and that you are as healthy in body as you are strong in spirit.
>
> 3 John 2

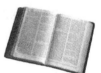

For His glory,

Kirk Evan Rogers

TheEdenAxiom@faithwriters.net

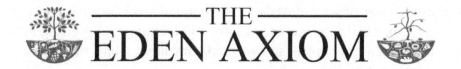

THE ── EDEN AXIOM

Appendix: For Further Study

The following is a list of experts in the field who I believe have helpful things to say about diet and health, and whom I trust to be generally accurate. Some of them disagree on some points, so obviously not all of them are always right. I have listed each one's website, plus for most of them one or more video lectures which give the gist of their views. There are other resources from most of these referenced in the footnotes throughout this book. I have also listed a few key videos and other resources which will help you better understand the subjects dealt with in this book.

Dr. Caldwell Esselstyn M.D. – The heart attack proof diet

Dr. Esselstyn's website:

http://www.dresselstyn.com/

Making Heart Attacks History – TED talk :

https://www.youtube.com/watch?v=EqKNfyUPzoU

Dr. John McDougall M.D. – Starch based diet

Dr. McDougall has been healing patients for about 40 years with a plant based diet. He has a wealth of helpful information on his website, including a searchable archive of many years of newsletters which contain explanations of the latest diet and health research, and hundreds of recipes for plant based meals.

Dr. McDougall's website:

https://www.drmcdougall.com/

Food We Were Born To Eat – TED talk:

https://www.youtube.com/watch?v=d5wfMNNr3ak

Death by Dairy:

https://www.youtube.com/watch?v=TJvrlwnEqbs

Dr. Michael Greger M.D. – Plant based diet

Dr. Greger's website:

http://www.veganmd.org/

Maximum Nutrition - Transitioning Towards a Plant Based Diet – Lots of great practical tips on preparing wholesome yummy foods:

https://www.youtube.com/watch?v=Y9nNa81dSoY

Dr. Greger's nutrition research videos:

http://www.nutritionfacts.org/

Dr. Greger reads all English language clinical nutrition journals and presents some of the info in easy-to-understand (and often humorous) terms in 3-5 minute videos which he posts every 2 or 3 days at nutritionfacts.org. If you subscribe, the link to the latest video will appear in your inbox. You can search by keyword and topic through his thousands of videos on the website.

The following three videos are about an hour long each. In them Dr. Greger gives some amazing scientific evidence for the importance of a plant based diet, how it can prevent and treat most of the main causes of death and suffering.

Uprooting the leading causes of death:

http://nutritionfacts.org/video/uprooting-the-leading-causes-of-death/

More than an apple a day: Combatting common diseases:

http://nutritionfacts.org/video/more-than-an-apple-a-day-preventing-our-most-common-diseases/

From table to able: Combatting disabling diseases with food:

http://nutritionfacts.org/video/from-table-to-able/

Dr. Dean Ornish M.D. – "Spectrum diet" to undo heart disease

In the *Lifestyle Heart Trial,* Dr. Ornish conducted groundbreaking research back in the late 1980s and 1990s proving the connection between coronary artery disease and diet.

Dr. Ornish's website:

http://ornishspectrum.com/

<u>Newsmax interview with Dr. Ornish</u> – Good summary of Dr. Ornish's philosophy of diet, with some helpful practical tips for eating whole food plant based:

https://www.youtube.com/watch?x-yt-ts=1422579428&v=WSUfgej-CF0&x-yt-cl=85114404

Dr. Colin Campbell – *The China Study*[464]

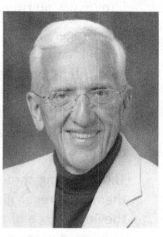

In *The China Study*, Dr. T. Colin Campbell, Professor Emeritus at Cornell University, details the connection between nutrition and heart disease, diabetes, and cancer. Recognized as the most comprehensive nutritional study ever conducted on the relationship between diet and the risk of developing disease, *The China Study* cuts through the haze of misinformation and examines the source of nutritional confusion produced by government entities, lobbies, and opportunistic scientists.[465]

---

[464] Campbell, <u>Order page for The China Study: The Most Comprehensive Study of Nutrition Ever Conducted And the Startling Implications for Diet, Weight Loss, And Long-term Health</u> http://smile.amazon.com/China-Study-Comprehensive-Nutrition-Implications/dp/1932100660/ref=sr_1_1?s=books&ie=UTF8&qid=1418049278&sr=1-1&keywords=the+china+study
[465] Campbell, <u>About *The China Study*</u> http://www.thechinastudy.com/the-china-study/about/

Dr. Campbell's website:

http://nutritionstudies.org/about/

The Remarkable Health Benefits of Nutrition:

https://www.youtube.com/watch?v=XEuRMm-a6mo

Dr. Joel Fuhrman – Nutritarian diet

Dr. Fuhrman promotes a plant based diet which he calls the "Nutritarian diet." It is based on his health equation: H=N/C (health = nutrients/calories). Thus the "nutrient dense" concept is central (see **Chapter 11**). His book Eat to Live! was a New York Times bestseller. Many have found his approach to be very helpful in losing weight and achieving good health.

Dr. Fuhrman's website:

http://www.drfuhrman.com/

Dr. Neal Barnard – Reversing diabetes diet

Dr. Barnard's website:

http://www.nealbarnard.org/books/diabetes/

Tackling diabetes with a bold new dietary approach – TED talk:

https://www.youtube.com/watch?v=ktQzM2IA-qU

Dr. Nicholas Gonzales – Diet and supplements to combat cancer, including pancreatic cancer

Dr. Gonzales' website:

www.dr-gonzalez.com/

Radio interview with Dr. Gonzales:

http://www.dr-gonzalez.com/kat-james-092113.mp3

Dr. Michael Klaper, M.D. – Nutrition-based medicine

Dr. Klaper has practiced medicine for over 40 years. For most of his career he has been healing patients in the context of a whole food plant based diet. His lecture A Diet for All Reasons – Food That Kills was one of the first that really got my attention and forced me to consider the wisdom of continuing to include meat and dairy in my diet.

Dr. Klaper's website:

http://doctorklaper.com/

A Diet for All Reasons – Food That Kills:

https://www.youtube.com/watch?v=52a3qrZKic4

From Operating Table to Dining Room Table:

https://www.youtube.com/watch?v=KatsJk0oBUI

Physicians Committee for Responsible Medicine – Dr. Barnard is the president of this organization of doctors and other health care professionals which support the attaining and maintaining of good health by eating a plant based diet.

http://www.pcrm.org/

Summary of the four plant food group "Power Plate" diet:

http://www.pcrm.org/pdfs/health/4foodgroups.pdf

Dr. Joseph Mercola – I have quoted Dr. Mercola several times in this book. He has a lot of good and helpful things to say. However, I disagree with some of his material. For example, he promotes the eating of dairy, eggs, and meat, though he is quick to emphasize the importance of choosing organic and free range. He also sells a lot of stuff, which may relate to the subject he is writing about. He doesn't give a strong sales pitch, but still the tendency to be influenced by profit can't be ignored. So be discerning when reading Dr. Mercola's articles – though discernment is of course needed no matter what you are reading! (Yes, it is true that the whole food plant based crowd also sells books and other products.)

Forks Over Knives – This documentary presents material similar to what I have included in this book. Drs. Esselstyn, McDougall, and Campbell are featured. Highly recommended! Note, this film is not available for free streaming or download; it is probably available on Netflix,

Amazon Prime, etc.

Forks Over Knives trailer:

https://www.youtube.com/user/ForksOverKnives

Plant Positive – This Youtube channel has many videos which provide in-depth analyses of low carb and paleo diet philosophies, showing their scientific flaws. They also provide an interesting historical perspective on nutrition, and irrefutable proof that a whole food plant based diet is the most sensible, healthful way to eat.

https://www.youtube.com/user/PrimitiveNutrition/playlists

Kaiser Permanente – This "integrated managed care consortium" has published a very good booklet, **The Plant-Based Diet – a healthier way to eat.** It is quite remarkable that such a mainstream physician-influenced outfit would "get it" so well when it comes to diet and health! I recommend this booklet as a helpful resource for you and your family as you move toward healthier eating habits.

http://mydoctor.kaiserpermanente.org/ncal/Images/New%20Plant%20Based%20Booklet%201214_tcm28-781815.pdf

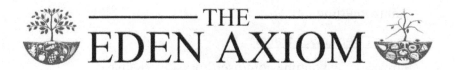

THE EDEN AXIOM

About the author

Kirk Evan Rogers was raised in Los Angeles, California. From a young age he took an interest in science, health and physical fitness. He took many courses in chemistry, biology, botany, and zoology during his years at college, and has been an avid reader on a variety of science topics every since.

Kirk attended church while growing up, but while in high school he rejected the church's beliefs, becoming an atheist by the time he entered college.

But when Kirk learned about the many ancient prophecies of the Old Testament which were fulfilled in the coming of Jesus Christ to earth, he knew God must be real, and His Word must be true in its entirety. Thus, when he read the Good News of Jesus' love for people, and what He had done to secure their salvation, Kirk put his faith in Jesus and became a Christian.

Challenged by the claim of God on his life, and Jesus' command to His followers that they spread His message to those who had never heard it, Kirk began to prepare for missionary service. He attended Bible college, and then a missionary training course.

Kirk and his wife Yolanda have served as church planters among a minority people group in Guinea, West Africa, since 1991. Kirk's ministry involves linguistics, Bible translation, Bible curriculum development, Bible teaching, discipleship, and literacy work. Kirk and Yolanda also do their best to help their African neighbors learn to eat a more healthful diet!

Kirk and Yolanda met at Bible college and married in 1986. They raised their four children in Africa. Their oldest, Colin, is now a missionary in South America, along with his wife Megan and son Judah. Cameron is a U.S. Marine. Colton and his wife Ashton, as well as Kayla and her husband Luke, are preparing for missionary service.

NOTES

Made in the USA
Las Vegas, NV
29 October 2023

79904980R00213